The Men's Health BIG BOOK

GETTING ABS

By **ADAM BORNSTEIN** and the Editors of *Men's Health*

RODALE.

© 2012 by Rodale Inc.
Photographs © 2012 by Rodale Inc.
All rights reserved. No part of this publication may be reproduced or transmitted in any form or by any means, electronic or mechanical, including photocopying, recording, or any other information storage and retrieval system, without the written permission of the publisher.

Rodale books may be purchased for business or promotional use or for special sales. For information, please write to: Special Markets Department, Rodale, Inc., 733 Third Avenue, New York, NY 10017

Men's Health is a registered trademark of Rodale Inc.
Printed in the United States of America

Rodale Inc. makes every effort to use acid-free ∞, recycled paper ♻.

Book design by Tara Long
With George Karabotsos, design director for *Men's Health* and *Women's Health* Books

Photography by Beth Bischoff
Grooming by Rachael Gray
Styling by Anna Su

Illustrations by Kurt Walters

Library of Congress Cataloging-in-Publication Data is on file with the publisher
ISBN: 978-1-60961-874-2

Distributed to the trade by Macmillan
2 4 6 8 10 9 7 5 3 1 paperback

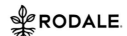

We inspire and enable people to improve their lives and the world around them.
Rodalebooks.com

Contents

Acknowledgments		**iv**
Introduction:	How to Win the Abs Game	**vi**
Chapter 1:	Six-Pack Secrets	**8**
Chapter 2:	All Your Abs Questions Answered	**20**
Chapter 3:	The Real Reason You Can't See Your Abs	**32**
Chapter 4:	Eat Your Way to Six-Pack Abs	**52**
Chapter 5:	The Secret to Shredded Abs	**66**
Chapter 6:	Abs-olutely Awesome Meals	**80**
Chapter 7:	Abs for Every Eater	**92**
Chapter 8:	The Abs Workout	**100**
Chapter 9:	The Best Abs Exercises Ever Created	**126**
Chapter 10:	Revolutionize Your Training	**336**
Chapter 11:	The Best Abs Workouts Ever Created	**346**
Index		**384**

Acknowledgments

I always feel that the acknowledgments are the toughest section to write, as I know that it's impossible for me to thank everyone that made the creation of this book possible.

Thank you to Maria Rodale and the Rodale family for providing an ongoing platform for health and wellness. To *Men's Health* editor-in-chief David Zinczenko, I'm grateful that I not only had the opportunity to work at *Men's Health,* but also to continue my relationship with the brand so that I could write books that truly offer tons of useful stuff. Same goes for Steve Perrine, publisher of Rodale Books. You'll always have the distinction of being the guy that had believed in me and gave me the opportunity to write books.

An infinite amount of appreciation must also be paid to all the editors at *Men's Health.* I've said it once and I'll say it again: The lessons I learned from you are invaluable and have allowed me to communicate more effectively and help more people. Thank you.

Thank you to Debbie McHugh for your continued faith in me and being an incredible, supportive friend. To Jeff Csatari, I appreciate your vision and help making this project happen. And Mike Zimmerman—truly one of the most talented editors and writers I've ever worked with—thank you for editing this project and making the process even more enjoyable. Beth Bischoff, your photos are top-notch as usual. Erin Williams, your copy editing (once again) makes me look like I've mastered the English language. And of course the design team lead by George Karabotsos—there wouldn't be a book without you.

Special thanks goes to John Romaniello for his guidance, support, and great workout knowledge. Jason Ferruggia, you've become a great influence and an even bigger motivator. And much appreciation to Alan Aragon, Mike Roussell, and Chris Mohr—you helped me load this book with more nutritional information than I thought possible.

To the many contributors that made this book that greatest compilation of fitness information and workouts ever assembled: Jim Smith, Martin Rooney, Eric Cressey, Matt McGorry, Kevin Neeld, Mike Robertson, Bill Hartman, Robert Dos Remedios, Rob Sulaver, Tony Gentilcore, Mike Whitfield, Craig Ballantyne, BJ Gaddour, Nick Tumminello, Roger Lawson, JC Deen, and Jon Goodman—you are all men of fitness genius.

Neema Yazdani—let your success be a model for others to follow.

Ted Spiker: You're such a great mentor that I decided to follow your lead and tackle the ever-desirable abs. Thanks for your continued guidance.

And I can't forget Dan Brian, Jeremy Reed, and Michael Kirby—my Demand Media and Livestrong.com family. This project does not happen without your support. Thank you.

Mom and Dad—you continue to inspire my even though I think I drive you crazier as I get older. Thank you for loving me and continuing to teach me about how to be healthier.

Josh, Aaron, and Jordan—I wish everyone could have brothers like you.

And Rachie: I could write an entire book about you, but no matter how hard I try, there will never be enough words to express how amazing you are and how much I love you.

Thank you all. I continue to be humbled by each and every one of you.
Now let's uncover some abs.

Introduction
How to Win the Abs Game

Unlocking the secrets of a six-pack starts by acknowledging the impossible as possible: You can build muscle and burn fat at the same time.

The name of this book

could have easily been "Project: Impossible."

About 2 years ago, I went searching for five men who were willing to try a new approach to exercise and nutrition. We're not talking about your typical "test-a-new-program-and-earn-a-free-T-shirt" gimmick. This was the real deal. As part of a 4-week program, I teamed with some of the smartest minds in exercise and nutrition to build a workout and diet program that was designed with one simple goal: to help men uncover their abs. This wasn't about guaranteeing a six-pack or making you look like a cover model. I just wanted guys to lose fat and look good. The initial 4-week phase was so successful that it became the foundation of the book you now hold in your hands.

How to Win the Abs Game

I use the word "impossible" because even I wasn't sure it'd work. After all, this wasn't any type of test. But after years of learning some of the best strategies that work for athletes and celebrities, I wanted to get back to the heart of health—helping ordinary people. So I targeted the "average" guys, the ones who care about their health, but have limited time and unlimited expectations of what they should look like. Every guy has his own better body desires: Some want to add some muscle, others need to lose fat, and there are those who are trying to prove that age really is just a number. These men can be active or sedentary, but all enjoy pizza, drink beer (preferably several bottles), and can't seem to figure out a way to uncover their abs.

You're one of these men. And so am I.

About 4 years ago, I found myself in the same position you're probably in now: frustrated and convinced that genetics control appearance. Despite my background and years as a fitness editor at *Men's Health*, I wasn't able to crack the code. That was until I transformed my body and slashed my body fat in half—down to a measly 6 percent—while increasing my strength and adding 5 pounds of muscle. (The transformation was documented in a story in *Men's Health*.) The crazy part: This occurred while working nearly 70 to 80 hours a week. Only the genetically blessed seemed to get these types of results. But "genetics" and "blessed" were words that were never combined when describing

me. I was once 30 pounds overweight, could only bench 65 pounds when I was in college (which the best man at my wedding shared with everyone in attendance, and now you know my dark secret, too), and I have suffered enough broken bones and torn ligaments to earn a pat on the back from Evel Knievel. But then I discovered that anyone— and I mean anyone—can have a lean, hard body.

Now it's time for you to find out how.

If you picked up this book, you're about to learn what the men of "Project: Impossible" discovered—that a rock-solid core and a lean midsection live within you. But this book comes with a warning: The knowledge you'll find here is not for the stubborn. As we know, men are programmed to be right. All. The. Time. We argue with our buddies, fight with our wives, and even try to outsmart our bosses. Unfortunately, we also continually challenge our bodies and fail to listen to what they're trying to tell us.

And that is: What you're doing isn't working.

You want to be lean and muscular. You want biceps that pop, abs you can show off, and a diet you can follow while still eating like a man. And yet your body always seems to be harder to understand than Sophia Vergara with a mouthful of marbles. No matter what workout you try or how many protein shakes you slug each day, the results don't feel right, look right, or match your efforts.

But you're a man, and you don't quit. You just kick it up a notch. Maybe you join a gym or start running sprints. You experiment with a new diet or bump up your workouts to six times a week. But your body works like a bad business deal: big investment, small return. At some point, your drive for ABS turns into WTF?

That frustration has led you to this book and your final stand in the war against fat. You're stuck and are facing a point of no return. You can accept a fate you don't want—or fight back with something new. Something different. And something completely supported by science and real-life results.

That's why we created *The Men's Health Big Book: Getting Abs*. Contrary to what you might think, your body wants to be lean and muscular. And no matter what you've experienced, you are not destined to have a beer belly and your metabolism isn't plotting against you to pack on the pounds.

This book is about providing you with a road map for transforming your average body into fighting shape, so that you can battle all of the daily stressors in life and come out on top. It doesn't matter if you're a 20-year-old guy who just discovered exercise or a 50-year-old looking to recapture his glory days. In a matter of weeks, you'll find that the prime of your life is not something you experience but something you achieve.

The Truth about Weight Loss

How will this time be any different? Because we're changing the game. Much of the diet and fitness advice you need is overplayed, overhyped, and inaccurate. You are taking pieces of information and trying to create a Frankenstein approach to your body.

That doesn't work. And if you doubt me, look in the mirror and convince me of something else.

Here's something most programs don't tell you: Your body is designed to incinerate the hard-to-lose fat. You know those areas as man boobs, love handles, and beer belly. But the real problem is that you've been fed a steady diet of misinformation about what your body needs in order to look its best. And we can tell you that radical, dramatic steps are the last things your body needs. You need something stable and sustainable.

The Men's Health Big Book: Getting Abs is a proven plan based on the information provided by the best fitness and nutrition experts and the latest research. You know what we discovered? If you drop the stubborn act and change your strategy based on a few simple guidelines, you can switch your body into a fitter, healthier mode. It will burn more calories and build more muscle, and you'll look amazing.

I'm guessing this is not the first time you've heard this speech. So before you hit the BS-button, consider that for once you're dealing with a more realistic approach to your body.

How to Win the Abs Game

On this plan, you'll be eating foods that you never thought would be on a diet plan. You can booze with the boys without worrying about how many calories are in a bottle. (You will still have to worry about hangovers, though.) You can even indulge in guy-grub like burgers and fries and still flatten your belly. In fact, Greek researchers found that those who don't indulge while on a healthy eating plan are more likely to gain weight. That's the type of digging we've done to create the most comprehensive guide to unlocking a better you. All you need to do is keep reading, to find out how.

New Plan, New You

Chiseled, Adonis-like bodies don't come from your local supplement store. If they did, we'd all look the way we want. And who hasn't tried the do-whatever-it-takes approach to losing weight? But not only does that lead to a shortage of cash, it also bends our will. In fact, a UCLA study notes that nearly 70 percent of people don't believe that exercise and diet can help them lose weight. That's a scary number for a nation that's already losing the battle against obesity. It's no wonder scientists estimate that the obesity trend won't slow down until the year 2050! And by that time, it's estimated that nearly half the country will be overweight. Do you want to be a statistic or do you want to help reverse the trend?

We can tell you that exercise and diet work. We've seen it with our own eyes, in scientific journals and in real life.

Change starts by realizing extreme behaviors are not the solution. After all, that's where our battle of the bulge went wrong in the first place. Let's go back to the 1980s. That's when dietary fat was identified as the root of all evil and cardio was elevated to the best form of exercise. Next thing you knew, the entire country was gorging on fat-free foods and going on slow jogs.

Fast-forward 30 years and those decades of eating fat-free, sugar-loaded foods have expanded our tummies. And long-slow cardio results in—you guessed it—long, slow weight loss. In a Purdue University study, rats that consumed a mix of low-fat diet chips plus regular high-fat chips gained significantly more fat than rats that only consumed high-fat chips. Why? The researchers speculated that not only did the added sugars add to weight gain, but the low-fat foods tricked the rats' bodies and prevented them from shutting off hunger signals, tempting the rats to eat more. In addition, Louisiana State University researchers found that the average number of calories burned during exercise dropped by 100 calories during the past 20 years, even though people were spending more time in the gym. So it should come as no surprise that the prevailing "best" approach to fat loss has resulted in obesity rates skyrocketing to all-time highs. And more importantly, it has left you more frustrated than ever.

While we've learned a lot in the last 30 years, people are still relying on the same information of the past. It's time to turn a new page, debunk old myths, and set the record straight: You can have flat, toned abs if you follow the lessons of *The Men's Health Big Book: Getting Abs*. Here's why:

1. You Have More Control

Most fitness plans are inflexible. They are based on a preset routine that doesn't consider your lifestyle. Work, family, friends, and other obligations can make eating healthy and exercising difficult. So much so, according to the Centers for Disease Control and Prevention, that people who turned these interruptions into excuses were up to 76 percent less likely to lose weight than those who figured out ways around them. In other words: You need to find techniques that won't result in failure, or else you're destined to eventually stop trying.

One of the biggest reasons why *The Men's Health Big Book: Getting Abs* works is because you can create your own schedule. You choose how many meals you want to eat, the days you want to exercise, and when you want to booze with your boys and feast on a plate of wings.

You want to eat six meals a day? Go for it.

Your schedule won't allow you to eat snacks? Just have three big meals.

You don't have an hour to exercise? No worries, we have complete body-shaping workouts that will take 20 minutes or less.

This is the first program that takes into consideration your priorities and offers the tips you need to look your best.

2. You Have More Freedom

You want to know the real diet secret? Build your plan around the foods you love! Let's be realistic: If the only things you eat are pizza and ice cream, you might have to adjust your plan (for the sake of your health most of all). For everyone else, we insist that you keep your favorite foods as part of your diet. The truth is, the negativity surrounding most foods is inaccurate. You can eat white rice and white bread and still lose weight. Pasta doesn't trigger any fat receptors that guarantee a gut. And gym sessions do not have to last hours upon hours in order for you to head to the beach shirtless this summer.

We'll teach you how to load up—the right way—on the food your body craves. You'll be eating what you like, along with what you need, and have more energy and faster fat loss. The plan is designed to guarantee that you never become tired of what you're eating. When that happens, there's no desire to break from it and spiral toward the same frustrating end. By knowing what you can eat—rather than focusing on what you can't—you'll discover the endless meals that can help you lose weight and keep it off.

3. You Have a Proven Formula

You can't out-exercise a bad diet. That's the most important rule of any success-ful plan. But a great diet without an exercise plan is incomplete. Your body needs to be active—both inside and outside the gym. Researchers have

How to Win the Abs Game

found that each 10 percent rise in sedentary time is associated with a more than 1-inch increase in the size of your waist. What's more, British scientists found that of the subjects they studied, the waist measurements of people who got up most often were more than 2 inches smaller than those of people who got up the least.

But you need to do more than just use the stairs at your office to rev up your metabolism and pack on new muscle. *The Men's Health Big Book: Getting Abs* will teach you how to upgrade your workout to the most efficient plan ever created. You'll learn how the best way to build your six-pick means limiting direct abs work. And how adding just 3 days of resistance training per week is enough to help you eat less and turn your body into a fat-burning machine 24 hours a day, 7 days a week.

Your Fittest Life Starts Here

You'd think that a successful diet and exercise plan would be easier to find. After all, we have more information at our disposal than ever before. But all that information creates a different problem: misinformation—and lots of it. That's why you've found yourself struggling to find the solution. Not anymore. We've done the work for you. We've interviewed the top experts, read all of the research, and found the best way to create real results.

We know that your body is important to you, and we understand that you only have so much time to think about your health. Our goal is to make healthy living attainable and fun.

As a bonus, you'll uncover hundreds of additional tips, tricks, and benefits. We've debunked the biggest diet myths, so you'll never veer off track with your eating or exercise. "The Lean Guide to Eating" shopping list (page 65) will make every trip to the grocery store a simple and rage-free experience. We've even included the most pressing concerns and issues that readers have sent directly to *Men's Health*. You'll finally have your questions answered. It's like having your own personal diet coach answering all of your questions—without shelling out the Benjamins.

We know that living healthy can seem difficult. We understand that many of you have struggled with your goals, whether it's dropping 100 pounds or just trimming the last 10. This book was developed for you. We put our brand behind this title because we know it'll work, using the same winning formula found in the pages of *Men's Health*. It's why we're excited to share this revolutionary new approach to helping you look lean and powerful.

This book is about cutting to the chase and providing you with exactly what you want: advice that walks the walk, and allows you to talk the talk. You'll eat better, exercise smarter, improve your sex life, and see changes to your overall health. It's the total package. Best of all? No matter what you look like or what you've experienced, you finally have a proven guide to help you find your abs.

Did You Make the Right Choice?

Few things are worse than picking up a book thinking that it'll offer you what you want, only to make it to the end and realizing you completely wasted your time. So to put your mind at ease, if you fit any of the following criteria then this book is for you.

- You want workout programs that have actually been tested and will provide results.
- You want variety in your training that will prevent you from becoming bored and hitting a plateau.
- You want to know why certain exercises work and others don't.
- You want to know what foods you can eat, what foods to avoid, and a list of the best (and worst) supplements for your body.
- You want to know if you should take protein powder and how much.

- You want a detailed formula that will help you lose fat *and* build muscle at the same time . . . or you just want a flexible plan without the math. This book offers both.
- You want workouts you can do in 10 minutes, workouts you can do on the road, and workouts you can do when you don't have any equipment on hand.
- You want to fix your posture and reduce aches and pains.
- You want to learn how to do the exercises *correctly* so that you can stop being injured.
- You want workouts that are hard and will challenge you to become a better version of yourself.
- You want a plan that won't have you living at the gym—but instead will give you the body that looks like you train 7 days a week.
- You want abs.

If any of these wishes describe you, then you've come to the right place.

Chapter 1
Six-Pack Secrets

Eighteen instant tips that will sculpt your body and eliminate your gut.

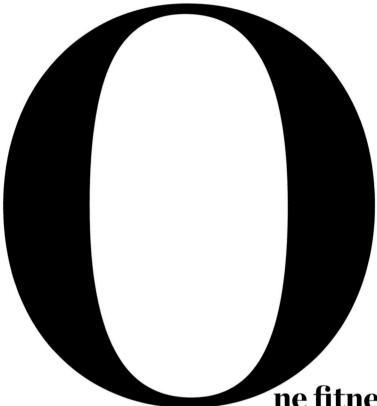

One fitness target is universally understood by all guys—abs. No matter how you look at them, a chiseled core represents good health, a fit body, and sex appeal. But finding your abs isn't much different from hunting for the perfect woman: You want to believe she exists, but every new choice seems to be crazier than the last.

At some point, you start making excuses because of constant roadblocks: bad genetics, a hectic work schedule, and the typical Sunday football menu of burgers, wings, and beer (the same way the dating excuses line up, Seinfeld-style, like "She eats peas with a fork" or "She's a low-talker"). The reality? The excuses are a bunch of bull. Any man can choose to lie down when it seems hard to reach his goals—or he can take control of his destiny.

9

Six-Pack Secrets

That's why it's time to put you back in charge of your body and arm you with all the information that makes it easier than ever to drop fat. Any man can see his six-pack, and the time has come to give you the keys to your own hard-body plan.

If you need inspiration, look no further than Neema Yazdani, a 30-year-old account manager for a major hardware company. Despite spending his high school days as a cross-country runner, and making the rec center his second home during college, Neema never quite reached his personal fitness goals. And his frustrations weren't limited to fat loss and seeing those mythical abs.

Neema struggled for years to put on muscle, despite hours in the gym. In fact, at one point, he was working out 5 days a week and still no luck. And it wasn't for a lack of variety. He hit the weights, did cardio, took supplements, and even tried a no-carb plan that left him starving for more food. Sure, he made some gains, added some weight, and looked like a guy who'd hit the gym. But he never looked the role of someone who lived in the gym and ate right. The harder he worked, the less he seemed to achieve; and his resolve was tested even more when he started a new job and had to spend more time at work.

His situation made him a perfect test subject for our approach: a regular guy who had tried everything and had less time than ever to commit to his health. Neema's results were the reason we created this book. He added 10 pounds of muscle to his body while simultaneously losing 4 percent body fat. But wait. Isn't building muscle and losing fat at the same time impossible? Many experts would have you believe that, but while Neema's results may appear shocking, they were typical for everyone who tried the diet and exercise program in *The Men's Health Big Book: Getting Abs.* Most impressively? Neema can now see his abs (much to the delight of his girlfriend, Megan).

Like most guys, you might be trying too hard and overthinking the process. Too many diets and too much exercise have resulted in information overload, which probably has you staring wistfully at yourself in the mirror and wondering why the hell nothing seems to be working. Before you hit the eject button, you need to realize that having a great body isn't about making endless sacrifices or following an unbearable plan. It's about understanding how tiny daily changes result in unbelievable transformations. We've seen the overweight become thin, men in their fifties shed their love handles, and regular guys who still eat pizza get—and stay—ripped.

Sure, some men seem to be born with an eight-pack and naturally flat abs. It's about as irritating as those born into megawealth. But you don't have to be born rich to make a lot of money, and you certainly don't need to be born with a six-pack to have a defined stomach.

Here's what you need to know: Your body is the most sophisticated natural machine. It burns calories to help you perform all of your daily tasks, like standing up, thinking, and sleeping. This daily maintenance is called your basal metabolic rate (BMR). Everyone has a BMR, but the bigger you are, the faster your metabolism works. Think about that: The more weight you carry, the better your metabolism.

On the surface, that doesn't make sense. After all, skinny people have better metabolisms, right? Well, not exactly. Think about it another way. Say you have two cars, an Audi and a Hummer. Which needs more fuel? The Hummer does, because it's much larger and has more demands. Your body is no different. Everything you do, from powering your heart to moving from point A to point B, requires energy. That's why the larger you are, the harder your body needs to work and the more calories you burn. Your body wants to be an Audi; you just have to be willing to trade in for a new model.

Consider this: Your metabolism isn't holding you back, and your body isn't hardwired to look a certain way. You can control your ability to lose weight. Simple, small adjustments to your diet, exercise, and other behaviors will make a surprisingly big difference and transform your body.

■

How easy can it be to see your abs?

Here are 18 instant changes you can make that will help your flat belly dreams become a reality.

1. Sleep more

Here's a truth that every man can appreciate: The best thing you can do for your body is to spend more time in bed. Researchers from Harvard University studied more than 68,000 people and found that those who sleep less than 6 hours a night weighed 5.4 pounds more and were 15 percent more likely to be overweight than those who slept more than 7 hours a night. The weight gain is no coincidence: Sleeping less actually changes how you react to images and thoughts of food. After just one night of bad sleep, you experience increased activity in your brain's reward center. That means when you see food, your brain triggers an increased desire to eat food—and a lot of it. The result:

Six-Pack Secrets

Those who sleep less eat an average of 220 more calories per day, say researchers from the University of Chicago. What's more, researchers from the Netherlands found that men who were sleep deprived were rated as less attractive and less healthy-looking by random observers.

QUICK FIX: Aim for 8 hours of sleep a night and never settle for less than 7. And don't mess around with this. We all know that sleep is probably the first thing you sacrifice. But there's a reason we listed this as the first tip. Sure, not getting enough sleep will make it extremely difficult to see your abs. Even worse? Sleeping less than 7 hours will lead to an early death, say Italian researchers. In fact, when you sleep 6 or fewer hours, you increase your chances of premature death by 12 percent. I'm a gambling man, but there are certain risks not worth betting on. Life is one of them. Sleep well and live longer.

If you're not a morning person, find the latest time possible you can wake up and be ready for work, and then work backward 7 hours. This is the latest you should go to bed every night. Set your alarm far away from your bed so you actually have to leave your pillow to turn it off. When you wake up in the morning, turn off your alarm and head straight to the shower. Don't worry. You'll learn that you won't miss hitting the snooze button six times.

2. Eat the way you want

For the past decade, you've heard that you need five or six meals per day for fat loss. The rationale was simple: When you eat, your body requires energy to burn away the calories. So the reasoning went that more meals would equal more calories burned. Only one problem—it's not how frequently you eat, but rather what you eat that impacts how many calories you'll burn during mealtime. So if you consume 2,000 calories in a day, it doesn't matter if it's in three, six, or 20 meals. You'll burn the same amount of calories, assuming that the foods you eat are the same.

QUICK FIX: There's no need to feel forced to eat more or less frequently. In an attempt to burn more calories, you might have been accidentally overeating and sabotaging your weight loss goals. With the diet plan in The *Men's Health Big Book: Getting Abs,* you'll understand what you need to eat. Then it's up to you to decide the times and frequency that work best.

In order to do this, take a week and journal when you feel most hungry. Then adjust your eating patterns accordingly. As you'll find out, breakfast is not more important than dinner, and snacks are not a necessity. You might find yourself hungriest at work, which means snacks are a great option. Play by your rules—and the ones we provide in this book—and not only will you stop being hungry, you'll also drop more weight.

3. Snack smarter

While the number of meals you consume doesn't matter, the size of your snacks does. According to Purdue University researchers, snacks have become meals, and meals have become feasts. In the last 30 years, snack sizes have increased from 360 to 580 calories. That's a

THE
ABS
BENEFIT
57
Percent less likely men with lean bellies are to die of heart disease

whopping 220 extra calories per snack. And when you consider that the average man snacks twice a day during the workday, you're looking at almost 500 extra calories per day. That number might seem innocent enough in isolation, but so does online poker. Just as your online debt can skyrocket after a few hours of Texas hold 'em, so can your waistline. In just 1 week, two oversize healthy snacks per day can contribute to an extra pound of fat.

QUICK FIX: Enjoy your food, but do it wisely. The lean, nutritious snacks in the meal plan will help you crush your cravings and whittle down your waist. Your best bet is to use one hand to solve your cravings. (Mind out of the gutters, fellas.) If a portion does not fit into your hand—whether it's some almonds, a chicken breast, cheese, or some fruit—then the portion is probably too much. If it's a packaged food, take 10 seconds and read the label. You're usually looking for something with 200 to 300 calories per serving, about 15 to 20 grams of protein, and with the same amount of carbs as protein (or less).

4. Eat more, drink less

Want to instantly cut weight? Conduct a quick inventory of what you eat and drink every day, and then remove all of the beverages not named water. Now add up the calories. If you're like most men, you'll find that you can cut your non-meal calories by more than 50 percent, according to the *American Journal of Clinical Nutrition*. In fact, 65 percent of Americans indulge daily in calorie-rich beverages, and those drinks are oftentimes the real culprit behind your weight loss struggles—not your metabolism. The problem is so bad that in 2011, Americans drank an average of 53 gallons of soda a year ... per person. That's enough sugar to make Willy Wonka diabetic and more than enough to turn your abs into a potbelly.

QUICK FIX: Stick to water, coffee (watch the creamers), teas, and calorie-free drinks to help keep your slim-down plan on track. Remember that any sugar drink—whether it's soda or a fruit juice—should be considered the equivalent of a dessert. And beer? You can indulge, but moderation is always key. Admit what you already know: Drink a lot in one night and you'll end up stuffing your face with piles of food as well (name a time that didn't happen).

5. Lift weights more often

The calorie tracker on the elliptical might make running seem like a fat loss genie, but all is not as it seems. That's because the more miles you log, the more efficient your body becomes at running and the fewer calories it burns. In other words, running may initially help you drop some pounds, but your progress will flatline as soon as your body adjusts to your exercise regimen. Plus, running long distances on a regular basis takes a physical toll (in the form of injuries, like runner's knee), which can seriously dampen your enthusiasm. Ultimately, all that pain and boredom can cause many people to burn out. Even worse, they give up the exercise routine altogether.

THE ABS BENEFIT

40

Percent less likely men are to die of cancer when they are at a healthy weight

THE ABS BENEFIT

12

Percent less likely men are to have a stroke when they lower their body fat percentage by just 2 percent

Six-Pack Secrets

WEIGHTS VS. MACHINES— WHICH IS BETTER?

Your local gym isn't necessarily designed for success. Why? Most gyms are filled with machines. And while you can experience a great workout hitting the latest machine circuit, it's an inefficient and dangerous way to exercise, say Drake University researchers. While it's true that you can use more weight with machines, you'll experience greater muscle activation with free weights. You see, free weights work your body harder with less weight. That means you can have a better, more efficient workout, without putting unnecessary stress on your body. Your best path is to use dumbbells and your own bodyweight to get back in shape.

QUICK FIX: Start lifting bodyweight and heavy metal. Just 3 days a week of resistance training will keep you burning calories and will offer the metabolic boost you need to slash fat and look hot in whatever outfit you choose.

Head to the gym three times a week, but don't make the cardio your first priority. Instead, use The Abs Workout in Chapter 8 to put your body on the fast track to rapid fat loss.

6. Lift heavier weights

Not only should you be lifting weights, you should also be focusing on the larger dumbbells. That's because researchers at Washington University School of Medicine in St. Louis discovered that the more iron you lift, the more fat you burn. In fact, the researchers found that heavy weights burn more calories during your workout and then increase your sleeping metabolism by 8 percent. That's right. You burn more calories just by lying on your back and dreaming of Scarlett Johansson. That 8 percent doesn't sound like much on a daily basis, but it can add up to more than 5 pounds a year.

QUICK FIX: When you perform The Abs Workout, don't be afraid to use bigger weights as you get more comfortable and improve your strength. Each time you reach the goal rep range, increase the weight and keep pushing yourself to become better.

7. Eat more fish (oil)

University of Pennsylvania researchers found that omega-3 fatty acids might be the secret ingredient to burning fat and gaining muscle at the same time. The scientists believe that omega-3s help fight against cortisol—the stress your body produces that makes it easier for you to store fat. By shutting down your cortisol production, you keep the extra weight off your hips, thighs, and stomach, and have an easier time adding lean, calorie-shredding muscle.

QUICK FIX: Take fish oil daily, whether it's a supplement or a whole food source like salmon or sardines. Alan Aragon, MS, a *Men's Health* nutrition advisor, recommends 2 to 3 grams of fish oil per day.

8. Load up on protein

Every time you eat a meal and don't consume protein, you're telling your body that you don't want to burn more calories. Here's why: Protein helps control your blood sugar, keeps you fuller, reduces hunger, and burns more calories during the digestion process so you can stay lean and strong and still enjoy your favorite foods. Also, it's harder for protein to be turned into fat. So if you're ever going to overeat, protein is your meal of choice.

QUICK FIX: Carbohydrates are not evil. But when you eat them alone, they set off a series of events—such as a rise of insulin—that can sabotage your healthy eating habits and cause you to crave more food and store more fat. So whether you're snacking or eating a meal, include some protein, and you'll drop fat and defeat stress. For meals, a 6-ounce portion (fish, chicken, beef) is reasonable. For snacks, think smaller: a handful of nuts, a stick of string cheese, or a cup of Greek yogurt or cottage cheese.

9. Don't fear the fat

If science has proven anything during the last 10 years, it's that eating fat helps you become slim. In fact, the Institute of Medicine recommends that fatty foods make up 20 to 35 percent of your total calories. This, of course, isn't an invitation to head over to the nearest fast-food joint. The fats you want to include in your diet are primarily saturated fats—from milk, red meat, and pork products—and monounsaturated fats (MUFAs) like nuts, avocados, and healthy oils.

A report published in the *British Journal of Nutrition* found that a MUFA-rich diet helped people lose small amounts of weight and body fat without changing their calorie intakes. Another report found that a breakfast high in MUFAs could boost calorie burn for 5 hours after the meal, particularly in people with higher amounts of belly fat. What's more, dieters who took a high-fat approach needed 25 fewer days to lose 10 pounds than those who used a high-carb approach, according to researchers at Johns Hopkins. And that was on a diet of 30 percent fat!

Even better: Fatty foods actually improve your HDL (good) cholesterol, which can help clear your arteries and prevent heart disease. And finally, a higher fat diet tends to lead to less consumption of carbohydrates, meaning you have fewer insulin spikes. The less you spike your insulin, the more you can control your hunger and reduce fat storage.

QUICK FIX: Fat is your friend! As long as you are staying away from fried foods, trans fats, and partially hydrogenated oils, the healthy fats you eat will make you leaner. According to the latest research, about 30 to 40 percent of your daily calories should come from fat. Opt for beef, pork, poultry, eggs, fatty fish (like salmon), cheese, and nuts. For your complete abs shopping guide, check out "The Lean Guide to Eating" in Chapter 4.

10. Eat real foods

Despite their low-calorie, low-carb, or low-fat claims, the "diet" foods at your grocery store might be the worst thing for your body if you're trying to lose weight. The reason is quite simple: Diet foods try to trick your brain. They provide you with the taste of a high-calorie meal without all the calories, but are filled with chemicals, artificial sweeteners, and preservatives. Unfortunately, your brain isn't fooled, and it leaves you craving more food, which causes you to overeat. Diet foods are usually packaged and processed, meaning they aren't filled with as much high-quality nutrition as the foods that come from natural sources. So not only are you gaining weight, you're also depriving your body of the most potent sources of nutrients that protect your general health. Even worse, diet sodas and artificial sugars may increase your risk for metabolic syndrome, which includes higher levels of belly fat, blood sugar, and cholesterol, according to scientists at the University of Minnesota.

THE
ABS
BENEFIT

40

Percent less likely men are to develop arthritis of the hips or knees when they drop 5 pounds of belly fat

THE
ABS
BENEFIT

69

Percent decrease in development of type 2 diabetes when you have lower body fat

Six-Pack Secrets

QUICK FIX: **Stick to whole, unprocessed foods. As a general guideline, try to shop around the perimeter of your grocery store. That's where you'll find more fresh produce and fewer prepackaged items. For all your shopping needs, use "The Lean Guide to Eating" shopping list (page 65).**

11. Enjoy your food!

It's not just what you eat—the way you eat might be the best way to curb your hunger. Eating fast makes you gain weight, according to Japanese researchers. In their study, they found that people who ate faster gained more weight than those who didn't. But if you want to flip the off switch on your insatiable appetite, all you need to do is slow down and enjoy. According to a study in the *American Journal of Clinical Nutrition,* people who take smaller bites and chew their food for nearly 10 seconds eat less food compared to those who scarf their bites in 3 seconds or less. That's because your satiety isn't just based on the amount of food you put in your stomach. In fact, the longer you keep food in your mouth, the fuller you feel.

What's more, it takes your stomach about 20 minutes to process food and then signal to your brain that you're full. The slower approach will not only leave you more satisfied, but also help keep you from overeating before your body has a chance to tell you that it's satisfied, say University of Rhode Island researchers.

QUICK FIX: **We don't expect you to bring a timer to your meals, so instead focus on how** much you chew your food. Chewing releases more flavor to your tastebuds, which will make all of your meals more savory and enjoyable. Plus it's a much nicer, calmer ritual to actually enjoy your food instead of gulping it down like a starving dog.

12. Worry less, eat less

Take a deep breath before you head into the kitchen to cook your next meal. As you know, the more stressed-out you are, the more comfort food you crave. But now scientists have figured out why: Stress activates ghrelin, a hormone that makes you feel hungry. When you're stressed before you eat, it alters the levels of dopamine (a feel-good hormone) in your system, suggest researchers from the University of Texas Southwestern Medical Center. The result: You don't achieve satisfaction from your meal, which leaves you craving more food.

QUICK FIX: **While a stressful day may feel impossible to overcome, the stress in your body is like a light switch: It turns on and off very easily. Simply find a distraction that calms you down—turn on the game, listen to music, call a friend—and within 5 to 10 minutes, your stress level will decrease so you can enjoy your meal without doubling back for more.**

13. Enjoy dessert

Go ahead, treat yourself—keep it small and frequent. When you're trying to lose weight, the worst thing you can do is ban all indulgences, which creates a feeling of withdrawal. German researchers discovered that this mentality makes it harder to stick to a plan and more likely that you'll pack on the pounds. A more effective approach is one that allows you to satisfy your cravings in controlled portions. Recent research from the University of Alabama found that when overweight people ate small desserts four times a week, they lost 9 more pounds than those who enjoyed a larger splurge whenever they wanted. The small sweets provide the psychological edge that allows you to stay motivated, without derailing your eating plan.

QUICK FIX: Within any diet, 10 to 20 percent of your calories can be directed toward a little treat, says nutritionist Alan Aragon. The key is watching the portion size, so that a cup of ice cream doesn't turn into an entire bowl. You'll learn more about how to make dessert a regular part of your diet in Chapter 5.

14. Eat with your gym crew

People who work out together should dine together. Eating with those who have a similar goal helps you lose pounds faster, according to a study in the journal *Obesity*. Once again, it's all mental. When you're with people who are also trying to lose weight, the social expectation creates a different attitude toward food (for example, you won't have to worry that everyone will be ordering chocolate lava cake for dessert). It's like weight loss osmosis. The good intentions of your fellow eaters rub off on you, and it makes the entire dietary process easier.

QUICK FIX: Try to make plans with buddies on a similar track to weight loss success. Reward yourself with a trip to a fun new restaurant, with those who will encourage you to make the right menu choices.

15. Shake up your diet

The stuff you see in the window of your local GNC isn't just for serious weight lifters. Protein powder can shrink your gut. This efficient source of protein is low in calories, maintains your hard-earned muscle, and helps you lower your body fat percentage. The most efficient kind of protein is whey. According to a study in the *Journal of Nutrition*, participants who took whey protein for 23 weeks had less body fat and a smaller waist than those who consumed soy protein. In fact, dieters who included whey protein in their eating plan doubled their fat loss compared to those who ate the same number of calories but didn't drink any shakes. Consider protein powder the little bit of extra magic that will finally reveal your abs.

QUICK FIX: Include a whey protein shake once a day or at least a few times a week. But don't feel that you can only have a shake before or after your workout. You can also substitute a shake for breakfast or a snack. Just make sure that shakes are always a secondary option to whole food sources. You'll find some great shake and smoothie recipes in Chapter 6.

THE ABS BENEFIT

21

Percent less likely men will experience erectile dysfunction if they exercise

Six-Pack Secrets

16. Add the big D

Here's something unexpected to add to your fat loss cocktail: vitamin D. That's because taking supplemental vitamin D can help you lose more fat. In a recent study, Canadian researchers found that people who take supplemental vitamin D store less body fat and burn more fat. Turns out, it plays a vital role in the hormones that cause your body to hold on to fat in your belly. So the more vitamin D, the more eager your body is to burn away your excess cheeseburgers. The magical vitamin also appears to reduce production of cortisol, the stress hormone that causes you to store belly fat.

QUICK FIX: While you can receive vitamin D from foods or even the sun, we recommend taking an additional 2,000 to 4,000 IU of vitamin D per day to receive the health benefits. If you want to avoid the supplemental route altogether, eat fish (such as salmon), dairy products (like yogurt), eggs, and mushrooms.

17. Make your goals personal

Setting goals is one of the most important parts of creating a successful plan—just make sure that you keep your intentions to yourself. While a good social support system is important, making your goals public can actually hurt your progress, according to research performed at New York University. When you tell your friends of your plans, their recognition can be interpreted as an accomplishment, and that feedback can decrease your motivation, according to the researchers.

QUICK FIX: When you start *The Men's Health Big Book: Getting Abs,* it's essential that you write down your goals. Don't just think them; prescribe an actual set of quantitative and qualitative goals. Take "before" pictures. By documenting your starting point, you'll create more internal motivation that will push you toward your goals. But until you reach your benchmarks, keep your specific objectives to yourself.

18. Do your body good

Looking for an abs power food? Try the original protein shake: milk. Scientists from Canada found that people who eat a high protein diet that consists of dairy gain more muscle and lose more fat compared to other diet combinations. The reason: Milk contains whey and casein, a powerful combo that delivers protein to your body in two phases, quickly and over time. This helps it reach your muscles fast and last longer than other forms of protein—keeping you feeling full and satisfied.

QUICK FIX: If you're not allergic or sensitive to dairy, add 8 to 16 ounces of milk to your diet to experience the benefits of the powerful protein. And if you're lactose intolerant, be sure to check out Chapter 7 for other smart options.

OH, AND LET'S NOT FORGET . . .

3 Big Reasons You Don't Have Abs

If there are repeated mantras in this book, it's because the information needs to be hammered home. Why? It's too easy to sabotage yourself, and research has shown again and again that the following habits are the fastest way to prevent—or erase—gains.

Beer is your best friend

Yes, this might be the *most* obvious answer, but it's also the most commonly overlooked. Listen, we're not going to tell you to stop drinking alcohol, but there are few things in this world that will kill your six-pack dreams faster. They're liquid calories, and the hops in beer have been linked to increases in estrogen, which makes your body soft. Those beers are a gateway for wings, pizza, and more beer. So you have to choose: You can have one type of six pack or the other.

Your workout sucks

While we might all wish it were true, every workout isn't designed to help you see your six pack. On the surface it might all seem the same: You lift weights, maybe add in some cardio, and then end with abs. But even if every workout includes an abdominal focus, that doesn't make it an ab-centric workout. For that, you need a special blend of exercises, rest periods, and planned progress to strip away your face and reveal the ripples in your midsection. Anyone that says all workouts are created equal doesn't know what they're talking about.

You train, but you don't "diet"

Guys like dieting about as much as they enjoy watching *Top Model* or visiting the proctologist. But neither of those facts changes the truth: You can't out-exercise a bad diet. Most guys do work hard in the gym, but then follow by eating what they want, when they want, and however much they desire. It doesn't matter how good your genetics are, without a smart approach to eating you will have trouble seeing your abs.

Chapter 2
All Your Abs Questions Answered

The ultimate Q&A session on carbs, tricky supplements, and the exercises that will carve your core.

What's the fastest way to lose fat?"

Simple. Bust your ass in the gym and follow a good diet. Did you expect something more complex?

Good, because actually, ass-busting won't get the job done. And there are plenty of good diets, but eating "healthy" foods doesn't guarantee that you'll lose weight, either. You see, in order to make the most of your gym time, you need to pick the right type of exercise and increase your intensity. That means prioritizing resistance training, pushing yourself to use heavier weights, and limiting your rest periods. Say good-bye to 5-minute chats with your buddies between sets. You want to be in and out of the gym fast—45 minutes is ideal, 60 max—and that's what will crank up your metabolism. Mix in a steady blend of squats, deadlifts, presses, and rows, and you have the ingredients you

All Your Abs Questions Answered

need for a body transformation. And that's exactly what you'll find in The Abs Workout in Chapter 8.

As for your diet, use the quick fixes you learned in the previous chapter to simplify your approach. Eat protein, limit processed foods, and don't over-snack. You'll find that the best fat loss diets tend to be lower in carbohydrates—but low carbs *doesn't* mean no carbs. Instead, put a bigger emphasis on protein and fats, and fill the gaps with carbs. We'll show you exactly how starting on page 53.

Now that you know there is a "fastest" way to burn fat—and that we'll be providing the solution—let's show you the rest of what you need to know to see your abs and keep them for good. We took some of our readers' most commonly asked questions, sent them to our smartest experts, and combined them into one chapter of information you can understand and use to your advantage.

I'm losing pounds but I don't look any different. What's wrong?

Technically, nothing is wrong. I know plenty of guys who would sacrifice a month of drinking if they could get the scale to downshift. (Ironically, that's exactly what most need to do.) But the key to actually seeing your abs isn't a matter of pure weight loss. You want to eliminate the excess fat that is currently invading your body, and build up some muscle to show off.

If you're just losing pounds but look the same, usually this means you're not weight training or eating enough of the right foods, says Alan Aragon, MS, a nutritionist in Westlake Village, California, and a *Men's Health* advisor. Doing both is the key to eliminating fat and building muscle—as opposed to just seeing a different number on the scale—and that's when you'll look like you have a new body. Resistance training burns calories during your sessions and stimulates your metabolism afterward. Make sure you get enough protein after a workout by having either 6 ounces of meat or 2 scoops of protein powder; each option yields about 40 grams of protein.

How often do I need to exercise to lose fat?

It might sound surprising, but you don't need to exercise to lose fat. You can shed your unwanted pounds by making sure you eat fewer calories than you burn, says Aragon. (This should show you the importance of a good diet.)

However, if you avoid exercise, you won't retain as much muscle, which means it'll be harder for you to eliminate your beer gut and have flat, sexy abs. You can lose weight without exercise, but if you don't retain or build muscle, your metabolism won't be as efficient, which means you'll have to eat even less food to see the same results. You can do better than that: A sensible exercise program will help stoke your metabolism, which will help you burn more fat, which will help reveal your six-pack. You're reconditioning your body as a metabolic engine.

So how much exercise does it take to achieve that? Take note, gym haters, it's really not that huge of a commitment. With just 30 minutes a day, 3 days a week, you can eat the foods you want and fast-track your weight loss. You'll find all the exercises you need starting in Chapter 9.

Do I need to count calories?

Counting calories is mainly a way of staying consistent with an eating plan that will allow you to lose weight, says Aragon. But that doesn't mean you need to do it to get results. In fact, we've created a no-calorie-counting method that sparks fat loss. The foods in this diet are flexible so you can choose your meals. But they also focus on foods that are energy dense, such as protein-filled foods, fruits, and vegetables. You'll be able to eat more of these foods and feel full, without expanding your waistline. You'll eat better, and, without realizing it, you'll be dropping pounds, too. For the ultimate guy's grocery list, check out "The Lean Guide to Eating" shopping list on page 65.

Do carbs give you a belly?

In a word, no. Your belly comes from eating too many calories. If you overeat, you'll store fat, regardless of what foods those calories come from, says Aragon. The leanest, healthiest populations on the planet typically eat more carbs than protein or fat. Controlling weight gain is more about total calorie balance than any particular food.

Now, that said, some people find it easier to control their weight when they reduce or avoid carb-heavy foods that they have a tendency to overindulge in, adds Aragon. And some people have sensitivities to processed grains and gluten, which make the fat loss process more difficult. But if you can control your intake and don't have sensitivities, enjoy the carbs. The best way to prevent overeating is to make sure that most of your carbs come from raw fruits and vegetables, while leaving a small portion for desserts.

Are protein shakes okay to drink when trying to lose weight?

Of course. Don't be fooled by the marketing slapped on most protein containers. While it'd be great if a powder could be Viagra for your muscles, protein powder is usually very low in calories, with most brands clocking in between 100 and 120 calories per serving. Not exactly the calorie bomb that will kill your abs plan. You can absolutely benefit from protein shakes, especially if you have a tough time hitting your protein requirement through regular whole foods. Just make sure you keep a close eye on the ingredient list of your favorite shake. There's a big difference between a protein powder and a "weight gainer" formula: One is just protein and the other is filled with excess carbs, fats, and calories and designed for those who are working extra hard to pack on the pounds and bulk up fast.

All Your Abs Questions Answered

Will eating smaller meals control my hunger?

Your meals are like the sports teams you represent: It's all personal preference, and don't let anyone else dump on your choice. Some people do great with a grazing pattern, while others prefer more substantial meals with less frequency. But there's a catch: When people are eating fewer calories than they're used to, they tend to prefer eating two to three larger meals rather than four to six small ones throughout the day, says Aragon. As for more frequent meals being better for your metabolism? That's just a myth that's been recently disproved by science. Canadian researchers proved this in 2010 when they compared folks eating three meals versus six meals and found no difference in participants' fat loss when the exact same foods were consumed.

How do I know what fat is okay to eat?

There's no need to avoid any particular type of fat, except for partially hydrogenated vegetable oils, which contain the harmful type of trans fat. Recent research has shown that saturated fat is actually good for you and isn't linked to heart failure or cardiovascular disease, says Aragon.

In fact, your diet probably doesn't include enough fat. (Marketers have done a very good job of brainwashing us about the benefits of "fat-free" versions of manufactured foods, which basically means the salt and sugar content has been boosted to make up for flavor loss.) The standard American diet lacks omega-3 fatty acids, which can be found in fish like salmon and sardines. Aside from that, the majority of the fats you eat should come from whole, minimally processed foods like meats, dairy, eggs, vegetables, fruits, nuts, seeds, avocados, grains, and olive oil.

Can I just do cardio, or do I need to lift weights to see my abs?

Answer that question with another question: Do you want the body of a man or a boy? Pumping a little iron is the most important part of any plan that you hope ends with you sporting a six-pack. When you add resistance training to your routine, it can speed up the weight loss process by making your muscles more efficient fat-burning furnaces, says Aragon. What's more, it's also good for your bone health and cardiovascular health, as well as optimizing glucose control so your body processes carbohydrates better. Plus, in addition to sculpting your abs, you'll build definition in your entire body and be able to eat more food. How many more reasons could you possibly need?

Can I have dairy and still lose my gut?

Even if you can't rock a manly 'stache, there's nothing wrong with sporting the milk version. In fact, researchers from the University of Tennessee found that dairy may help eliminate belly fat when you're on a weight loss plan. You can even enjoy higher-fat cheeses and yogurts. The trick is, make sure you don't eat too much. Cheese and milk are both high in calories, so keep a close eye on your portion size—and enjoy.

What foods are the worst for ruining defined abs?

Your focus shouldn't be on the worst foods but instead on the best plan. A great eating plan—like the one you'll find in this book—highlights the healthy, nutritious foods that make dropping pounds as effortless as texting. Understand, it's impossible to judge foods in isolation from the rest of your diet. What matters most for shedding belly fat boils down to calories in versus calories out. It might be tempting to call a certain food, like a candy bar, "bad" for your abs. But if that candy bar is part of a diet that's dominated by whole and minimally processed foods, and eating it doesn't blow your calorie load for the afternoon, it could actually be "great" for your abs. Those small indulgences are often what helps you adhere to your program. This is why cheat meals actually work: Virtually no foods are off-limits as long as they're a small portion of what you eat.

I sit at a desk all day. Is there anything that I can do at work to improve my abs?

Get up from your desk as often as you can. A minimum of every half hour, try to at least stand up and stretch, then walk around, take a trip to the restroom, or take a lap around the office, says Aragon. This process is important because it increases your non-exercise activity thermogenesis (NEAT). Your NEAT plays a big role in the number of calories you burn, so even small movements like fidgeting or tapping your heels can contribute to your overall transformation. This will also help prevent your desk job from altering your posture, which can play a role in your slowed metabolism (not to mention an aching back!).

And here's a radical idea: These days, a majority of the editors in the *Men's Health* office now have "standing rigs" at their desks, which allow them to stand and work at their computers for as long as they want (some stand all day). All you need is a way to raise your screen and keyboard. You'll burn more calories daily, improve your posture, and never, ever fall asleep at your desk.

Should I take supplements to see my abs?

Most fat loss supplements are a waste of money, and most of them have risks that outweigh the minimal gains of fat loss, says Aragon. The most potent fat loss supplements contained caffeine and ephedrine, but that combination was banned from the market after too many reports of adverse, dangerous effects. The truth is, the actual fat loss caused by any supplement is minor and is even less significant in people who are overweight or have a substantial amount of weight to lose, says Aragon. Bottom line:

All Your Abs Questions Answered

The best and only real way to see your abs is to focus on two things: what you eat and how you exercise.

Is it okay to have artificial sweeteners?

This is an area of big debate among nutritionists, but there's no scientific evidence that artificial sweeteners will make you fat. If you can avoid them, you should. That said, some people will still include them in their diet. For those who do, make sure you don't abuse diet soft drinks, which are filled with fake sugars, says Aragon. A good rule of thumb is to limit your intake of artificial sweeteners to 3 to 4 servings per day at most, whether it's from a diet soft drink or some other artificially sweetened product. If your diet consists mainly of real foods, you can enjoy a little sugar, whether it's artificial or not.

Isn't running the fastest way to lose weight?

It depends: How fast are you running? No question, running is a great form of exercise, and it can be very good for your overall cardiovascular health. But long, slow jogs are not an efficient way to blast away your fat, says strength coach Eric Cressey, CSCS, owner of Cressey Performance in Hudson, Massachusetts. If running is your preferred form of exercise, then stick to interval or fartlek training (yeah, yeah, I know, I said "fartlek"). This form of exercise has you working at a high level of intensity for short periods of time, followed by quick rest periods. Overall, your cardio workouts will be shorter but much more effective.

However, if you want to shed pounds fast, you'll want to spend the bulk of your exercise time performing resistance training. Adding muscle helps you burn more calories, even when you're not exercising. Bottom line: Resistance training doesn't just take body fat off—it keeps it off.

Can I get flat abs by just doing crunches?

You want to lose belly fat as fast as possible, right? To do that, you need exercises that activate the most number of muscle fibers, says Cressey. Crunches simply don't cut it. When you perform multi-muscle and multi-joint exercises, you're actually working your abs whether you realize it or not. This is why movements like squats, deadlifts, lunges, chinups, and pushups are so effective. They work the muscles you feel (legs, arms, chest, back, shoulders) and your abs simultaneously. Any workout that incorporates these moves will keep your core working overtime and ensure that you'll see a flat belly in no time.

Think of it this way: Compound exercises are actually compound movements, and what do you encounter during your day-to-day activities? Compound movements. Whether it's picking up a toddler or reaching to put something up on the top shelf, compound movements prepare you for what life throws your way. And a little bit of strength goes a long way in making your life easier, such as preventing nagging issues—like throwing out your back or having sore knees—that occur naturally when you ignore these types of exercises. These exercises will create such incredible changes to your body that you'll not only be happy with your newfound strength, but also be thrilled every time you walk past a mirror.

So does that mean squats and deadlifts are enough, or do I also need to do direct abs work?

Relying on compound exercises to develop the core muscles is only one piece of the puzzle, says Jim Smith, CSCS, strength coach and owner of Diesel Strength & Conditioning. Compound exercises such as squats and deadlifts utilize the core as it was intended: to stabilize your torso, protect your spine, and transfer force. But if your core is too weak, then you won't be able to transfer force and you'll struggle to improve at the exercises. That's why targeting your core directly must be integrated into your workout to train weaknesses that aren't always easy to spot.

My doctor has warned me that I'm a candidate for a hernia. Is there a good way to work the lower abs?

Abs-olutely, and thanks for reminding readers that our abs have functionality beyond making women want to rub our bellies. All men are at risk for hernias, especially if they're starting from scratch physically. A regular hernia is a protrusion of intestine through a weakness in the lower abdominal wall. A "sports" hernia is a tearing of abdominal muscle where it attaches to the pubic bone in the pelvis. Both types are caused by underconditioned abdominal muscles.

So here's the deal: While you can never fully isolate a muscle group, Spanish researchers discovered that specific exercises can individually target the upper and lower regions of rectus abdominis (the six-pack) to a greater extent. For example, exercises like the Reverse Crunch (page 323) can engage the lower abs, says Smith. Luckily, you can find variations in Chapter 9 to completely train the entire region.

Is there one abs exercise that I should definitely be doing?

Your core is complex because it's involved in virtually every movement. Sometimes you'll be flexing (like Med Ball Slam, page 325), other times stabilizing (Plank, page 282), and then there are times when you need to resist movement (anti-rotation exercises like the Cable Core Press, page 321).

But if you're looking for the most bang for your training time, says Smith, it's hard to beat the Dumbbell (or kettlebell) Getup (page 227). Getups require you to stabilize your core in multiple planes of motion and have stability through an unrestricted full-range movement. Who cares about stability? Your six-pack. And when

All Your Abs Questions Answered

ABOUT THE EXPERTS

Alan Aragon is a nutritionist with more than 18 years of success in the fitness field. He earned his master's degree in nutrition with top honors. Aragon is a continuing education provider for the Commission on Dietetic Registration, National Academy of Sports Medicine, American Council on Exercise, and National Strength and Conditioning Association. He maintains a private practice designing programs for recreational, Olympic, and professional athletes including the Los Angeles Lakers, Los Angeles Kings, and Anaheim Mighty Ducks. Aragon is a contributing editor and resident weight loss coach of *Men's Health* magazine, and runs a research review that can be found at http://alanaragon.com.

Eric Cressey is president and co-founder of Cressey Performance, a facility located just west of Boston. He is a Certified Strength and Conditioning Specialist (CSCS) through the National Strength and Conditioning Association and received his master's degree in kinesiology, with a concentration in exercise science, through the University of Connecticut Department of Kinesiology.

you're doing an exercise where your abs must support and stabilize every movement to prevent you from falling over, they work harder and build more muscle that you can use and see. Translation: shredded abs.

Can I work my abs every day?

Training the muscles in your core is just like training any other muscle group. They require stimulation to develop and time to recover in order rebuild. For most people, this means only training your abs three or four times per week. If you want to train your abs—or any body part—every day, you need to look at two things: the intensity of your last workout and the recovery techniques you use between workouts, says Smith. In order to make progress, you must vary the levels of intensity from workout to workout, so that you give yourself time to recover and you don't affect your performance in a subsequent training session. When training abs in successive sessions, try to target different core movement patterns with each workout. This will ensure you improve progressively and don't overtrain with each workout.

Everyone says I need low body fat to see my abs. I'm skinny but still can't see them. What's wrong?

Your body is like a statue: You don't simply chisel away stone and make greatness appear. You actually have to create the fine details that turn it into a work of art. So while it is true that you

need to attain a low body fat percentage to see a nice set of abs, that's just part of the equation. You have to develop those muscles, too. Crunches are fool's gold for that. Because your rectus abdominis (the six-pack muscles) is responsible for movement that is generated at your hips, exercises like hanging knee raises and ab rollouts help maximize activation of your muscles so that once you burn away your fat, your abs are ready to pop.

I've been told not to eat late, but usually I'm starving after my shift. What should I do?

Your body isn't on a 24-hour clock. What counts is whether you burn more calories than you ingest by the end of the day (or better yet, the week), says Aragon. If your cravings surface at night, any combination of fruit, nuts, nut butter, or dairy (such as milk, yogurt, or cheese) makes a perfect pre-bed snack. Just watch your portion size.

If I sit on an exercise ball instead of a chair at my office, will I lose weight?

Sitting on a ball might help strengthen your core, but it won't help you burn a significant number of calories. The misconception comes, in part, from studies on non-exercise activity. Fidgeting, a common example, is often cited as a way to help burn extra calories. Mayo Clinic researchers found a significant increase in energy expenditure if you fidget while standing. But that effect is not as pronounced if you fidget while seated, says Aragon. So any difference between ball sitting and chair sitting is probably too small to have a real impact, calorie-wise.

But there are other little ways to move around that do keep you more active: walking over to a co-worker's desk instead of e-mailing, standing up while talking on the phone, or just taking a brief lap around your office every so often. (And check out a standing desk, like I previously mentioned.)

I always gorge after a workout. Bad habit?

Depends on your definition of "gorge." Are we talking large meal or John Belushi in the Animal House cafeteria? Postworkout is actually the best time to have the largest meal of your day—as long as it's a reasonable size and not a hot dog eating contest (48-ounce steaks are a lousy idea, too). Eating well post-workout helps replenish your body's spent fuel reserves, and food can help aid your muscle recovery. Also, when your body is in a recovery state, incoming calories and nutrients stand a better chance of being absorbed by muscle tissue instead of being stored as fat.

Your strategy: To curb uncontrollable hunger after a workout, make sure you're filling up on beef, poultry, or fish. Solid foods are more filling than liquid foods, and protein is the most filling of all. Pair some of that meat with whole food, high-fiber carbohydrate sources, such as beans, because fiber can also help you feel fuller faster.

3 Abs Myths Busted

If you listened to all the flawed abs advice out there, you'd be doing upside-down crunches until you passed out. Some people tell you to do crunches, some say planks, and others insist that you avoid both entirely. The truth is, there's a place for almost every type of abdominal training, but not all of them will have you ready to hit South Beach. Here's how to make the most of every rep, no matter what exercise you do.

Myth #1: **High-rep workouts make your abs grow.**

Reality: Your progress will plateau if you do the same exercises, regardless of reps.

You need to intensify and vary your workouts, and include exercises that train your abs to stabilize your bodyweight. Technically, every exercise you perform could be considered a stabilizing movement. After all, your abs help support your spine and hips. But there are some exercises that force more stabilization and thus make your abs work harder. Compare a plank to your traditional situp. Sure, your abs are doing some work on situps. But so is your lower back (I know you've felt that twinge), and momentum usually starts taking over at some point. On the other hand, what's holding you up on a plank? It's your abs, which are supporting your bodyweight and preventing your body from collapse. Do a plank with only one arm or one leg, and suddenly you realize just how much stability—or lack

An accomplished author, Eric has written more than 200 articles and five books. He also co-created four DVD sets that have been sold in more than 50 countries. You can find his work at http://ericcressey.com.

Jim Smith is a strength coach and owner of Diesel Strength & Conditioning (http://dieselsc.com). Smith is a highly respected, world-renowned strength and conditioning specialist who has been called one of the most innovative strength coaches in the fitness industry. Training athletes, fitness enthusiasts, and weekend warriors, he is dedicated to helping them reach beyond their potential. Smith holds multiple national fitness certifications, including Certified Strength and Conditioning Specialist (CSCS) and Russian Kettlebell Certification (RKC), and is a member of the United States Weightlifting Association (USAW). He is a consultant and lecturer, and speaks at seminars all over the country. He is the author of several strength-, power-, and muscle-building manuals and has produced best-selling DVDs covering all aspects of strength training.

All Your Abs Questions Answered

thereof—makes your abs burn with each passing second.

Your plan: Add either more challenging variations of bodyweight exercises or weighted abdominal exercises once the unweighted versions become too easy. Matt McGorry, CFT, a trainer at Peak Performance in New York City, recommends the triple plank. This combo—a front plank followed by a left-side plank and a right-side plank—forces you to contract your abs for long intervals, which helps carve your midsection. Start by maintaining each plank for 15 seconds and work up to 60 seconds. When you hit that level, start adding sets, resting only 30 seconds between them. If planks on the floor are too easy, put your feet on a small box.

But don't forget: "No amount of abs work can take the place of a well-planned diet and a total-body workout," McGorry says. Abs won't magically appear as you work out; they show when you've built all the muscles in your body and cut the fat around your midsection.

Myth #2: Abs exercises heal lower back pain.

Reality: Some abs exercises make back pain worse.

Hang with us for a second on this one. You've probably heard that a strong core helps prevents back pain. Luckily, the rumor mill didn't screw that one up. Your core actually includes multiple muscles, including your six-pack, your lats (the back muscles that extend like wings from your shoulder blades down to your lower back), your lower back, and even your glutes. When all of those muscles are strong, they serve to protect your back.

But how you build those strong muscles makes a big difference in whether you experience back pain. When you bend your spine during crunches or situps, you risk injuring it, says Stuart McGill, PhD, a professor of spine biomechanics at the University of Waterloo in Ontario. Doing those exercises isn't the best way to target your abs anyway, because you're really just repeatedly bending the disks in your back, not forcing your abs to resist motion. That's why Dr. McGill suggests exercises that encourage spinal alignment and stability, such as planks. Your abs do all the work to keep you stabilized and lower your risk of back injury. (If you have back pain, see a physician before starting any abs regimen. As we said, some abs exercises can make back problems worse.)

Yes, a six-pack is one of our goals, but make sure you approach this journey the right way. Exercises that prevent movement are especially good for building lateral abdominal strength, which is what helps your body stay in proper form under pressure (like when you play sports or do squats and deadlifts). Dr. McGill suggests the suitcase carry: Hold a heavy dumbbell in one hand and then walk increasingly long distances while maintaining perfect posture. This actually burns more calories than crunches do and isn't nearly as tedious!

Myth #3: **Rotational exercises are best for building your obliques.**

Reality: Rotational exercises don't build obliques well at all and can harm the spine in some cases.

Your obliques surround and accentuate your abs and protect them from damage when you rotate your body quickly. So while exercises like twisting side to side while holding a weight can help you build your obliques, they may not be the best way to build foundational strength, and they can force your spine to rotate under stress, says McGorry.

Instead, use heavy compound exercises—like squats and deadlifts—to make your obliques work harder to keep your spine aligned. For more challenge, add unbalanced moves such as a single-leg lunge or a deadlift with one dumbbell. These types of exercises require your body to adjust to uneven stress while your spine is in its neutral position, which further stabilizes your core and builds your obliques (as long as you maintain proper form).

That's not to say that all rotational exercises should be avoided. You'll find many in this book, including movements like chops, lifts, and Russian twists. With these exercises, the secret is to make sure that your rotation occurs at the hips, not in the spine, and that you use your abs to help resist movement rather than create it. When you combine all of these exercises—as you'll do in the workouts ahead—you have the perfect recipe for a bulletproof set of abs.

Chapter 3
The Real Reason You Can't See Your Abs

(It's not what you think.)

This chapter will set your body straight for good.

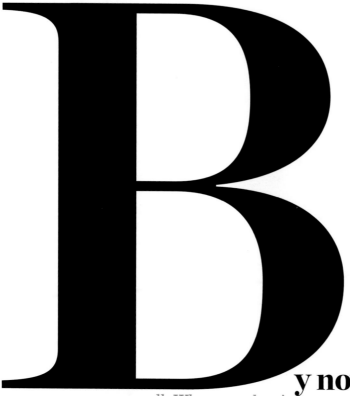

By now, you know the drill quite well. When you begin your quest to uncover your abs, the mission is a simple two-pronged attack: improve your diet and lift weights. You might start with the simple stuff like removing sugar from your diet, eating more fruits and vegetables, and cutting out the booze with your buddies—at least from Monday to Friday. Then you start hitting the gym. Maybe you crunch, maybe you don't. A few rounds of cardio, bench press, bench press, and a few curls, and you're on your way to a six-pack.

But as you soon find out, the two-part mission is a strategic failure. Even if you drop some fat with your new eating plan and build muscle to change the look of your body, you're still likely to fall short of the chiseled abs you see on the cover of this book. Why? (Or, depending on your frustration level, Why, dammit?)

The Real Reason You Can't See Your Abs

You neglected to add a third component to your plan. In reality, it's the one area that almost every guy overlooks, but it's what separates the successes from the "I lost a bunch of weight but still can't see my abs" group. The answer: Improve your posture.

This isn't about sitting up straight in a chair or not slouching on the couch (although you'll want to avoid both of those). Your posture affects everything you do in life—from how you look to how you breathe to how effectively you can train your muscles. You could be in phenomenal physical condition, but if you have a posture problem like, say, an anterior pelvic tilt that pushes your lower body outward, your lean body can look like it has a big belly.

Listen, becoming lean takes consistent hard work. And staying lean requires more of the same dedication. But nothing will derail your plans quicker than poor posture, nagging pains, and unnecessary injuries, says Kevin Neeld, CSCS, exercise scientist, and director of athletic development for Endeavor Sports Performance.

Almost every issue that slows a man's workout progress can be linked to a structural problem that needs to be addressed.

Shoulder problem that won't let you bench press? Posture problem.

Hip pain while squatting? Posture problem.

Back pain? I think you see the point.

Think of it this way: Good posture

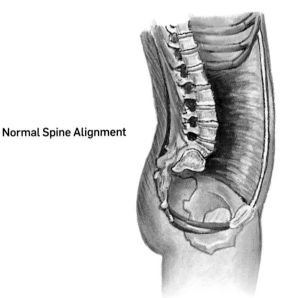

Normal Spine Alignment

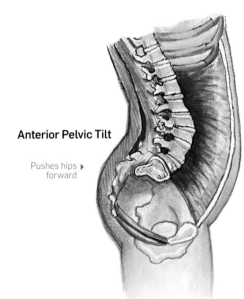

Anterior Pelvic Tilt

Pushes hips ▶ forward

◀ Creates the illusion of a belly

means great progress. Your posture plays an integral role in how you train and what you gain. At any time, the quality of your muscle is determined by the position of the bones in which it interweaves, says Neeld. In other words, the position of your bones dictates the capacity and capabilities of your muscles. If you want to build more muscle and shred more fat, your body must be properly aligned to unleash its true potential. Otherwise, all of your hard work will only produce a fraction of what is possible. Your muscles might not be weak because they are poorly developed; rather, it might be because they are in a poor position to do their job correctly.

Unfortunately, that's not the entire story. Poor posture can also limit your ability to recover, says Neeld. When your body isn't in optimal alignment, certain structures (like the lower region of your spine) are placed under excess tension. And while tension on your muscles is good in the gym, it's bad for recovery because it doesn't allow your muscles to shut off and recuperate.

This is bad news for your abs. When your body is in a state of constant tension, it sends off an alarm, much like getting in a fight with your wife or girlfriend. And while a stressful relationship will result in a night or two of sleeping on the couch, the constant stress on your body can make it harder for your body to adapt and change. If you have stress in one area that's causing pain, your body needs to focus on helping it recover. While this is good for your pain, it's bad for your abs and the rest of your muscles in your body. The pain is a distraction that takes away from the rest of your body to recovery. That's why bad posture is so problematic. It keeps your body in a constant state of stress that never allows everything else to function optimally.

The end result? No matter how hard you work, your metabolism can slow to a crawl and your muscle growth can be locked in place.

Remove the Barriers

If you're serious about getting lean, you have to fix your posture. Think of movement as a continuous flow from one posture to another. With every movement, whether you're walking your dog, sprinting around a track, or going for a new personal record on the squat, there is an optimal alignment for your body based on the demands placed upon it, says Neeld. A failure to find this alignment, at the very least, is an extremely inefficient use of energy; at worst, it will push you closer to injury and impair your ability to change your body.

Luckily, fixing your posture is a relatively simple process. But it's one that requires dedicated effort and focus. Follow this plan designed by Neeld, who is an expert in corrective exercise, to help set your body straight. Not only will you improve your posture, you'll also correct your form on all exercises so that your muscles can work as designed. And when that happens, this essential third component of your abs plan will make your lean body dreams a reality.

The Real Reason You Can't See Your Abs

Optimal Movement for Optimal Results

The key to maximizing your results, and minimizing the risk of having a setback related to pain or an injury, is good form. You hear that all the time from trainers, but what you're about to read is the secret formula for incredible workout results. If you master these seven major exercise movement patterns, you'll apply the principles of posture just discussed, and you'll notice the difference immediately. Use this guide to identify your problem and set your body on a better path.

Lower Body Pushing

Includes almost all squat variations, such as front squats, sumo squats, and one-leg squat.

Common Error

While this pattern has plenty of room for error, one of the most common movement mistakes is not maintaining a neutral lumbar spine (lower back) throughout the motion.

Signs

When you overextend or round your lower back on these exercises, you put excessive stress across the area and are likely to develop back pain.

General Coaching Cues

When performing a lower body pushing pattern, keep the following cues in mind:

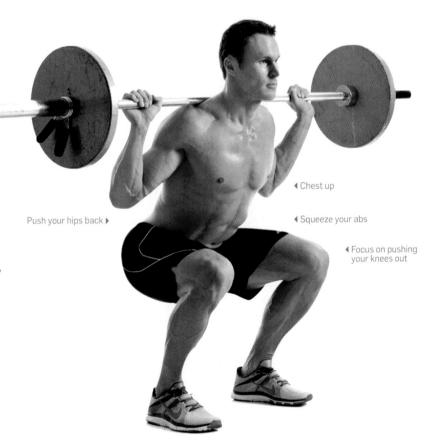

Push your hips back ▶

◀ Chest up

◀ Squeeze your abs

◀ Focus on pushing your knees out

THE ABS SOLUTION

Movement in your lower back is usually an issue of hip mobility or stability (or both). These two exercises will help open up your hips and activate your glutes for better movement.

DIAGONAL HIP ROCK TO STEP

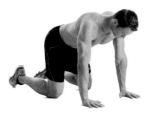

- Begin on all fours with your hands beneath your shoulders and your knees beneath your hips.

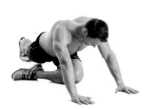

- Keep your back flat as you reach diagonally back with one leg. Pause in this position for a second to feel a stretch in the outside of your front hip.

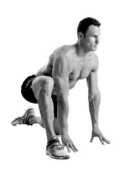

- Then step forward with that leg so your foot is flat on the ground outside your hands. Pull your chest forward so that it extends beyond your hands, and pause for a second to feel a stretch in the front of your back hip and the bottom of your front leg. Return to the starting position and repeat with your other leg. Repeat for 6 to 8 reps on each side.

BACKWARD MONSTER WALK

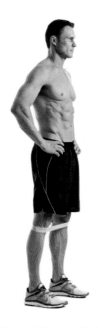
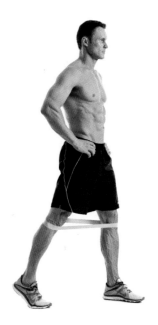

- Start with your feet shoulder-width apart, hands on your hips, and a mini-band wrapped around your legs just beneath your knees. With your hips level, prevent your knees from caving inward and take a step back with one leg so that the toes of that foot are even with the heel of your front foot.

- Now take a step back with the other leg, and continue stepping backward for 15 to 20 yards. You should feel the muscles on the outside and back of your hips engage.

The Real Reason You Can't See Your Abs

Lower Body Pulling

Includes deadlift variations, such as straight and trap bar deadlifts, stiff-legged deadlifts, cable pull-throughs, and box squats.

Common Error

A common movement flaw is not maintaining your neck and upper back position throughout the movement. This pattern is one of the more difficult to master.

Signs

When you create movement through your neck or upper back during these exercises, you place excessive stress on your spine. These movement dysfunctions can lead to pain along the inside of your shoulder blades, through your neck and up into your head. The next time you perform any of these exercises, pay attention to the position of your neck and upper back. Once you lock yourself in place—meaning that your neck and back are aligned with your spine—there shouldn't be any movement. Rounding your shoulders or pulling them too far back, or lifting your head, is a recipe for disaster, especially as you become stronger and lift more weight.

General Coaching Cues

When performing a lower body pulling pattern, keep the following cues in mind:

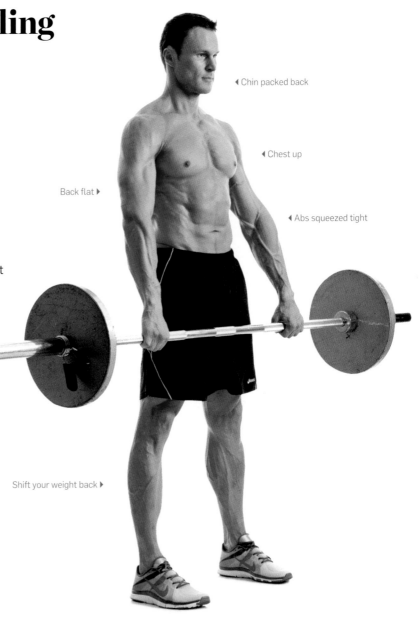

◀ Chin packed back

◀ Chest up

Back flat ▶

◀ Abs squeezed tight

Shift your weight back ▶

THE ABS SOLUTION

You need to teach yourself how to "brace" your spine. That is, you create complete tension throughout your upper back and neck while moving. The movement isn't the hard part; it's maintaining complete stability and staying locked into place while doing anything that is dynamic.

LYING SCAP AND CHIN RETRACTION

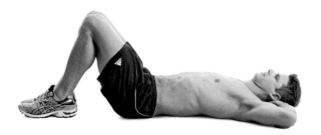

- Lie on your back with your knees bent and feet flat on the ground. Interlock your fingers behind your head.
- Keeping your hands behind your head, squeeze your shoulder blades together so your elbows move toward the floor. You should feel your shoulder blades squeeze together in the back, as if you were trying to hold a pencil with them. From here, imagine growing tall through the back of your neck as you pull your chin in. You should feel your neck stretch in the back.
- Hold this position, with your elbows pulled into the ground and chin pulled in, for 5 seconds. Relax and repeat for 4 to 6 reps.

DUMBBELL FARMER'S WALK

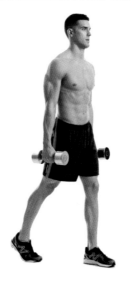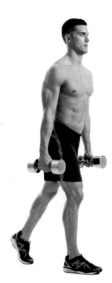

- Grab a pair of heavy dumbbells and hold them at your sides at arm's length.
- Now walk forward (or in a circle) for the prescribed time or distance.
- If you feel like you could have gone longer, grab heavier weights on your next set.

The Real Reason You Can't See Your Abs

Lower Body Split Stance/Lunge

Includes exercises like split squats, rear foot elevated split squats, stepups, and forward, lateral, and reverse lunges.

Common Error
Poor knee control. What you typically end up with is excessive forward movement and your knees collapsing toward each other.

Signs
When your knee moves too far forward over your ankle, it redistributes your bodyweight from your hips to your knee, which often aggravates pain through the front of the joint. In general, your knee should stay within a range directly above your ankle to directly above your midfoot during these exercises.

General Coaching Cues
When performing a lower body split stance or lunge pattern, keep the following cues in mind:

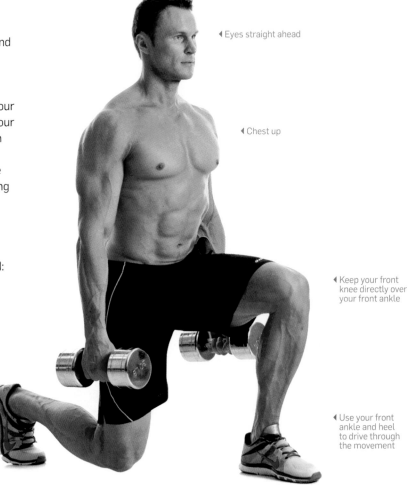

◄ Eyes straight ahead

◄ Chest up

◄ Keep your front knee directly over your front ankle

◄ Use your front ankle and heel to drive through the movement

THE ABS SOLUTION

Undesirable knee movement is generally initiated from poor foot or hip control. These two exercises will improve your ankle mobility and strength in the muscles that give you more control when you're standing on one leg.

3-WAY ANKLE MOBILIZATION

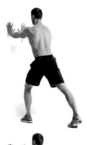

- Set up in a split stance with your front foot about 4 inches away from a wall and your back foot about 2 to 3 feet behind the front. Place your hands on the wall for support.

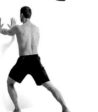

- Keeping the heel of your front foot down, slowly drive your front knee forward as far as you can. Pause for a second and return to the starting position. Repeat for 5 reps.

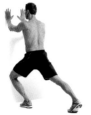

- Now drive your knee forward and inward slightly so that it passes over your big toe. Repeat for 5 reps.

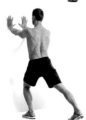

- Finally, drive your knee forward and outward slightly so that it passes over your pinky toe. Repeat for 5 reps and then switch legs. You may feel a stretch in your calves as you drive your knee forward.

MINI-BAND RESISTED SINGLE-LEG STANCE

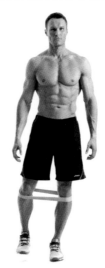
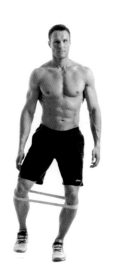

- Stand with your feet shoulder-width apart with a mini-band around your legs just below your knees.
- Lift one foot off the ground a few inches and sit down into a quarter squat position with the other leg.

- Aim the knee of the squatting leg outward so that it points toward your pinky toe. You should feel the outside of that hip engage. Hold this position for 10 seconds, then return to the starting position.
- Repeat for 3 reps on each side. Progress to lower depths until you're able to reach a half-squat position.

Upper Body Horizontal Pulling

Includes all rowing variations, such as bent-over rows, one-arm dumbbell rows, low pulley rows, standing cable rows, and inverted rows.

Common Error

You don't pull your shoulder blades together correctly during pulling movements. With any type of row, good form begins with stable shoulders.

Signs

Pain in the front or top of your shoulder is a symptom of instability (and impending injury). The next time you perform any rowing movement, pay attention to whether your shoulder blade is pulling all the way back with each rep. Is your upper back rounding? Is the weight pulling you forward instead of you pulling it back with proper form?

General Coaching Cues

When performing an upper body horizontal pulling pattern, keep the following cues in mind:

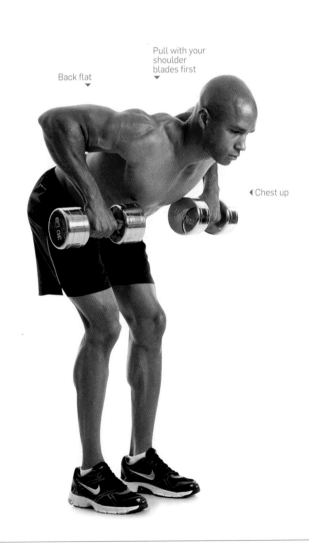

Back flat

Pull with your shoulder blades first

◄ Chest up

THE ABS SOLUTION

Whatever the reason, when you attempt to row a weight, you start by rounding your shoulder blade forward so that you can pull your elbows all the way back. This is bad. The two exercises below will help improve extension and the strength of the muscles that pull your shoulder blades back.

STANDING HIPS FLEXED TS AND WS

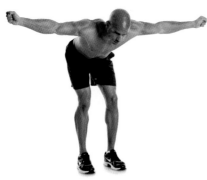

- Stand with your feet shoulder-width apart and bend forward at the waist so your torso is parallel to the floor. Let your arms hang down to the floor and rotate them so that your palms face forward. Lift your arms up as high as you can—thumbs pointing toward the ceiling—to form a T with your torso. Squeeze your shoulder blades together as you lift your arms. Pause for a second.

- Keeping your thumbs up toward the ceiling, pull your elbows into your sides to form a W. Pause for a second before returning to the T position and then back down. Repeat for 8 reps.

QUADRUPED EXTENSION-ROTATION

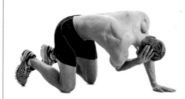

- Set up on all fours with your hands beneath your shoulders and your knees beneath your hips. Place one hand behind your head. Rotate your head away from the side of the raised arm and follow through with the arm so that your elbow pulls across your body and under the opposite arm.

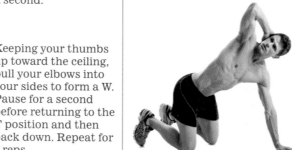

- Hold for a moment, then reverse the movement and follow through so that your elbow is pointed up toward the ceiling. Your hips and lower back should remain stable throughout the motion. Repeat for 6 to 8 reps, and then switch sides.

The Real Reason You Can't See Your Abs

Upper Body Vertical Pulling

Includes all chinup and pullup variations.

Common Error
Your shoulder blades round forward because of an inability to pull your shoulder blades down and back, and hold them in that position, while you perform vertical pulling exercises.

Signs
The next time you perform any chinup variation, note the position of your shoulder blades. When you begin in the "dead hang" (with your arms extended), your shoulder blades should be pulled down and back. In this position, the tops of your shoulders are far away from your ears. When you pull your chest up toward the bar, most men have a tendency to shrug their shoulders upward. However, even in the top position, the distance between your shoulder and your ears should remain the same.

General Coaching Cues
When performing an upper body horizontal pulling pattern, keep the following cues in mind:

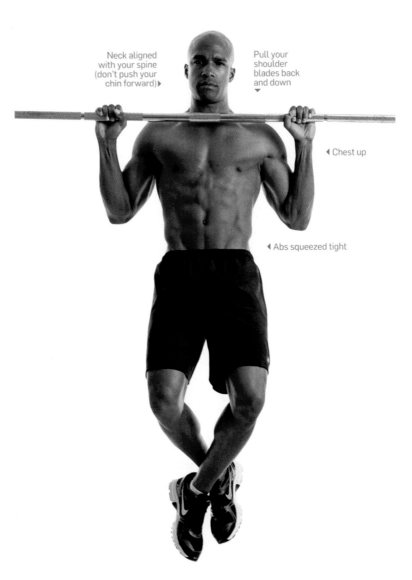

Neck aligned with your spine (don't push your chin forward) ▶

Pull your shoulder blades back and down ▼

◀ Chest up

◀ Abs squeezed tight

THE ABS SOLUTION

Your shoulders generally round forward at the top of chinup movements because your middle back lacks range of motion and the muscles that pull your shoulder blades back are weak. These two exercises will help pull your shoulder blades back and down.

MED BALL EXTENSION WITH BREATH

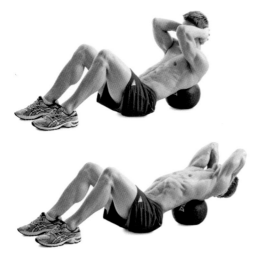

- Lie on the floor with your knees bent, feet flat on the floor, and a small, hard medicine ball (about the size of the ball you'd use in dodgeball) in your midback, between the bases of your shoulder blades. Interlock your fingers behind your head and point your elbows toward the ceiling.

- Exhale, slowly opening your elbows and lowering them outward as your back extends over the ball. Stop and hold the movement just before your lower back arches and your ribs flare in the front. From this position, take a deep breath in through your nose and feel your thoracic spine and chest open up. Exhale through your mouth as you return to the starting position. Repeat for 8 reps.

WALL SLIDE

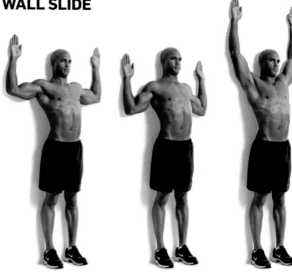

- Lean your head, upper back, and butt against the wall. Place your hands and arms against the wall in the "high-five" position, your elbows bent 90 degrees and your upper arms at shoulder height. Hold for 1 second. Don't allow your head, upper back, or butt to lose contact with the wall.

- Keeping your elbows, wrists, and hands pressed into the wall, slide your elbows down toward your sides as far as you can. Squeeze your shoulder blades together.

- Slide your arms back up the wall as high as you can while keeping your hands in contact with the wall. Lower and repeat.

The Real Reason You Can't See Your Abs

Upper Body Horizontal Pushing

Includes all bench press and pushup variations.

Common Error

During horizontal pushing exercises, there's a tendency for your shoulders to shift down toward your torso at the bottom of the movement, rather than remaining locked in place. Not only does this lead to most shoulder injuries that guys suffer on the bench press, it also limits the amount of power you can generate, which results in a bench press number that you have to hide from your buddies.

General Coaching Cues

When performing an upper body horizontal pulling pattern, keep the following cues in mind:

Signs

The next time you perform any horizontal pushing exercise, note the position and movement of your shoulder blades as you do it. Are your shoulders completely locked into place so that it feels like you're rowing the weight toward your chest and tucking your elbows in at your sides? Or do you feel your shoulders move as your elbows flare out to the sides? Do you feel weak and unstable as you transition out of the bottom? These are signs that you likely have a poor setup and movement pattern.

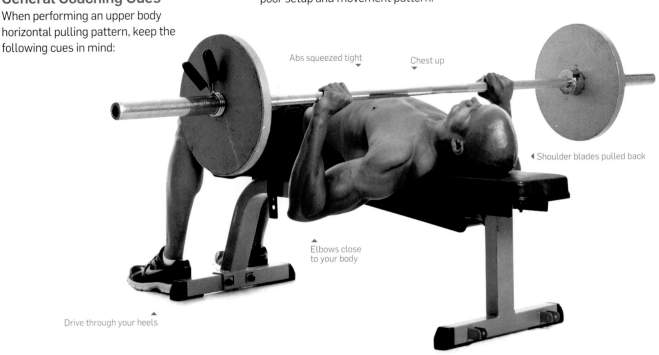

Abs squeezed tight

Chest up

◀ Shoulder blades pulled back

Elbows close to your body

Drive through your heels

THE ABS SOLUTION

If your shoulder blades retract properly, they will come together at the bottom of horizontal pressing movements to allow your arms to extend to a greater degree, which allows you to achieve full range of motion. The exercises will help improve range of motion and the strength of your multiple muscles that connect in your shoulders.

SCAP PUSHUP

STABILITY BALL FRONT PLANK WITH MINI ROLLOUT

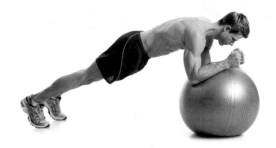

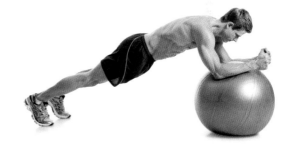

- Start in a pushup position. Keep your elbows locked and slowly pull your shoulder blades together without letting your lower back break form.

- Once your shoulder blades are together, lower yourself to the floor, pause, then press back to the starting position, allowing your shoulder blades to relax at the top. Repeat for 8 to 10 reps.

- Set up in a plank position with your feet shoulder-width apart and your forearms on a stability ball. Squeeze your shoulder blades together and hold.

- Without losing this position, slowly push the ball a few inches away from you until you feel your core engage. Pause for a second and then return to the starting position. Repeat for 8 to 10 reps.

The Real Reason You Can't See Your Abs

Upper Body Vertical Pushing

Includes all overhead pressing variations, like shoulder presses, as well as inverted overhead pushups.

Common Error
With overhead pressing movements, the most common issue is excessive arching of the lower back.

Signs
This might be the most obvious problem to detect, though many guys aren't even aware they're doing it. The next time you press overhead, use a mirror to get a look at the arch in your lower back. It should be natural with a slight S-shaped curve.

But when preparing to press overhead, many men press their hips back excessively and jut their stomachs out to try and create more stability. This is what's known as an anterior pelvic tilt, where the back of your hips sit significantly higher than the front.

General Coaching Cues
When performing an upper body horizontal pulling pattern, keep the following cues in mind:

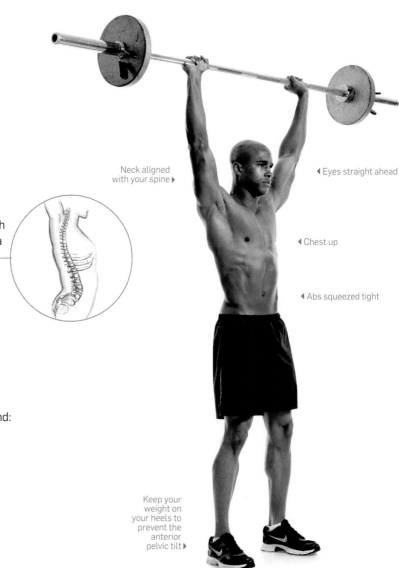

Neck aligned with your spine ▶

◀ Eyes straight ahead

◀ Chest up

◀ Abs squeezed tight

Keep your weight on your heels to prevent the anterior pelvic tilt ▶

THE ABS SOLUTION

Leaning back and excessively arching your lower back could be compensation for inadequate mobility through the upper back and shoulders—or a demonstration of inadequate core support. Address both issues and build more shoulder strength.

WALL SNOW ANGEL

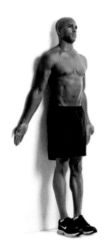
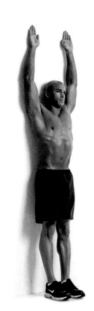

- Stand with your back against a smooth wall and your feet about 6 to 8 inches away from the wall. Raise your arms into an overhead position so that the backs of your hands and forearms are resting on the wall.

- With your forearms pressing lightly against the wall, squeeze your shoulder blades together and slide your arms in a big arc all the way down to your sides. Pause for a second to feel the muscles on the insides of your shoulder blades engage, then return to the starting position. Repeat for 8 to 10 reps.

ONE-ARM WAITER'S WALK

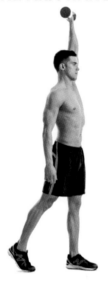
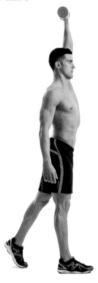

- Stand with your feet shoulder-width apart and one dumbbell in your left hand. Raise the dumbbell overhead and hold it with your arm straight up. Look straight ahead, keep your chest out and your back straight, and squeeze your shoulder blades together.

- Now walk in a straight line for 25 paces (you can make turns if space is an issue). Pause, lower your arm, then switch hands, and walk back for a total of 50 paces. You should feel your grip and shoulders working. Avoid letting your lower back arch and resist any side bending throughout the exercise. If you can't maintain proper form throughout, use a lighter dumbbell.

The 24-Hour Rule:
Save Your Posture Outside the Gym

Training smarter can go a long way toward preventing injury and melting more fat. But your hard work in the gym can be reversed if you don't take care of yourself outside the weight room. It's the infamous 24-hour rule. If you spend 1 hour in the gym, it's important you don't spend the other 23 causing unnecessary damage, says Neeld.

People spend the majority of their non-training time in one of three positions: standing, sitting, or lying. The goal is to minimize unnecessary muscle activity and imbalanced stress across your joints. The following guidelines are meant to help put your body in a more efficient position, no matter what you're currently doing.

Standing
Neutral Position
- Feet are pointed straight ahead or out slightly. Weight is evenly distributed across the entire foot; make sure you're not leaning to one side so that one foot takes on more weight.
- Ankles, knees, hips, shoulders, and ears are all in line.

Common Flaws
- Weight is shifted forward on the feet or more to one leg than the other.
- Upper back is slouched.
- Head is positioned forward of the spine.

Quick Fix
Perform three quick, small jumps. (Yes, it might look a little funny at a dinner party, so have a good story ready and waiting.) The jumping should help align your feet and reestablish your balance, which will snap your body back into preferred and ideal posture.

Sitting
Neutral Position
- Feet are flat on the ground, pointed straight ahead or out slightly.
- Hips are flexed to roughly 90 degrees.
- Weight is evenly distributed on both sides of your butt.
- Hips, shoulders, and ears are all in line.
- Face and eyes are oriented straight ahead.

Common Flaws
- One leg is crossed over the other.
- Weighted is shifted to one side more than the other.
- Upper back is slouched.
- Head is positioned forward of the spine.
- Arms are not supported.

Quick Fix

Place both feet on the floor, raise your arms overhead, and then pull your arms down and drive your elbows down and back. (image you're performing a chinup). The arms overhead will help lengthen your spine, and pulling your shoulders back should help open up your chest and prevent the hunched-over desk syndrome.

Lying
Neutral
- Side-lying position will have the shoulders, hips, knees, and ankles stacked directly above the opposite side.
- Knees and hips are slightly bent.
- Ankles, hips, shoulders, and ears are all in line.
- Pillows under the head, between the arms, and between the knees support neutral alignment.

Common Flaws
- Lying on your face or back, which applies undesired torque on the neck
- Lying on your side with one shoulder and/or hip rotated relative to the opposite side
- Lying on your side with your body curled up in a fetal position
- Lying on your side with your neck under- or over-supported

Quick Fix

For a week, try going to sleep on your side with a pillow squeezed between your legs. You'll train your body to sleep in the correct position, and by improving your sleep quality, the new position should become second nature.

It's important to note that while some postures are more desirable than others, the best posture is a changing posture. In other words, you don't want to be stuck in the same position for hours on end. That means you should stand up and move a little at least once every hour. Your body naturally adapts to the positions it spends the most time in. Regularly breaking these cycles with movement and stretching can help ensure you don't structurally or functionally adapt to a position that is going to limit your performance or set you up for injury.

Chapter 4
Eat Your Way to Six-Pack Abs

The world's greatest (and simplest)
hard-core eating plan.

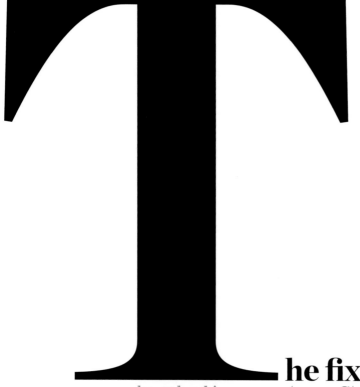**he fix to all** of your dieting woes can be solved in one sentence: Stop looking for a one-size-fits-all solution. That was the message of a 20-year study on weight loss conducted at the Harvard School of Public Health. The researchers concluded that dieters who only focused on how much they ate—rather than the types of foods they consumed—were more likely to fail at losing weight.

The reason: Restrictive dieting isn't sustainable and causes stress, which increases the likelihood of long-term failure. That's not to say that removing certain foods doesn't work. Or that counting calories isn't an effective way to easily drop pounds. It is. In fact, it's so effective that a Kansas State University professor proved that by counting calories, he could eat a diet consisting of Twinkies and chips and still lose 27 pounds—in just 2 months!

Eat Your Way to Six-Pack Abs

(Take that, Slim-Fast!) The experiment showed that how much food you consume is still the most important factor in the weight loss equation. It also proved that any food—if you can call Twinkies food (they have more than 40 ingredients and can survive multiple apocalypses)—could be part of a weight loss plan. And while the empty-calorie diet might leave your tastebuds satisfied and your buddies impressed, it won't help you live longer, fight aging, and build muscle (see "The Truth about Processed Foods" on page 58). Your goal isn't to minimize how much food you eat. It's to make sure you're filling your body with quality foods that will help you lose weight and add healthy, nutritional benefits.

Even though the numbers game works, some guys just want an easier, less mathematical way of melting fat. You don't need scientists at Harvard to tell you that counting calories can be more annoying than Joan Rivers. And we know that studying nutrition labels and carrying a scale to every meal isn't exactly great for your social life. Knowing what to eat should be simple and shouldn't create any stress. That's what causes bad eating habits in the first place. So we devised a series of simple rules that offer all the benefits of counting calories, without much mental stress.

If you want to experience success like never before, all you have to do is make these four simple rules your mantra. Say them out loud a few times. Learn them by heart. They are the Hard Body Rules.

And pretty soon, they'll become as much a part of your daily routine as checking out your hot new reflection in the mirror!

HARD BODY RULE #1
"I will lift heavy weights"

When it comes to weight loss, you can't out-exercise a bad diet. But when you combine the best workout strategies with good eating habits, you can transform your body in ways you never thought imaginable. Since the beginning of time, cardio has been touted as the best way to strip away pounds—and to meet women who like to run in sports bras. Problem is, while running on the treadmill might burn a lot of calories, it's not the most efficient way to burn fat. If your goal is to have a rock-solid body that will actually encourage the bra-runner to pay attention to you, weight training is the way to go. Lifting weights doesn't target the number on the scale; it specifically works on eliminating body fat. For maximum fat loss, increasing your intensity is the best approach.

Need proof? Scientists at the University of Connecticut found that dieters who lifted weights lost nearly 40 percent more fat than those who did traditional cardio, even though the total amount of exercise time was the same. I'll say it again: Weight training keeps your internal furnace burning for days after you complete your last rep. According to the National Center for Health Statistics, just three sessions a week of strength training can reduce your body fat by 3 percent in just 10 weeks—even if you don't change anything in your diet. It might not seem like much, but that can translate to 3 inches off the pony-keg you call your belly. What's more, your new muscle will literally transform your body into a fat-burning furnace. A study in *Medicine & Science in Sports & Exercise* found that after 6 months of lifting weights—just 3 days a week—the participants boosted their metabolism by 7 percent.

To really understand the body-transforming impact of weight training, consider this groundbreaking study in the *Journal of Strength and Conditioning Research.* The authors found that men who completed strength training programs—like the one you'll find in this book—burned an average of 100 more calories in the 24 hours after their workout than they did when they hadn't lifted weights. At three sessions a week, that's 15,600 calories a year, or more than 4 pounds of fat—without having to move a muscle. (It doesn't even count the hundreds of calories you scorch during your exercise routine.) That means you're losing weight just sitting around doing nothing! That's something even the longest run or most restrictive diet can't offer.

Of course, that should be reason enough to pick up a dumbbell. But the benefits of weight training are even sweeter: Weight training is designed to provide faster results with less time in the gym. Not only do you have to work out fewer times per week (we'll recommend a minimum of three times), you'll also have shorter sessions. That's because intensity is much more important than duration for eliminating fat. So you can spend a fraction of the time in the gym and still kiss your tummy good-bye. In fact, research has shown that 8 to 12 minutes of intense intervals can burn as many calories as 25 to 30 minutes of constant moderate exertion exercise. Does that mean you only need to exercise for 8 to 12 minutes to see your abs? Unfortunately, no. But don't be surprised when you abandon the cardio machines, pick up a few dumbbells, spend less time in the gym, and suddenly don't even recognize your own body.

These facts seem clear, so why do so many guys still gravitate toward the cardio area (besides the women)? Because the gym is filled with liars. You know them better as the treadmill, elliptical, and stairclimber. While these machines are great forms of exercise, they make you feel like you're working harder than you are. Canadian researchers discovered that cardio machines can significantly overestimate your caloric burn—sometimes by hundreds of calories.

Right now, you might be thinking, why run? If you enjoy it, hey, do it. Traditional cardio is still good for your body and your heart, and it does burn calories. But if you're tight on time (and we know you are), and you want the most bang for your workout buck, then weight training should always be your priority. Think of your exercise as a prioritized

Eat Your Way to Six-Pack Abs

list: As long as weight training is at the top and always crossed off, you'll be one step closer to your new body.

We recommend that you lift weights 3 days a week, which will work your muscles, stoke your metabolism, and give you the body you want faster than ever. Researchers at Ball State University compared participants who performed cardio to those who used resistance training as their primary form of exercise. While both groups lost the same amount of weight, the group that lifted weights burned nearly 5 pounds more fat than the aerobic group. Why? Because the group that used weights burned almost pure fat, while the cardio group was losing muscle. Your workout will be structured the same way. In just 30 to 45 minutes per workout, you'll unlock the body you've always wanted.

HARD BODY RULE #1

"I will eat greens. Every. Day."

Here's a rule you probably never thought you'd hear suggested in a diet plan: Eat as much as you want. But that's exactly what we want you to do with vegetables. Whether you prefer spinach, peppers, asparagus, or exotic offerings like bok choy and kale, pack your plate high with as many shades of green and varieties as you like. Vegetables are packed with so many supernutrients that they have been linked to almost every health benefit imaginable—heart health, cancer prevention, a boost in mood and energy, even a revved-up sex life.

The biggest benefit, however, is weight loss. A study in the *American Journal of Clinical Nutrition* found that men who included veggies in every meal were able to eat 25 percent more food but lose an additional 3.5 pounds. How? Vegetables help you lose fat by keeping you more satisfied, so you're less likely to overeat. (And they have fewer calories.) Greens are low in calories, high in volume, and nutrient dense. So you can eat a lot of them, feel full, and not have to worry about other foods sneaking into your diet and sinking your healthy eating plan.

What's more, a 20-year review of dietary behavior by the *New England Journal of Medicine* found that people who added just 1 serving of veggies daily made a positive impact on weight loss. And Pennsylvania State University researchers found that when study participants made sure to include vegetables in every meal, they cut their caloric intake by 11 percent and lost more weight. Need more proof? You'll experience it right here in The World's Greatest Hard Body Plan. If possible, we recommend that you eat your vegetables at the beginning of each meal for the biggest effect. This way, you'll fill yourself up with good stuff that won't pack on the pounds. After all, much of the overeating that occurs happens because you're still hungry and trying to find anything to feed your pangs. Veggies will do the trick.

Is it a cheap ploy? Yes. But will you complain when you can still eat steaks and have washboard abs? Probably not. Just choose your favorite vegetables from the list on page 65, and you'll lose more weight and never feel hungry again. So enjoy!

HARD BODY RULE #1
"I will make protein my wingman."

When it comes to ripped abs, protein is your secret weapon When you consider that Johns Hopkins University linked a high-protein diet to lower blood pressure, less body fat, better cholesterol levels, improved triglycerides, and the prevention of diabetes, obesity, and osteoporosis, it's no wonder we're in favor of protein. But if you're like most men—even those who love steak and wings—you're not doing a good enough job using this crucial weight loss tool.

Your plan of attack: Eat protein in every meal and snack. Focusing on protein fights off hunger and makes your stomach unlikely to bulge since protein is less likely to be stored as fat. That's because protein is harder to digest, so you burn more calories just eating the food. This process also helps ensure you eat less. Men who made sure their diet was at least 30 percent protein ate almost 450 calories less per day and lost 11 pounds more than those who ate less protein, according to a study published in *Nutrition & Metabolism*.

So whether it's burgers, chicken, or eggs, you'll be eating a constant source of nature's ultimate abs superfood. Need more convincing? British researchers found that emphasizing protein in each meal leaves you feeling fuller, accelerates fat loss, and maintains your muscle mass, which is key to shedding pounds and revealing your most chiseled body ever.

HARD BODY RULE #1
"I will trade empty calories for real carbs."

If there's one "food group" you should limit on this plan, it's sugar. Your fix: Eat more fruit. Fruit—nature's sweet reward—provides plenty of carbs for energy, but has less impact on your blood sugar than processed sweets and other carbohydrates. This is crucial to help you avoid the cravings and binges that occur when your blood sugar rises quickly and then crashes. Ideally, the majority of your carbs will come from fruits. That doesn't mean you won't have grains, beans, or other carbohydrate sources and the occasional treat, but they will be a secondary source. Limit yourself to just a couple servings daily of sugars and processed carbohydrate sources, and consume the rest of your carbs from fresh produce. You'll soon find you don't even miss your old sugary snacks!

THE ABS BENEFIT

10
Pounds of fat lost by high-protein dieters who didn't exercise, over just 16 weeks, according to Canadian researchers

150
Calories per day from sugar recommended by the American Heart Association. That's equal to 9 teaspoons. A can of soda alone is equal to 8 teaspoons.

Eat Your Way to Six-Pack Abs

The Truth about Processed Foods

On any diet, calories are king. If you eat more than you burn, you will gain weight. But the types of foods you eat do make a difference to your metabolism, your ability to gain muscle, and your need to eat more or less food. Processed foods (like cakes and cookies) that are high in refined carbohydrates and sugars cause bursts in your blood glucose and raise your levels of insulin. This sends a chemical signal to your brain that makes you crave more food. As a result, you listen to your body's "need" (even if you're not really hungry) and continue to eat more at your current meal—and the next, say Syracuse University researchers. It's dietary double jeopardy: You eat more than you need, and you don't receive any nutritional benefit.

This is why fruits and vegetables need to make up the majority of your carbohydrates. They actually do what food is supposed to do—leave you satisfied. These natural sugars don't play tricks on your mind or your body, and as a result you'll be able to eat to your heart's content without any guilt or the fat to show for it.

This doesn't mean that you have to completely trash all of your favorite indulgences, though. Like anything in life, moderation is the key to finding balance. "You don't need to completely remove processed foods from your diet, but keep them to a maximum of 10 to 15 percent of your daily calories," says nutritionist Alan Aragon, MS. When you eat more than that, you risk creating a diet that doesn't provide you with the vitamins, minerals, and nutrients your body needs. While it might not seem that important, research has found that a diet high in processed foods increases your risk for cardiovascular diseases and metabolic syndrome, says Aragon—not to mention extra flab around your waist.

What's more, eating processed foods actually slows down your metabolism, which is why you want to follow our suggested guidelines. Researchers from Pomona College found that meals consisting of processed foods burn significantly fewer calories than a less-processed meal. So instead of burning calories, you're storing more of what you eat as fat. In fact, a 20-year review conducted by the *New England Journal of Medicine* unlocked the reason why so many people gain weight: processed foods. The researchers found that processed foods—like potato chips, cookies, and french fries—cause people to gain up to 17 pounds over a 20-year span. If your plan is to never feel hungry and still reshape your body, then replacing the processed snacks in your diet can be the small change that finally helps you reveal that six-pack.

Ignite Your Weight Loss

Science shows that it's not how often you eat but what you eat that makes the biggest difference. And as long as you're fueling up with the right foods, your metabolism doesn't know the difference between three meals or six in a day. The best plan of attack is to find what works for you. If you want six meals one day and three the next, go for it. As long as your choices are in line with the Hard Body Rules, eat as frequently—or infrequently—as you'd like.

In this plan, you'll eat three main meals per day (breakfast, lunch, and dinner) plus additional snacks. You can eat the snacks as separate meals, or you can add them to any of the main eating times to create a bigger meal. Finally—a diet where you are in control.

BREAKFAST
Breakfast is designed to get you started off on the right food. That means a plentiful offering of dairy options like yogurt or milk, protein from eggs or a protein smoothie, and your choice of grains or fruit.

LUNCH
The foundation of lunch is lean protein like chicken or tuna. Combine that with your favorite vegetables or a side salad to help you power through your afternoon.

DINNER
Your evening meal is packed with more protein, but this time you can go for something a little fattier, like steak, salmon, or trout. These fats will help you stay full. Once again, pile your plate high with veggies, such as grilled zucchini, asparagus, and squash, or sauté some spinach and broccoli.

SNACKS
This is where the fun begins and you really take control of your daily menu. Remember, snacks can be eaten separately at any point in the day, or they can be added to any meal. Each day, add healthy fat sources like nuts, a small source of protein such as deli meat, and some smart carbs like a piece of fruit or grains such as a bowl of cereal.

230
Calories more per day that people eat on low-protein diets compared to their high-protein counterparts, according to Australian researchers

5 WAYS TO EAT LESS

Use smaller utensils. According to a Rhode Island at Kingston study, people who opted for smaller cutlery consumed 70 calories less per meal.

Eat slower. When you take more time to chew, you're able to savor the texture and taste of food. Not only will this make your meal more enjoyable, it gives your body the time it needs to register a full belly (generally 15 to 20 minutes). Those who eat quickly tend to pack in more food.

Be a social eater. If you talk to your friends or family when you eat, you prolong the length of your meal. The longer your meal lasts, the less likely you are to overeat. Plus, the mental distraction helps prevent overindulging, according to researchers at Flinders University in South Australia.

Make it a hot meal. Adding spices to your meal helps you chew your food more thoroughly and drink more water—one of the keys to a better eating plan.

End with black tea. The green version might receive all the love, but black tea actually decreases your blood sugar after a meal for up to 2.5 hours, according to a study in the *Journal of the American College of Nutrition.* The benefit: You'll feel fuller faster and stay satisfied longer.

Eat Your Way to Six-Pack Abs

4 Weeks to Abs

Follow this eating plan, which incorporates all of the Hard Body Rules and the foods you need to fill up and slim down.

Week 1

Monday	Tuesday	Wednesday	Thursday	Friday	Saturday	Sunday
Meal 1 1 cup plain Greek yogurt ½ cup blueberries ¼ cup sliced strawberries	**Meal 1** Strawberry-Banana Protein Smoothie (page 91)	**Meal 1** Mexican scrambled eggs (3 eggs, chopped tomatoes, onions, spinach, bell peppers, ½ cup shredded cheese, ¼ cup salsa) 1 orange	**Meal 1** 2 slices whole grain toast 2 tablespoons almond butter 1 cup 1% milk	**Meal 1** Eggs and cheese sandwich (2 scrambled eggs and 1 slice melted cheese placed on a toasted English muffin)	**Meal 1** Strawberry protein pancakes (Mix 1 scoop vanilla protein powder with 1 egg, ½ cup milk, ½ cup oats, 1 teaspoon salt, 1 teaspoon baking powder. Blend and pour on a griddle. Slice up 1 cup strawberries and place atop the pancakes)	**Meal 1** Smoked salmon scramble (3 eggs, ¼ sliced onion, 3 ounces salmon, capers) Grapefruit
Meal 2 6 ounces sesame-crusted ahi tuna served over a bed of mixed greens, drizzled with balsamic vinaigrette	**Meal 2** 6 ounces baked salmon with peach-mango salsa 1 cup sliced cantaloupe Steamed spinach	**Meal 2** ½ cup shirataki noodles with 6 ounces ground turkey, roasted spinach, and mushrooms	**Meal 2** 6 ounces grilled chicken with arugula, baby spinach, walnuts, cucumbers, mint leaves, and mandarin oranges	**Meal 2** 6 ounces tuna steak marinated in 2 tablespoons soy sauce, 2 teaspoons wasabi, and 1 tablespoon rice wine vinegar Side salad with mixed greens	**Meal 2** Tuna melt sandwich (1 5-ounce can tuna, 2 slices multigrain bread, ½ sliced avocado, 1 slice Cheddar cheese)	**Meal 2** 6 ounces seared trout topped with herbs and drizzled with olive oil Steamed broccoli
Meal 3 6–8 ounces Cajun-rubbed top sirloin with grilled zucchini, onion, and steamed spinach	**Meal 3** 6–8 ounces grilled chicken breast, cooked in olive oil, topped with ½ avocado Grilled asparagus and squash	**Meal 3** Kebabs with 2 ounces shrimp, 6 ounces chicken, onion, and red and green bell peppers Kale salad topped with ½ avocado	**Meal 3** 8 ounces grass-fed beef burger (less than 10% fat) with sautéed bell peppers, onions, and mushrooms	**Meal 3** Turkey chili (8 ounces lean ground turkey, diced tomatoes, black beans, corn, dried chili mix, ground flaxseed, ¼ cup water)	**Meal 3** 6 ounces grilled chicken and steak skewers, mixed with bell peppers, onions, and zucchini	**Meal 3** 8 ounces broiled salmon topped with lime, slow-roasted Roma tomatoes, and Broccolini Spinach and kale salad
Snacks Banana and almond butter 2–3 hard-cooked eggs	**Snacks** 1 apple 3 ounces hard cheese	**Snacks** 1 cup cottage cheese Handful of almonds	**Snacks** 3 strips turkey jerky 1 stick mozzarella cheese	**Snacks** 1 5-ounce can of tuna topped with salsa Handful of walnuts 1 apple	**Snack** Chocolate–Peanut Butter Smoothie (page 91)	**Snacks** 1 cup ice cream 1 cup mixed berries

Week 2

Monday

Meal 1
3-egg omelet with spinach, mushrooms, onions, bell peppers, and Cheddar cheese

½ cup oatmeal with cinnamon

Meal 2
6 ounces grilled chicken breasts marinated in 2 tablespoons teriyaki sauce and 1 tablespoon water

Roasted butternut squash and walnuts

Meal 3
8 ounces pork chops glazed with Dijon mustard

Sweet potatoes and broccoli

Snacks
1 cup plain Greek yogurt with ½ cup blueberries and blackberries

Handful of almonds

Tuesday

Meal 1
2 strips bacon and 2 fried eggs

Grapefruit

Meal 2
Chicken fajitas (6 ounces sliced chicken breast, onion, green and red bell peppers, 1 jalapeño chile pepper, cilantro, cumin, 1 whole wheat tortilla)

Meal 3
8 ounces cedar plank salmon seasoned with salt and pepper and drizzled with olive oil

Side salad with cucumber, artichoke, broccoli, sprouts, and tomatoes

Snack
Chocolate–Peanut Butter Smoothie (page 91)

Wednesday

Meal 1
Supercereal (cereal of choice with more than 3 grams of fiber, topped with sliced bananas and 1 tablespoon chia seeds)

3 hard-cooked eggs

Meal 2
6 ounces grilled salmon with a spinach and arugula salad

Meal 3
Turkey meatballs (8 ounces extra-lean ground turkey, 1 clove garlic, 4 saltine crackers, ¼ onion, ¼ cup tomato sauce)

Grilled bell peppers, butternut squash

Snacks
1 cup plain cottage cheese

½ cantaloupe

Handful of almonds

Thursday

Meal 1
½ cup oatmeal, cinnamon, ¼ cup raisins

2–3 links chicken sausage

Meal 2
Soba noodle chicken pad thai (¼ cup soba noodles, 6 ounces chicken, peas, carrots, water chestnuts, and ¼ cup diced peanuts; add a sauce of 2 teaspoons Sriracha and 2 tablespoons soy sauce when finished cooking)

Meal 3
4 ounces grilled calamari and 4 ounces grilled shrimp served over sautéed Swiss chard and shallots

Snacks
4 strips beef jerky

¼ cup quinoa

Friday

Meal 1
Breakfast burrito (3 scrambled eggs, 1 whole grain tortilla, shredded mozzarella cheese, 2 ounces shredded chicken, sliced tomato, onions, bell peppers, avocado)

Meal 2
6 ounces roasted halibut with ½ cup fava beans, yellow squash, and diced shallots

Meal 3
Spicy beef and chicken stir-fry (4 ounces lean steak, 4 ounces chicken, spinach, bell peppers, onions, mushrooms, snap peas, bean sprouts, 2 tablespoons soy sauce, and as much Sriracha as desired)

Snacks
Apple and 1 tablespoon almond butter

1 cup milk

Saturday

Meal 1
Protein berry smoothie (2 scoops vanilla protein powder, 6 ounces almond milk, strawberries, blueberries, blackberries, 1 tablespoon chia seeds, 1 cup spinach, 4 ice cubes)

Meal 2
Spinach wrap filled with 6 ounces sliced chicken breast, bell peppers, black olives, arugula, feta cheese, and ¼ cup hummus

Meal 3
Spaghetti squash with 4 ounces scallops and 4 ounces shrimp topped with ½ cup garlic-infused marinara

Steamed peas

Snacks
2 hard-cooked eggs

1 stick cheese

Sunday

Meal 1
Mexican scrambled eggs (3 eggs, chopped tomatoes, onions, spinach, bell peppers, ½ cup shredded cheese, ¼ cup salsa)

1 orange

Meal 2
Tuna melt sandwich (1 5-ounce can tuna, 2 slices multigrain bread, ½ sliced avocado, 1 slice Cheddar cheese)

Meal 3
8 ounces Cajun-rubbed top sirloin with grilled zucchini, onion, and steamed spinach

Snacks
1 cup cottage cheese

Handful of almonds

Eat Your Way to Six-Pack Abs

Week 3

Monday	Tuesday	Wednesday	Thursday	Friday	Saturday	Sunday
Meal 1 Power protein oatmeal (½ cup oatmeal, 1–2 scoops protein powder, 1 cup berries) 1 cup almond milk	**Meal 1** Spicy omelet (3 eggs, 1 link spicy red pepper chicken sausage, spinach, 2 mushrooms, 1 tablespoon grated Cheddar cheese, ½ cup salsa) 1 cup V8 juice	**Meal 1** Strawberry-Banana Protein Smoothie (page 91)	**Meal 1** Spinach, mushroom, and cheese omelet (3 eggs, 1 teaspoon salt, 1 teaspoon black pepper, ¼ cup Cheddar-Jack cheese, spinach, mushrooms)	**Meal 1** 2 scrambled eggs 2 strips bacon 1 cup mixed berries (strawberries and blueberries)	**Meal 1** Pineapple-banana breeze (1–2 scoops vanilla protein powder, 6 ounces almond milk, ½ cup pineapple chunks, 1 banana, 1 teaspoon vanilla extract, 4 ice cubes; blend and serve)	**Meal 1** 1 cup plain Greek yogurt 1 cup fresh cherries 2 hard-cooked eggs
Meal 2 Wild salmon salad (6 ounces wild salmon, arugula, romaine, cherry tomatoes, ¼ cup pecans, mandarin oranges)	**Meal 2** Portobello and salmon kebabs mixed with onions and red, yellow, and green bell peppers Steamed kale and cauliflower	**Meal 2** Chicken spinach Parmesan (6 ounces chicken breast, 1 tablespoon Parmesan cheese, 1 clove garlic, ¼ cup marinara sauce, spinach) ½ cup quinoa	**Meal 2** Turkey melt (6 ounces sliced turkey breast, 2 slices sprouted grain bread, 1 slice cheese, 1 teaspoon ground red pepper, tomato, lettuce, chopped celery)	**Meal 2** Romaine lettuce, 1 hard-cooked egg, 3 ounces sliced chicken, cherry tomatoes, small handful of sliced almonds, 1 teaspoon rice wine vinegar	**Meal 2** 6 ounces grilled chicken breast, ½ avocado Grilled asparagus and zucchini	**Meal 2** 6 ounces grass-fed beef burger on a bed of kale
Meal 3 Chicken stir-fry (6 ounces chicken, snow peas, spinach, scallions, mushrooms, chestnuts, ¼ cup peanuts) served over ½ cup brown rice	**Meal 3** 8 ounces broiled flank steak Mixed salad with baby spinach, carrots, cucumber, radish, and sprouts	**Meal 3** 8 ounces grilled steak with chimichurri sauce (1 tablespoon water, 2 tablespoons red wine vinegar, 2 minced cloves garlic, 1 teaspoon salt, ground red pepper, black pepper, olive oil)	**Meal 3** Chicken fajitas (8 ounces grilled and sliced chicken marinated in Cajun seasoning, ½ cup black beans, ½ cup salsa, ½ avocado, and a small flour tortilla)	**Meal 3** 8 ounces grilled chicken sautéed in lime-butter sauce (2 limes, 1 tablespoon butter) 1 cup steamed spinach 1 cup mashed butternut squash Steamed asparagus	**Meal 3** Grilled shrimp and scallops (4 ounces shrimp, 4 ounces scallops) ½ cup cooked quinoa Steamed broccoli and carrots	**Meal 3** Fish tacos (8 ounces grilled halibut, 2 small corn tortillas, ¼ sliced avocado, 2 tablespoons salsa, ½ cup shredded romaine, 1 cup red and yellow bell peppers, sliced onions, ½ sliced jalapeño chile pepper)
Snacks Handful of almonds 2 ounces hard cheese 1 apple	**Snacks** Protein pudding (1 tablespoon almond butter, 1 scoop protein powder, and 3 ounces almond milk; freeze for 1 hour and serve) 1 banana	**Snacks** 1 ½ cups grapes 1 slice mozzarella cheese 3 ounces ham, sliced	**Snacks** 1 cup cottage cheese 1 cup sliced strawberries	**Snacks** 3 ounces beef jerky 4 ribs celery with 1 tablespoon peanut butter	**Snacks** 1 stick cheese Handful of walnuts	**Snacks** Berry bliss smoothie (4 ounces almond milk, 4 ounces water, 1 scoop vanilla protein powder, ½ cup blueberries, ½ cup strawberries, ¼ cup blackberries, 4 ice cubes; blend and serve)

Week 4

Monday	Tuesday	Wednesday	Thursday	Friday	Saturday	Sunday
Meal 1 2 servings Smoked Salmon and Scrambled Eggs on (spelt) Toast (page 83)	**Meal 1** Huevos Rancheros (page 83)	**Meal 1** Flat Green Chile and Goat Cheese Omelet (page 84)	**Meal 1** Spinach and Feta Frittata (page 83)	**Meal 1** Peanut Butter Strawberry Wrap (page 84)	**Meal 1** Egg and Avocado Breakfast Sandwich (page 84)	**Meal 1** Eggs and cheese sandwich (3 scrambled eggs and 1 slice melted cheese placed on a toasted English muffin)
Meal 2 Peruvian Seafood Stew (page 84)	**Meal 2** Berry Goat Cheese Salad (page 85)	**Meal 2** Tangy Turkey Ciabatta (page 85)	**Meal 2** Chipotle Glazed Steak with Black Bean Salad (page 86)	**Meal 2** Grilled Chicken and Pineapple Sandwich (page 85)	**Meal 2** Better-for-You Egg Salad (page 86)	**Meal 2** Special Shrimp Salad (page 86)
Meal 3 Asian Salmon Burgers (page 87)	**Meal 3** Chicken Lettuce Cups (page 87)	**Meal 3** Chili-Spiced Fish Tacos (page 88)	**Meal 3** Beef, Vegetable, and Almond Stir-Fry (page 88)	**Meal 3** Chicken with Walnuts and Spinach (page 88)	**Meal 3** Hoisin-Orange Glazed Chicken (page 89)	**Meal 3** Pork Gyros (page 89)
Snack Mixed Fruit Breakfast Smoothie (page 90)	**Snack** High-Protein Blueberry Yogurt Shake (page 90)	**Snacks** Mint Chocolate Chip Smoothie (page 91)	**Snack** Chocolate–Peanut Butter Smoothie (page 91)	**Snacks** 1 apple 2 hard-cooked eggs	**Snack** Strawberry-Banana Protein Smoothie (page 91)	**Snacks** 1 cup cottage cheese Handful of almonds

How Often Do I Need to Eat?

More nutritional information is available to us today than ever before, yet we still can't seem to figure out the most basic question: How often do I need to eat to lose weight? There's no need to also worry about how often. So here's a fast tip: It doesn't really matter how frequently you eat. All that matters is what you eat.

The multiple meal approach started with a simple premise: When you eat food, you burn calories. As you might know, protein helps you burn the most calories, while a smaller percentage of the calories you eat from carbs and fats are metabolized. Researchers wondered, if we burn fat when we eat, why don't we just eat more often to burn even more calories? In principle, the idea was great. But once more numbers were crunched, the reality painted a different story. Assuming that the foods you eat are the same and the number of calories isn't any different, you won't get a metabolic boost from eating more often.

Let that sink in: You don't need to eat four, five, or six meals per day.

Now that's not to say multiple meals don't help you lose weight. They can—but not because of some metabolic magic. For some, eating more frequently is simply a personal preference.

But snacking can also lead to an expanding waistline. Researchers from the University of North Carolina examined eating habits from the last 30 years. They found that people eat, on average, 500 calories more per day and that the majority of those calories come from overeating on snacks. In fact, people eat more calories as a result of snacking than from increased portion sizes at mealtime.

On the flip side, eating less often can prove to be a more satisfying approach—assuming that hunger doesn't cause you to binge. Researchers from Kansas found that people on a diet who eat less frequently increase their feelings of fullness, while those who snack feel hungry more often. The researchers believe that more frequent meals might make it harder to break the overeating habits and that focusing on better food choices, at fewer meals, is an easier change.

Your best strategy is to follow the guidelines we've provided in The World's Greatest Hard Body Plan and then select the frequency that works for your lifestyle. You might find that one day you'll eat three meals and another you'll eat five or six. Every day, you'll have a snack allowance, and those snacks can be added to any of your main meals to create a large offering or taken between meals to keep you grazing all day long. The choice is up to you. You are in control.

Remember, there's no need to overthink eating as long as you are making sure that the majority of your foods come from proteins, vegetables, and fruits.

THE ABS BENEFIT

40

Percent of dieters who regain weight within 4 years, say UCLA researchers

SHOPPING LIST
The Lean Guide to Eating

PROTEIN SOURCES
(serving size = 4 ounces)

Canned tuna

Chicken breast

Eggs

Fish (all types)

Lean ground beef (preferably grass fed)

Lean pork (ham, bacon)

Lean turkey

Shrimp

DAIRY
(with serving size)

Cheese: 1 stick or slice

Cottage cheese: 6 ounces

Milk: 1 cup

Plain low-fat yogurt: 6 ounces (one single serving of prepackaged)

Sour cream: 2 tablespoons

STARCHES AND GRAINS
(with serving size)

Black beans: ½ cup

Bread (with 3 grams of fiber or more): 1 slice

Cannellini beans: ½ cup

Cereal (with 3 grams of fiber or more): 1 cup

Corn tortillas: 1 tortilla

Flour tortillas (with 3 grams of fiber or more): 1 tortilla

Garbanzo beans: ½ cup

Oats: ½ cup (uncooked)

Pasta: ½ cup (cooked)

Pita bread: 1 pita

Potatoes (regular or sweet): 1 medium-size potato (size of your fist)

FRUITS

Apples

Bananas

Blueberries: ½ cup

Cantaloupe: 1 cup

Grapefruit: 1 cup

Grapes: 1 cup

Kiwi

Oranges

Peaches

Pears

Pineapple: ½ cup

Raspberries: 1 cup

Strawberries: 1 cup

Watermelon: 1 cup

NUTS AND FATS
(with serving size)

Avocado: ½ tablespoon

Nut butters: 2 ounces

-Almond

-Cashew

-Peanut

Nuts: a handful (1 ounce)

-Almonds

-Brazil nuts

-Cashews

-Pecans

-Pistachios

-Walnuts

VEGETABLES
(unlimited)

Artichokes

Arugula

Asparagus

Bell peppers

Bok choy

Broccoli

Cabbage

Carrots

Cauliflower

Celery

Cucumbers

Green beans

Kale

Leafy greens

Leaks

Lettuce

Mushrooms

Onions

Spinach

Sprouts

Squash

Zucchini

YOUR DIET, YOUR WAY

We've provided you with the ultimate 4-week eating plan designed to put you on the fast track to six-pack abs. But that doesn't mean you can't make substitutions and eat your way, every day. Here's a quick cheat sheet that you can use to fuel your body with any food choice. Use "The Lean Guide to Eating" and apply your favorite foods.

THE BIG BOOK: GETTING ABS FLEXIBLE EATING GUIDE

Meal 1
2–3 servings protein
1 serving dairy
1 serving fruit or grain
Unlimited vegetables

Meal 2
2–3 servings protein
Unlimited vegetables

Meal 3
3 servings protein
1–2 servings healthy fat/nuts
Unlimited vegetables

Snacks (eat separately or add to any meal)
2–3 servings protein
1 serving healthy fat/nuts or 1 serving dairy
2–3 servings fruit or starches/grains

Chapter 5
The Secret to Shredded Abs

The 4-step plan that will strip away
fat and carve your core.

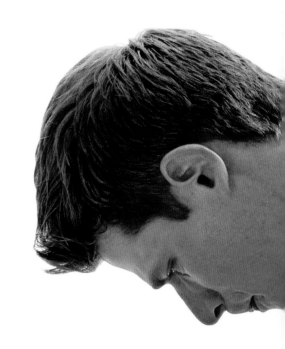

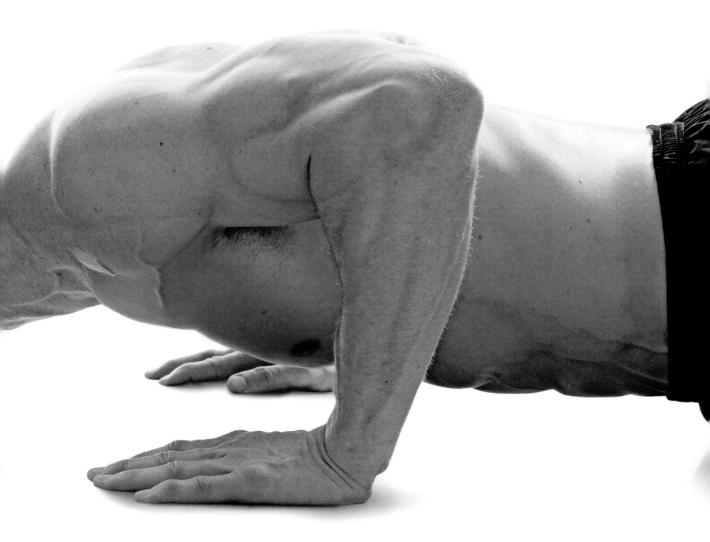

The Secret to Shredded Abs

You will have six-pack abs.

That's the first thing you need to convince yourself of before you start this plan. Like most guys, you probably find it hard to believe that you have a chance in hell at sculpting your core without swapping bodies with someone else. After all, it's not like you haven't tried to look great in the past. Hired a personal trainer and had your butt kicked 5 or 6 days a week? Been there, done that. How about diets that forbid you from eating after 6 p.m.? Yeah, tried them too. Maybe you've even made a few late-night purchases from the shopping network that you're not so proud of. It's okay—we don't judge.

That's not to say some of these options don't work. They do. In fact, a good trainer can be one of the best investments you can make for your body. But sometimes, to fight fat and win, you need an approach that doesn't require a complete lifestyle makeover and isn't full of promises you can't keep and demands you can't meet.

Consider this the flexible solution you need. This diet and exercise plan is based on cutting-edge research that utilizes the most effective fat loss strategies. In fact, the foods you'll eat on this program have been found to boost fat loss by more than 30 percent compared to the standard American diet.

And when combined with The Abs Workout, you'll transform your body into a calorie-burning machine that even works as you sleep.

Best of all, by following these tips, you'll eliminate the reason why most diets fail: frustration. Most diet and exercise plans offer you only one option for success. Suddenly, your flexible lifestyle is trapped in concrete. Between teaching yourself to like new foods and trying to find hours to exercise each day, you burn out. The supposed healthy plan becomes a threat to your comfort zone. This plan is different. The exercise and diet were designed around simple strategies that put you in charge of owning the body you want.

The Diet

There's a secret among the top nutritionists in the world. Most diets are created for short-term results. It's a cruel trick that has led to the endless cycle of deceptive weight loss and depressing weight gain. Your body is very good at losing weight—until it adapts and makes it seemingly impossible to burn off another pound. It's why each of your ex-diets ended up being more difficult than each of your ex-girlfriends.

If you want to keep eating the foods you like—and losing weight—you need to understand how the body processes food, and work with it, not against it. We understand if you want to swear off diets forever, but there's something else the nutritionists tell their clients: Diets work. That's why it's time to eliminate your fears and preconceived notions about going on a specific plan and not being able to eat like a man. We're here to show you how you can eat and still strip away pounds.

The nutrition experts at *Men's Health* understand the adaptation process and know how to prevent you from hitting the dreaded plateau that has been the beginning of the end for all your previous diets. This plan fills your body up with the right kinds of foods, so you burn calories more efficiently. The payoff: You can eat more food, burn fat faster, and still indulge in some of your favorite treats. If it sounds too good to be true, we don't blame you. But we've already seen the results. In fact, dieters in a study at UCLA followed a plan that included foods similar to what you'll find in this book. Not only did they lose more weight compared to a traditional diet, they also consumed more food and felt more satisfied from their meals. Sounds like your type of plan, right?

So dig in and enjoy this new approach to eating. It's a proven road map to tone up all your trouble spots and scorch belly fat, regardless of your shape, size, or age. We've created a plate that represents what you should consume at each meal. Your job: Simply select the foods you enjoy from each category and see results that last. That's it. No removing foods completely and living a life that's not the one you'd choose. Follow each of these guidelines and watch pounds melt away.

The Guidelines

The key to a good diet is remaining satisfied. That's why The World's Greatest Hard Body Plan is all about filling your plate. But sometimes it's difficult to know how much to eat without overeating. So we searched for a simpler way to fill your plate without having to count calories and created a system that's as easy as counting to four. Literally. These four steps, when utilized for each meal, will have you on the fast track to a flat belly. Follow these simple guidelines to ensure that you're always eating enough, seeing results, and never having to count calories again!

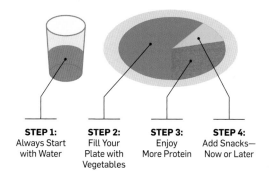

STEP 1: Always Start with Water **STEP 2:** Fill Your Plate with Vegetables **STEP 3:** Enjoy More Protein **STEP 4:** Add Snacks—Now or Later

STEP 1:
Always Start with Water

Few dieters realize that it's the small, simple tactics that create the greatest changes. Food is habitual, so it's best to determine the daily changes you can make that can become a part of your lifestyle. Few weight loss strategies are as easy—and effective—as drinking water. Everyone knows that a little H_2O is good for your body. But drinking water

The Secret to Shredded Abs

at the right time does more than hydrate. It can actually set you up for a day of fat loss without any effort.

In a recent study in the journal *Obesity*, dieters lost an additional 4.5 pounds when they drank 2 cups of water before each meal. That's why the leanest individuals start every meal with two glasses of water and continually drink throughout the day. A study in the *Journal of the American Dietetic Association* found that having 2 cups of water before breakfast can cut your daily food intake by 13 percent.

What's so special about water? Isn't it just, well, water? Once again, part of this is a cheap ploy to prevent your hunger from clicking into Hoover vacuum mode. Water can help you recognize when you're truly hungry. Oftentimes what you think is hunger is actually thirst. Dehydration is a bitch on many levels. It can make you eat when you don't need food. But a lack of fluid can also slow fat burning—another stealthy roadblock in your fat loss journey. Scientists at the University of Utah found that when you don't drink enough, your metabolism burns up to 2 percent fewer calories per day. When you're trying to fight back against a stubborn metabolism, the last thing you need to do is give your body any reason to store fat.

Additional research performed by German scientists revealed that 6 cups of cold water per day (2 cups before breakfast, lunch, and dinner) can raise your resting metabolism 50 calories a day. The research on the metabolic effects of water is mixed. And while 50 calories probably doesn't have you thinking, "Good-bye gut," it could potentially add up to 5 pounds in 1 year. Sounds a little better, right? Though the extra calories you burn drinking a single glass don't amount to much, making it a habit can add up to pounds lost without any effort.

Your Secret Move

Before each meal, consume 16 ounces (2 cups) of water. The water can be cold or hot. Feel free to mix your water with tea, preferably one without any calories or sweeteners. We recommend green tea because of its extra metabolism-boosting benefits. But black tea is great, and so is coffee.

STEP 2:
Fill Your Plate with Vegetables

You know that greens are good for you, but in truth they possess enough weight loss and health benefits to fill an entire medical encyclopedia. Eating more vegetables has been linked to better heart health, fighting off nearly every disease imaginable (including cancer), increasing positive emotions, creating more energy, and even revving up your sex life.

We know what you're thinking. "Great. A diet based on salads. Original and manly." We might not be the first to suggest vegetables, but on this plan your veggies are just the appetizer, not the main course. Here's why: A 20-year

The Best and Worst Fat Loss Supplements

By now you know there's no such thing as a magic pill that will instantly make your abs pop. But that doesn't mean certain supplements can't help make your fat loss plan a little more effective. You just need to be able to separate real science from marketing shams. Use this guide from nutritionist Chris Mohr, RD, PhD, owner of Mohr Results, Inc. (MohrResults.com), to help make the right additions to your exercises and diet plan.

BEST BUYS

Green tea
Commonly sold as green tea extract, the benefits seem to come from the combination of caffeine and something called epigallocatechin gallate (EGCG). All teas have catechins (a powerful antioxidant), but EGCG is extremely potent and can play a role in speeding weight loss. Specifically, caffeine and EGCG work together to increase calorie burn. Just don't expect a massive difference; some studies show that the calorie boost can be as little as 3 to 5 percent. But green tea is still beneficial to any diet plan because of its overall health benefits.

Raspberry ketones
This supplement is fairly new to the scene, and while most of the research has been conducted on mice, the results are too interesting to ignore. Raspberry ketones might release something called hormone sensitive lipase, which is an enzyme that has the ability to reduce fat accumulation by "freeing" fatty acids from within fat cells. If they're freed, then it might be easier to use your fat more readily and burn it as fuel.

Fish oil
Often thought of as a heart healthy supplement (which it is), there's actually some data that it may boost fat loss, too. In one study that looked at fish oil and sunflower oil in people who exercised and those who didn't, the participants supplementing with the fish oil had significantly greater fat loss and reduced body mass index (BMI) above and beyond the other group.

IGNORE THE HYPE

Conjugated linoleic acid (CLA)
Naturally found in whole fat dairy products, beef, and lamb, CLA skyrocketed to popularity after some promising preliminary data. Yet as time has passed, most research has found that CLA is not an effective fat loss tool. One study measured the effects of 5 grams per day of CLA versus a placebo in subjects who were resistance training for 7 weeks. The results showed the difference to be 0.8 versus 0.4 kilogram fat loss in the CLA versus placebo groups—or, as the researchers stated, "relatively small changes in body composition."

Chitosan
The promise of chitosan sounds amazing: By taking the supplement, you decrease the amount of fat absorbed from the foods you eat. And when you absorb less fat, you take in fewer calories and by default lose fat—all through the process of eating. Sounds great, if only it were true. Researchers have found an almost negligible increase in fat excretion in both men and women, meaning that the promise doesn't live up to the reality.

The Secret to Shredded Abs

review of dietary behavior by the *New England Journal of Medicine* found that people who added just 1 serving of veggies daily had a positive impact on weight loss. And Penn State researchers found that when the study participants included vegetables before every meal, they cut their caloric intake by 11 percent and lost more weight. Think about that: You're still eating (a lot) and you're losing. The vegetables help prevent you from overeating and indulging in the same crap that always kills your lean body plans. Remember, if you want better results, it's time to open your mind to something new.

Leafy greens happen to possess special nutritional qualities that allow you to eat as much as you want without gaining weight. After all, no one ever became fat on a diet of spinach, bell peppers, and mushrooms. In fact, a study in the *American Journal of Clinical Nutrition* found that you could eat more and reveal your hard-earned muscle. The researchers compared men who needed to lose weight. One group followed a reduced-calorie diet, while the other followed a similar approach but feasted on vegetables. The veggie group ate 25 percent more food (by volume) but lost more weight. How? They were loading up on vegetables, which decreased their hunger, and they ended up eating fewer calories.

That's why we suggest you start every meal with vegetables. It guarantees that you won't "forget" to eat this weight loss superfood, and eating them early in the meal can potentially make your fat loss more potent. Research has shown that high-fiber vegetables can rev your fat burn by as much as 30 percent. So by kicking off your meal with your favorite variety, you improve satiety and ignite more caloric burn during your meal. Whether you eat a starter salad or mix vegetables with your main course, this will be one of the most important steps in keeping you satisfied and helping the pounds vanish.

Your Secret Move

Pile your plate high with veggies and enjoy them before you begin your main meal. High-fiber veggies include artichokes, broccoli, Brussels sprouts, carrots, endive, green beans, jicama, peas, spinach, and squash. Remember, green veggies, bell peppers, onions, and a host of other options are "free food." That means you can literally eat as much as you want—but that doesn't mean you can pour as much salad dressing as you want. Start with 1 to 2 cups of steamed broccoli or spinach, a side salad, or some bell peppers, onions, and mushrooms drizzled lightly in olive oil.

STEP 3:
Enjoy More Protein

Yes, we're talking about protein again. But it's time for you to admit something to yourself: You probably don't eat enough protein. Sure, you might eat steak and throw back the occasional protein shake, but most men are still undereating the most powerful abs-friendly food group. No matter what you think, your body could use more of nature's most potent nutrient—and if there's anything you should overeat, it's probably protein. According to British researchers, emphasizing protein in each meal leaves you feeling fuller, accelerates fat loss, and spares your lean muscle mass.

Look at some of the fittest men in the world. All seem to possess a lean body secret—and it's not just because they can afford trainers and live-in chefs who prepare their meals (although that helps, too). Fit men understand that high protein intake is critical to losing fat and having bigger biceps, a sculpted chest, and head-turning abs.

Perhaps the biggest benefit of a high-protein diet is that you burn calories by eating. Your metabolism is increased when you eat. This process is known as the thermic effect of food (TEF). Every type of food affects your metabolism differently, but nothing is as powerful as protein. The TEF of protein is about 30 percent, meaning more than a quarter of the calories this nutrient provides are burned during digestion and processing. Carbohydrates have a TEF of 8 to 10 percent, and fat's TEF is just 3 to 5 percent. This is why consuming protein at each meal can keep your metabolism elevated and prevent larger meals from storing too many calories.

Whether you want to add mass or just be lean and strong, you need protein to build and preserve your muscle. As you build more muscle, your body will burn

more fat, which makes every dietary slipup (let's be honest, we don't expect you to completely ditch beer and pizza) a nonfactor.

While you might not be thinking in terms of saving your muscles, that's the difference between looking great at any age or just dropping pounds and becoming "skinny fat." Think about it: As you lose weight, you want to make sure you reveal solid, sculpted muscles. Eating protein helps make this possible, especially when it's consumed before and after your workouts. University of Syracuse researchers found that when you down protein around your weight training session, you blunt the effects of cortisol, the stress hormone that tells your body to store fat. As a result, you burn more fat not only during your workout, but for an additional 24 hours afterward.

Focusing on protein also keeps your stomach more satisfied and keeps it lean. When you overeat carbohydrates or fat, both nutrients are easily soaked up by your body and stored as fat. But protein is different. That's not to say protein can't make you fat, but when you need a little food therapy after a rough day, a high-protein meal is less likely to make you fat.

Your Secret Move
Here's where you can go a little crazy. There are lots of flavorful protein options just waiting to be enjoyed. Grill yourself a steak. Bake some chicken. Crack eggs or pan-sear your favorite fish.

THE DAILY DESSERT
(Or Beer...Or Pizza...)

So how does dessert fit in to all of this? Easy: Your daily desserts will come from your snack allotment. Remember, you can enjoy one small indulgence every day, whether it's a couple of cookies, pizza, or maybe a beer (or three). For the first two weeks, we'd recommend that you avoid dessert completely (if you choose to eat it) and focus on cleaning up your diet. This isn't necessary, but if you struggle controlling your junk food urges, this should help you adjust to the smaller portions.

Here's your guide to keep you lean and satisfied.

1 beer = 2 servings grains

½ cup ice cream = 1 serving fat

1 slice pizza = 2 servings starches/grains

1 small slice of cake/pastry = 2 servings starches/grains

The Secret to Shredded Abs

If you're a vegetarian, try hemp or seitan (called the wheat meat). Even if your favorite form of protein has some fat on it, don't worry (see "Eat Fat to Lose Fat" opposite). However, if you select a form of protein that's high in fat, make sure you limit how much additional fat you include with your meal.

STEP 4:

Add Snacks—Now or Later

The time has come to reinvent weight loss. Rather than repeating the mistakes of so many diets, we want to accommodate the most overlooked aspect of every weight loss approach: YOU. An eating plan should revolve around your preferences, your busy lifestyle, and your need to adjust to daily demands. And let's be honest, while all diet plans expect some give-and-take, few provide real flexibility required for long-term success. It's expected that you'll have to make changes to how you eat, but that doesn't mean you need to give up your favorite foods or be forced into an eating schedule that doesn't work for you. We're all familiar with late-morning starts altering our breakfast plans, unscheduled business lunches disrupting an anticipated meal, or nonstop travel making it seem impossible to eat healthy. That stops here.

We already mentioned that you can choose how frequently you eat. Whether you want six smaller meals or three big meals, you decide what you need, without having to worry that one option will be better for fat loss. That also

EAT FAT TO LOSE FAT

The health scare surrounding saturated fat and cholesterol was overblown.

That was Walter Willett's conclusion after reviewing 21 studies on high-fat diets. Willett, MD, DrPH, chairman of the department of nutrition at Harvard University, published a study that showed there is no evidence that dietary saturated fat is associated with coronary heart disease, stroke, or cardiovascular disease. This was the defining moment in a 30-year battle to determine if eating fat makes us fat.

The confusion began in the 1980s when obesity rates began to climb. The low-fat craze took over, and the next thing you knew, we all became fatter. The number of overweight people increased by 30 percent, while the amount of fat consumed decreased by 11 percent. So clearly, fat wasn't the problem. What people didn't realize was that not only is fat not bad, it's actually an incredibly potent weight loss tool.

Research now indicates that as much as 20 to 35 percent of your calories should come from fats. Fat-filled meals keep you full and burn calories. Researchers from Georgia Southern University found that eating a high-protein, high-fat snack increases your resting calorie burn for up to 3.5 hours. When it comes to understanding fat, your options can be broken down into two main groups: saturated and unsaturated fats. Both of them are good, and both possess a variety of benefits.

Monounsaturated fats—MUFAs
(pronounced MOO-fahs), for short—come from the healthy oils found in plant foods such as olives, nuts, and avocados. A report published in the *British Journal of Nutrition* found that a MUFA-rich diet helped people lose small amounts of weight and body fat without changing their calorie intakes. Another report found that a breakfast high in MUFAs could boost calorie burn for 5 hours after the meal, particularly in people with higher amounts of belly fat. And a study in the *American Journal of Clinical Nutrition* showed that people who swallowed 1.9 grams of omega-3s daily (you'd find twice that in a 4-ounce portion of salmon) reduced their body fat, lowered their triglycerides, and raised their HDL cholesterol.

Saturated fats—like those found in red
meat, eggs, and milk—used to be avoided. But now they are an essential part of a healthy diet. No food represents the benefits of fat better than eggs. If you're skipping the yolks, you're missing out on one of the best fat loss foods. A study in *Nutrition Research* showed that the fat in eggs helped reduce appetite for up to 24 hours. And British scientists discovered that dieters who ate eggs for breakfast instead of a bagel lost 65 percent more weight—without any negative consequences to their cholesterol or triglycerides. Research has also found that consuming calcium dairy foods, such as milk and yogurt, may reduce fat absorption from other foods, which makes it easier to stay lean.

Embrace fats in the form of avocados, butter, nuts and seeds, as well as olive and coconut oils. Cook your foods in these healthy fats, or add them to your meals for additional flavor, nutrition, and fat loss benefits. There are also many options for those lactose intolerant in the grocery aisle.

The Secret to Shredded Abs

means you can push back your breakfast to when you want, have a big lunch, or pack in more calories at the end of the day. Optimizing your meals—the frequency and the size of them—becomes possible with snacks. These are flexible foods that you can eat at any point in the day, and they are usually the foods that you enjoy the most. Think pasta, bread, and even dessert. As long as you follow the Hard Body Rules, you can have some fun with your diet.

You might be wondering what makes this approach to snacking any different than other plans. Simple: We've created a diet where you'll only eat a snack when it's needed. Because the foods you'll be eating will keep you satisfied longer, you'll find that you need to eat snacks less frequently. And when you do, they won't be sabotaging your weight loss plan. You see, the snacks have been strategically designed to only take up a small portion of your daily calories. They're enough to leave you satisfied and not craving some of your favorite foods—but not so calorie heavy that you'll derail your diet faster than you can say "Twinkie."

Here's how it works: Breakfast, lunch, and dinner will be the foundation of your eating plan. You decide when to eat them. If you want to eat breakfast at 6 a.m. or noon, or enjoy dinner at 10 p.m., that's up to you. Just make sure you structure each meal around the Hard Body Rules. That means start by drinking water, then consume veggies and fill your plate with protein and healthy fats.

From there, the fun and flexibility begins with "floating meals."

Ever feel like you needed just a little more food on your plate? Or you were curious about how much you could graze without gaining weight? Snacks, or floating meals, solve all of these issues. These are foods that you can add to any meal (breakfast, lunch, or dinner), or you can use these foods as daily snacks. That means if you want to add two or three mini-meals during the day, you simply select the foods you want from the floating meals allotment to keep yourself satisfied. If you're not much of a snacker but would prefer a bigger meal, you can take the floating meals and eat them in addition to one of your main meals. This way, you can eat more without taking a step back.

The plan is designed to always leave you feeling satisfied, and it takes into consideration that sometimes your hunger is unpredictable and the demands of your day dictate how you eat.

Your Secret Move

Add the following foods as snacks during the day or in addition to your main meals. These additions are optional, so if you're satisfied by breakfast, lunch, and dinner—or by just a few of the snacks—you don't need to eat more. The idea is that these foods will fuel your body, not your fat cells. So you can eat them if you're hungry, but keep in mind you only need to consume them if you're not satisfied. And always remember the first three rules: Drink water first, begin your

The Amazing Abs Formula

The diet plan you've been given is as foolproof as you'll find. But some guys don't want general guidelines—they need specifics. They are men who appreciate a detailed spreadsheet, the specs on a new car, and the science behind a new discovery.

Maybe you're one of those guys, the kind who thrives on more control. If that's the case, we have the plan that will make sure you're in charge of your body and your success.

We worked with *Men's Health* nutrition advisor Alan Aragon to develop an equation that will work with your body. We'll warn you: This plan is incredibly effective, but it requires counting calories and keeping a close watch on how much protein, carbs, and fats you eat each day. And you still must follow all of the Hard Body Rules, as well. If you want to go the extra mile, here is what every man must know about the ultimate abs diet plan.

STEP 1: Set up your daily caloric goal

**Goal weight
x
(workout hours per week + 9.5)
=
total number of calories**

EXAMPLE: Say you're 200 pounds and your goal weight is 180.
If you plan to work out 3 days per week using our program (see Chapter 8), do this:
Add 3 (workout hours) + 9.5 and then multiply the sum (12.5) by your goal weight of 180 pounds
Daily calorie goal = 2125

STEP 2: Set your nutrient goals
Here's how you can figure out exactly how many grams of protein, fat, and carbohydrates you should eat each day:

**Grams of protein
=
goal weight**

**Grams of fat
=
half of your goal weight**

**Carbs
=
daily calories – [(protein grams x 4)
+ (fat grams x 9)] ÷ 4**

IN THE SAMPLE SITUATION:
Protein = 180 grams
Fat = 90 grams
Carbs = 2125 – [(180 x 4) + (90 x 9)] / 4
2125 – [720 + 810] / 4 = 148 grams of carbs
Carb total = 148 grams

The reason is simple: Each gram of protein is equivalent to 4 calories. Each gram of fat is 9 calories. And since fat and protein are the cornerstones of this diet, once you figure out how many calories come from those foods, the remainder can be allotted toward carbohydrates.

Follow the Hard Body Rules, eat the foods you want to reach these nutrient goals, and you'll finally solve the abs equation.

The Secret to Shredded Abs

plate with veggies, and stack up on protein. And if your protein source is high in fat (like pork or a rib-eye steak), try to avoid adding nuts to the meal.

Your Snack Allowance
Vegetables: unlimited servings
Healthy fat/nuts/or dairy: 2 servings
Fruits or starches/grains: 1–2 servings
Protein: 2–4 servings

The Truth about Late-Night Meals

Breakfast has long been touted as the king of all meals. In fact, many researchers have hypothesized it's the most important meal of the day. A University of Massachusetts medical school study found that people who routinely skipped breakfast had a significantly higher incidence of obesity than those who ate eggs and an English muffin. But just because one meal is good doesn't mean the others are bad. Yet, somehow the importance of breakfast was translated as "A big dinner makes you fat." Fortunately for you, nothing could be further from the truth.

Cutting-edge research from scientists all over the world appears to have finally cracked the weight loss code. And the solution doesn't include banishing late-night eating. If you're serious about changing your body, these findings might be the key to unlocking new fat loss pathways. That's because your body's ability to gain weight is mainly about what you eat and how much, not when you eat. Your body isn't on a 24-hour clock. What counts is whether you burn more calories than you ingest by the end of the day (or better yet, the week).

Researchers from Israel wanted to test whether eating more at night actually led to more weight gain. What they found was groundbreaking. In the 6-month study, the scientists compared people who ate their largest meal at breakfast to those who ate their largest meal at dinner (8 p.m. or later). The participants who satisfied their late-night munchies not only lost more fat, they also experienced more fullness throughout the entire 6 months and saw more favorable changes to their fat loss hormones.

Consider some of the impressive findings. Compared to the morning eaters, those who ate at night:

- **Had fewer hunger cravings and were more satisfied with their meals**
- **Lost 11 percent more weight**
- **Had a 10 percent greater change in abdominal circumference**
- **Lost a whopping 10.5 percent more body fat**

What's more, a study conducted by the U.S. Department of Agriculture also showed some convincing evidence for nighttime feasts. When dieters ate 70 percent of their calories after 7 p.m. compared to earlier in the day, they preserved muscle mass and lost more body fat.

So how did we come to fear late-night meals and, even worse, carbs? It was a classic case of misunderstanding. Many people eat at night out of boredom or other emotions instead of hunger, and they wind up consuming more calories than they need for the day. Remember when we said that counting calories works? Well, nighttime eaters typically bust past their calorie goal, which leads to fat storage. But that doesn't mean your body processes food differently at different times of day. In fact, late-night meals actually do a better job of priming your hormones for fat loss and improving your sleep.

If you've ever experienced a stressful week at work or in your home, you know that a lack of sleep appears to instantly add pounds to the scale. And researchers from Wake Forest University discovered why: Too much or too little shut-eye might lead directly to weight gain. People who slept 5 hours or less each night gained nearly 2.5 times more abdominal fat than those who logged 6 to 7 hours. People with sleep deficits tend to eat more (and use less energy) because they're tired, say the researchers. And if you're sleep deprived and not just groggy, University of Chicago researchers report that lack of sleep can torpedo weight loss by slowing your metabolism, increasing your appetite, and decreasing the number of calories you burn. All the more reason to eat late (if you prefer), sleep better at night, and watch the pounds melt—and stay—off your body.

But the best reason to eat late at night has nothing to do with losing fat or sleeping better. It's a decision that's best for our social life. How many times have you gone out and sabotaged a perfect day of eating with a few drinks or a big celebratory meal? On this plan, you can eat out without the guilt. Simply save your carbohydrates for the last meal of the day and indulge. Not only will these carbs help you sleep better, they'll also fuel more fat loss. This doesn't mean you can't have carbs earlier in the day, but most people prefer a big dinner to a big lunch. And on this plan, we encourage this approach for amplified results.

Your Secret Move

It's time for you to let loose and have some fun with your eating plan. If you've been following The Abs Secret guidelines, you should be free to enjoy your final meal of the day. If you haven't used up your floating meals, this is where you can squeeze in more calories to help you sleep better, improve your metabolism, and stop those nagging cravings. We recommend that you save 1 to 2 servings of your carb allotment (like grains and pastas) for after your workout or dinner. Remember, carbs at night can be a great thing for your weight loss goals. But if that's not your preference, your results won't be slowed.

Chapter 6
Abs-olutely Awesome Meals

The unbelievably simple, muscle-building, fat-melting, show-off-your-stomach recipe guide.

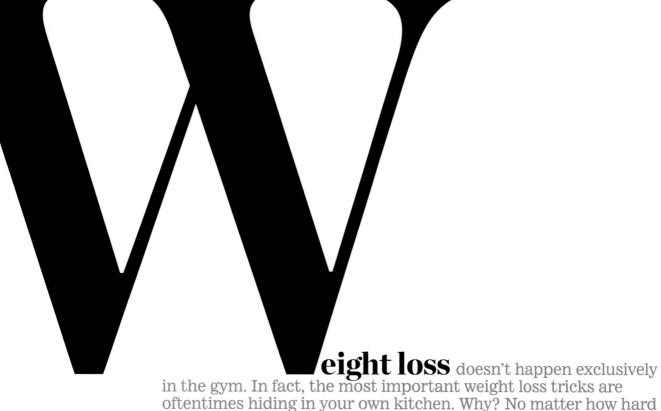

Weight loss

Weight loss doesn't happen exclusively in the gym. In fact, the most important weight loss tricks are oftentimes hiding in your own kitchen. Why? No matter how hard you exercise or how many calories you burn, the foundation of any good plan starts with your diet. And cooking your own food is the best way to stay on track. While eating out is an enjoyable and convenient experience it is a minefield of gut-bombs waiting to explode. Most restaurant foods are loaded with calories because they're cooked using methods you never would. A stick of butter here, a fistful of salt there, and, oh, an entire bottle of dressing for a kick. Next thing you know, your seemingly healthy meal is tipping the scale at more than 1,000 calories—and that's the "healthy" option.

Abs-olutely Awesome Meals

You don't need all the restaurant extras to create a satisfying meal. In fact, every man can become a master chef with a little bit of training. Doing so will help you enjoy all the benefits of a restaurant, while also paying less for a meal that won't derail your flat belly dreams. It all starts by reacquainting yourself with your kitchen. We've decided to make the process a little bit easier by providing some of the tastiest meals that are also easy to prepare and cook. How easy? Many of these options can be made in less than 10 minutes and don't exactly require training from a culinary institute. But if you're in the mood for something more advanced, we have options that will prove your master chef skills.

Regardless of your cooking experience or preferences, these meals can serve as the foundation of your new body. They're good for the home, on the go, or even for lunch at work. Try them out, experiment with your own changes, and discover your inner chef. It might be the smallest change you make, but it could be the difference maker that allows you to control your cravings and satisfy your appetite on fewer calories.

THE TOP 5 LEAN-BODY FOODS

Some meals pack a little extra nutritional punch. Include any of these on a weekly basis to help improve your cognitive functioning, skin tone, energy level, and calorie control.

Rainbow Trout
This fish has almost as much eicosa-pentaenoic acid (EPA) as salmon. This powerful omega-3 fatty acid might help prevent the stress chemical cortisol from boiling over and can help improve the health of your skin cells.

Blueberries
No berry is packed with more anti-oxidants than blueberries. They help counteract aging, reduce inflammation, fight off high blood pressure, and have even been linked with a boost in memory. One cup is all you need for the long list of benefits.

Pumpkin Seeds
They're not just great during Halloween season. Pumpkin seeds contain a boost of magnesium, which can help kick your energy and metabolism into a higher gear. Have them alone or add to eggs, yogurt, or cereal.

Ricotta Cheese
You know those whey protein shakes that come in big jars? This is the food equivalent. It's loaded with amino acids that can help you build muscle, burn fat, and recover faster from your workouts.

Dark Chocolate
According to the *Journal of the American Medical Association,* this healthy treat helps prevent stress from making your blood pressure surge. Dark chocolate has also been shown to ward off negative moods, meaning it's a healthier option than a bottle of Jack after a bad day.

BREAKFAST

SMOKED SALMON AND SCRAMBLED EGGS ON TOAST

Prep time: 3 minutes
Cook time: 7 minutes

1 slice hearty bread, such as sourdough, whole wheat, or spelt
1 egg
Salt
Pepper
1 ounce smoked salmon
1 red onion, thinly sliced (optional)
Capers (optional)
Fresh dill (optional)
1 lemon (optional)

• Toast the bread. Meanwhile, in a bowl, whisk the egg with salt and pepper. Pour into a nonstick pan and scramble. Lay the smoked salmon on the toasted bread and top with the scrambled egg. Finish with your choice of red onion, capers, dill, or a squeeze of lemon.

HUEVOS RANCHEROS

Prep time: 5 minutes
Cook time: 2 minutes

2 eggs
1 scallion, sliced
1 tablespoon diced cilantro
2 tablespoons shredded Mexican blend cheese
2 tablespoons salsa
1 medium whole wheat tortilla

• In a microwaveable bowl, stir the eggs with a fork until well blended and microwave for 2 minutes. Arrange all the ingredients on the tortilla, fold the ends, then roll.

SPINACH AND FETA FRITTATA

Prep time: 5 minutes
Cook time: 15 minutes

3 tablespoons olive oil
¼ cup chopped onion
2 cloves garlic, minced
1 pound baby spinach leaves
4 large eggs
4 large egg whites
¼ cup finely crumbled bread crumbs
2 tablespoons fresh basil
2 teaspoons grated lemon zest
½ teaspoon black pepper
1 cup crumbled feta cheese (4 ounces)

• In a large skillet, heat 1 tablespoon of the oil over medium heat. Add the onion and garlic and cook for 5 minutes.

• Add the spinach and stir until wilted. Remove from the skillet and keep warm.

• In a medium bowl, beat together the whole eggs and egg whites. Beat in the bread crumbs, basil, lemon zest, and pepper.

• In the same skillet, heat the remaining 2 tablespoons oil over medium heat. Stir the spinach mixture and the feta into the egg mixture, then pour into the skillet. Reduce the heat to low, cover, and cook until the top of the frittata is set.

• Cut into wedges to serve.

3 FAT-FIGHTING FOODS

Stock up on these foods to help you curb hunger and speed weight loss.

Grapefruit
In a study at the Nutrition and Metabolic Research Center at the Scripps Clinic in San Diego, people who ate half a grapefruit with each meal lost an average of 3.6 pounds in 3 months. The cause might be grapefruit's ability to counter an increase in insulin after you eat, and keep your blood sugar lower and your metabolism humming at a faster pace.

Raspberries and Blackberries
Berries are a stealthy source of fiber, which can help you stay full and eat less. Raspberries and blackberries both contain more than 8 grams per cup, which is almost a quarter of your daily allowance. Add them to any meal to help slow digestion, reduce your insulin response, and provide an antioxidant boost.

Yogurt
Your fat loss plan requires a double dose of calcium and protein—both of which are found in yogurt. This food is the perfect way to start your day, boost your afternoon slump, or end your day with dessert.

Abs-olutely Awesome Meals

PEANUT BUTTER STRAWBERRY WRAP

Prep time: 5 minutes
Cook time: 0 minute

1 whole wheat tortilla

2 tablespoons natural unsalted crunchy peanut butter

½ cup sliced strawberries

• Lay the tortilla on a work surface. Spread with the peanut butter. Cover with the strawberries. Roll into a tube. Slice on the diagonal into the desired number of pieces.

EGG AND AVOCADO BREAKFAST SANDWICH

Prep time: 4 minutes
Cook time: 4 minutes

2 large eggs, lightly beaten

1 tablespoon mashed avocado

1 small (3") bagel, halved and toasted

• Coat a small nonstick skillet with cooking spray and place over medium heat.

• Add the eggs and cook until set.

• Spread the avocado on half of the bagel. Top with the eggs and the remaining bagel half.

FLAT GREEN CHILE AND GOAT CHEESE OMELET

Prep time: 5 minutes
Cook time: 25 minutes

2 or more Anaheim green chile peppers (wear plastic gloves when handling)

½ tablespoon butter

1 onion, thinly sliced

½ teaspoon dried oregano (optional)

4 large eggs

½ teaspoon sea salt

¼ cup crumbled goat cheese

Whole wheat tortillas (optional)

• Preheat the broiler.

• Roast the chiles in the flame of a grill or gas burner (or as close as possible to a broiler flame) until the skins are bubbly and charred. Put them in a bowl, cover with a plate, and let them steam for about 10 minutes. Slip off the skins, cut off the stem end, and push out the seeds using the flat side of a knife. Tear or cut the chiles into strips.

• Heat the butter in an 8" nonstick ovenproof skillet over medium heat. Add the onion and oregano, if desired. Stir and cook gently. If the chile strips are still firm, add them to the skillet. Cook for 12 minutes, or until the onion has softened. Remove the chiles and onion from the skillet and cool slightly.

• Beat the eggs with the salt. Add the slightly cooled chiles and onion. If desired, add a bit more oregano. The skillet shouldn't need more butter, but if it seems dry, add about a teaspoon and swirl it around the skillet. Add the egg mixture to the skillet and cook over medium-low heat.

• As the eggs begin to set around the edges, lift them up with the tip of the spatula and let the wet egg flow underneath. Repeat this process until you can't do so easily any longer. Then sprinkle the goat cheese over the top.

• Once the eggs seem fairly well set, place the pan under the broiler so that the top can finish cooking and become golden. Slide the omelet onto a serving plate and, if desired, dust with extra oregano and serve with warm tortillas.

LUNCH

PERUVIAN SEAFOOD STEW

Prep time: 20 minutes
Cook time: 25 minutes

1 tablespoon olive oil

1 onion, chopped

1 jalapeño chile pepper, seeded and minced (wear plastic gloves when handling)

3 cloves garlic, minced

1 teaspoon ground cumin

1 can (15 ounces) reduced-sodium white beans, rinsed and drained

¾ pound small red potatoes, cut into ¼"-thick slices

½ bunch kale, coarsely chopped

1 bottle (8 ounces) clam juice

3 cups water

½ teaspoon salt

1 pound cod fillets, cut into 1" chunks

1 pound shrimp, peeled, deveined, and cut into 1" pieces

Lime wedges

Green Salad with Corn (recipe follows)

• In a soup pot, heat the oil over medium heat. Add the onion and cook, stirring frequently, for 6 minutes, or until golden brown. Stir in the pepper, garlic, and cumin and cook for 1 minute. Add the beans, potatoes, kale, clam juice, water, and salt. Bring to a boil. Reduce the heat to low, cover, and simmer for 12 minutes, or until the potatoes are tender.

• Stir in the cod. Return to a boil, then reduce the heat and simmer, covered, for 2 minutes. Gently stir in the shrimp and simmer, covered, for 2 to 3 minutes, or until the shrimp and cod are cooked through. Serve with the lime wedges.

Green Salad with Corn:
In a large bowl, combine 4 cups salad greens and ½ cup fresh or frozen and thawed corn kernels. Drizzle with 1 tablespoon cider vinegar and 1 teaspoon olive oil. Sprinkle with ⅛ teaspoon salt and toss.

• Makes 6 servings

BERRY GOAT CHEESE SALAD

Prep time: 15 minutes
Cook time: 10 minutes

Dressing
¼ cup sliced strawberries
1 tablespoon fresh orange juice
1 ½ teaspoons red wine vinegar
½ teaspoon orange zest
½ teaspoon sugar
2 tablespoons fat-free plain Greek yogurt
1 large pinch kosher salt

Salad
1 tablespoon pecans
3 cups baby spinach
½ cup halved strawberries
½ cup blueberries
1 yellow tomato, cut into eighths
2 purple radishes, thinly sliced
1 boneless, skinless chicken breast (6 ounces), grilled
1 teaspoon goat cheese crumbles

• For the dressing: Combine the strawberries, orange juice, vinegar, zest, sugar, yogurt, and salt in a blender or food processor, or whisk together until smooth.

• For the salad: Toast the pecans in a 400°F oven for 2 minutes. Remove from the oven and set aside. In a large bowl, combine the spinach, berries, tomato, and radishes. Drizzle with the dressing.

• Sprinkle with the pecans and goat cheese. Toss gently.

• Makes 2 servings

TANGY TURKEY CIABATTA

Prep time: 4 minutes
Cook time: 0 minute

1 tablespoon pesto
1 ciabatta roll
¼ cup baby spinach leaves
2 ounces sliced lean turkey
1 slice part-skim mozzarella cheese
3 pickle slices

• Spread the pesto on the ciabatta roll. Layer on the spinach, turkey, cheese, and pickles.

GRILLED CHICKEN AND PINEAPPLE SANDWICH

Prep time: 40 minutes
Cook time: 12 minutes

4 boneless, skinless chicken breasts (6 ounces each)
Teriyaki sauce
4 slices Swiss cheese
4 pineapple slices (½" thick)
4 whole wheat buns or lettuce wraps
1 red onion, thinly sliced
Pickled jalapeño chile peppers (wear plastic gloves when handling)

• Combine the chicken and enough teriyaki sauce to cover in a resealable plastic bag. Marinate in the refrigerator for at least 30 minutes and up to 12 hours.

• Coat a grill rack with nonstick spray. Preheat the grill. Remove the chicken from the marinade and place on the grill, discarding any remaining marinade. Cook over medium-high heat for 4 to 5 minutes on the first side. Flip and immediately add the cheese to each breast. Continue cooking until the cheese is melted and the chicken is lightly charred and firm to the touch.

• While the chicken rests, add the pineapple and buns to the grill. Cook for 2 minutes per side. (If you prefer lettuce wraps, skip this step.)

• Top each bun with the chicken, onion, pepper slices, and pineapple.

Abs-olutely Awesome Meals

SPECIAL SHRIMP SALAD

Prep time: 10 minutes
Cook time: 0 minute

2 ¼ tablespoons white wine vinegar

½ teaspoon salt

½ teaspoon chili powder

3 tablespoons extra-virgin olive oil

3 cups butter lettuce, torn into pieces

2 grapefruit, cut into segments

2 avocados, peeled and sliced

10 ounces precooked shrimp

1 scallion, including top, thinly sliced

4 teaspoons chopped cilantro

• Combine the vinegar, salt, and chili powder in a small bowl. Whisk in the oil.

• Put the lettuce on a serving plate or on 4 individual salad plates. Arrange the grape-fruit, avocados, and shrimp over the lettuce. Sprinkle with the scallion and cilantro.

• Drizzle with the chili dressing.

BETTER-FOR-YOU EGG SALAD

Prep time: 15 minutes
Cook time: 12 minutes

4 large eggs

8 ounces soft silken tofu

4 teaspoons brown mustard

½ teaspoon salt

⅛ teaspoon hot-pepper sauce

⅓ cup minced onion

¼ cup chopped parsley

• In a medium saucepan, place the eggs in cold water to cover by several inches. Bring to a boil over high heat. Remove from the heat, cover, and let stand for 12 minutes. Run the eggs under cold water until chilled. Peel, halve, and transfer to a large bowl.

• Add the tofu, mustard, salt, and pepper sauce and mash with a potato masher until some small chunks remain. Fold in the onion and parsley. Cover and chill until serving time.

CHIPOTLE GLAZED STEAK WITH BLACK BEAN SALAD

Prep time: 20 minutes
Cook time: 10 minutes

1 can (15 ounces) reduced-sodium black beans, rinsed and drained

1 cup frozen and thawed corn kernels

2 plum tomatoes, diced

1 avocado, diced

1 jalapeño chile pepper, seeded and finely chopped (wear plastic gloves when handling)

2 tablespoons chopped cilantro

2 tablespoons fresh lime juice

½ teaspoon salt

1 ½ teaspoons salt-free chipotle seasoning blend

1 teaspoon packed brown sugar

1 pound sirloin steak, trimmed of visible fat

• Combine the beans, corn, tomatoes, avocado, chile pepper, cilantro, lime juice, and ¼ teaspoon of the salt in a medium bowl. Set the salad aside.

• Coat a grill rack with nonstick spray. Mix the seasoning blend, brown sugar, and the remaining ¼ teaspoon salt in a small bowl. Rub the spice mixture over both sides of the steak.

• Grill or broil the steak, 4 minutes per side for medium rare, turning once. Let rest for 5 minutes. Thinly slice the steak and serve with the black bean salad.

• Makes 4 servings

RICE BOWLS WITH SHRIMP AND BOK CHOY

Prep time: 20 minutes
Cook time: 10 minutes

1 cup quick-cooking brown rice blend

3 tablespoons ponzu sauce

3 tablespoons unseasoned rice vinegar

2 teaspoons grated peeled fresh ginger

2 teaspoons packed brown sugar

1 teaspoon Sriracha sauce

4 teaspoons dark sesame oil

1 head bok choy, thinly sliced

1 pound cooked shrimp

2 carrots, shredded

1 cucumber, peeled, halved, seeded, and thinly sliced

⅓ cup fresh cilantro

• Cook the rice according to package directions without added salt or fat.

• In a small bowl, whisk the ponzu sauce, vinegar, ginger, brown sugar, Sriracha sauce, and 3 teaspoons of the sesame oil.

• In a large nonstick skillet, heat the remaining 1 teaspoon sesame oil over medium heat. Add the bok choy and cook for 3 to 4 minutes, stirring frequently.

• Place the rice in the centers of 4 bowls. Arrange the bok choy, shrimp, carrots, and cucumber around the rice. Drizzle with the dressing and sprinkle with the cilantro.

• Makes 4 servings

■ DINNER

POLENTA LASAGNA

Prep time: 25 minutes
Cook time: 1 hour

1 tablespoon olive oil

1 onion, chopped

1 carrot, finely chopped

3 cloves garlic, minced

1 bunch collard greens, coarsely chopped

½ cup water

1 tube (18 ounces) prepared polenta, thinly sliced

1 cup part-skim ricotta cheese

1 cup shredded part-skim mozzarella cheese

2 cups reduced-sodium marinara sauce

½ cup grated Parmesan cheese

Mushroom Salad
(recipe follows)

• Preheat the oven to 375°F. Coat a 9" baking pan with nonstick spray.

• In a large saucepan, heat the oil over medium heat. Add the onion and carrot. Cook for 5 minutes, or until softened. Stir in the garlic. Add the collard greens and water. Bring to a boil, then reduce the heat and cook, stirring frequently, for 10 minutes, or until the greens are tender and the water evaporates.

• Arrange one-third of the polenta slices on the bottom of the prepared pan. Add half of the collard greens, spreading evenly. With a teaspoon, spoon on half of the ricotta cheese (no need to spread it out). Sprinkle with half of the mozzarella cheese. Spoon on half of the marinara sauce. Repeat the layering once. Top with the remaining polenta slices and sprinkle with the Parmesan cheese.

• Bake for 35 to 40 minutes, or until hot and bubbly. Let stand 10 minutes before serving.

Mushroom Salad
In a medium bowl, combine 1 tablespoon lemon juice, 1 tablespoon olive oil, ⅛ teaspoon salt, ⅛ teaspoon black pepper, and a pinch of ground red pepper. Add 1 package (8 ounces) sliced mushrooms and 1 rib celery, thinly sliced. Toss to combine. Let stand for 10 minutes before serving.

• Makes 6 servings

ASIAN SALMON BURGERS

Prep time: 12 minutes
Cook time: 10 minutes

1 pound skinless salmon fillet, cut into chunks

¼ cup fresh whole wheat bread crumbs

1 large egg

2 cloves garlic, chopped

2 teaspoons reduced-sodium soy sauce

½ teaspoon dark sesame oil

2 scallions, chopped

4 tablespoons pickled ginger

2 tablespoons toasted sesame seeds

4 whole wheat buns, toasted

¼ cup baby spinach

• In a food processor, combine the salmon, bread crumbs, egg, garlic, soy sauce, oil, scallions, and 2 tablespoons of the ginger. Pulse until coarsely chopped. Form into 4 equal (3" diameter) patties. Sprinkle the tops with sesame seeds.

• Coat a large nonstick skillet with cooking spray and heat over medium heat. Put the patties, sesame seed side down, in the pan. Cook for 5 minutes. Flip and cook for 5 minutes longer, or until done.

• Place the burgers on the buns. Top with the spinach and the remaining 2 tablespoons ginger.

CHICKEN LETTUCE CUPS

Prep time: 15 minutes
Cook time: 8 minutes

2 teaspoons coconut oil

½ cup chopped sweet onion

1 ½ cloves garlic, minced

1 ½ cups minced gingerroot

½ cup water chestnuts

1 cup diced cooked skinless chicken

2 tablespoons low-sodium chicken broth

1 tablespoon reduced-sodium soy sauce

2 tablespoons rice wine vinegar

Pinch of black pepper

2 cups cooked brown rice

2 scallions, thinly sliced

4 Bibb lettuce leaves, washed

1 teaspoon black sesame seeds

• Heat the oil in a large skillet over medium-low heat. Add the onion and cook for 3 minutes. Reduce the heat to low. Add the garlic and gingerroot and cook for 1 minute. Add the water chestnuts and cook for 1 minute longer.

• Add the chicken, broth, soy sauce, vinegar, and pepper and stir well. Add the rice and cook for 3 minutes. Remove from the heat and stir in the scallions.

• Divide the chicken mixture equally among the lettuce leaves. Sprinkle with the sesame seeds and serve.

Abs-olutely Awesome Meals

CHILI-SPICED FISH TACOS

Prep time: 4 minutes
Cook time: 7 minutes

5 ounces barramundi fillet
Pinch of salt
Pinch of black pepper
Pinch of cumin
Pinch of chili powder
1 teaspoon olive oil
2 corn tortillas
½ cup chopped tomato
½ cup shredded green cabbage
1 tablespoon fresh cilantro
1 teaspoon lime juice

• Coat a grill rack with nonstick spray. Preheat the grill.

• Season the fish with the salt, pepper, cumin, and chili powder. Grill (or cook in 1 teaspoon olive oil over medium heat) for 5 minutes. Flip and cook for 2 minutes longer.

• Divide the fish between the tortillas. Serve with the tomato, cabbage, cilantro, and lime juice.

BEEF, VEGETABLE, AND ALMOND STIR-FRY

Prep time: 10 minutes
Cook time: 10–15 minutes

½ cup rice
1 pound flank steak, sliced ¼" thick
3 teaspoons reduced-sodium soy sauce
2 teaspoons toasted sesame oil
1 tablespoon grated fresh ginger
2 cloves garlic, minced
2 medium carrots, thinly sliced
1 medium onion, chopped
1 medium red bell pepper, thinly sliced
8 ounces snow peas
3 tablespoons sliced almonds
2 tablespoons hoisin sauce

• Cook the rice according to package directions.

• Meanwhile, toss the steak with 2 teaspoons of the soy sauce. Heat 1 teaspoon of the oil in a large nonstick or cast-iron skillet over medium-high heat. Add the ginger and garlic. Cook, stirring, for 30 seconds. Add the steak and cook, stirring occasionally, for 2 to 3 minutes. Transfer to a plate and set aside.

• Return the skillet to the heat, and add the remaining 1 teaspoon oil, the carrots, onion, and bell pepper. Cook, stirring occasionally, for 3 minutes, or until the vegetables start to soften. Stir in the snow peas and almonds. Cook, stirring occasionally, for 2 minutes.

• Add the reserved steak and juices, the hoisin sauce, and the remaining 1 teaspoon soy sauce. Cook, stirring, for 1 minute. Serve over the rice.

CHICKEN WITH WALNUTS AND SPINACH

Prep time: 16 minutes
Cook time: 38 minutes

1 tablespoon olive oil
⅓ cup chopped onion
1 cup chopped walnut pieces
1 cup chopped baby spinach
½ cup grated provolone
4 thin-sliced boneless, skinless chicken breasts (4 ounces)
¼ teaspoon salt
¼ teaspoon black pepper

• Preheat the oven to 375°F. Grease a baking sheet.

• Heat the oil in a medium skillet over medium-low heat and add the onion. Cook for 5 minutes, or until softened. Add ½ cup of the walnuts and cook for 1 minute. Increase the heat to medium. Add the spinach and cook for 2 minutes, or until wilted. Put the mixture in a bowl and stir in the cheese.

• Season the chicken with the salt and pepper. Divide the spinach mixture among the chicken slices and roll up to enclose. Coat the chicken with cooking spray and roll in the remaining ½ cup walnuts. Place on the baking sheet and bake for 30 to 35 minutes.

HOISIN-ORANGE GLAZED CHICKEN

Prep time: 10 minutes
Cook time: 15 minutes

2 navel oranges
¼ cup water
3 tablespoons hoisin sauce
2 tablespoons dry sherry
1 tablespoon reduced-sodium soy sauce
3 cloves garlic, thinly sliced
½ teaspoon five-spice powder
4 (5-ounce) boneless, skinless chicken breasts
1 bunch asparagus, cut into 2" pieces
4 cups broccoli florets
1 teaspoon dark sesame oil

• From one of the oranges, grate ½ teaspoon zest and squeeze ⅓ cup juice. Remove the peel and white pith from the remaining orange, and cut between the membranes to segment the orange.

• In a large skillet, mix the orange juice, orange zest, water, hoisin sauce, sherry, soy sauce, garlic, and five-spice powder over high heat. Bring to a boil and add the chicken breasts. Reduce the heat and simmer, covered, for 10 to 12 minutes, turning once, or until a thermometer inserted in the thickest portion registers 160°F and the juices run clear.

• Meanwhile, fill a large saucepan with 1" water and insert a vegetable steaming basket. Add the asparagus and broccoli and bring to a boil. Cover and cook for 3 minutes, or until the vegetables are crisp-tender. Transfer to a bowl and drizzle with the sesame oil.

• Transfer the chicken to a plate and cover with foil to keep warm. Bring the hoisin mixture to a boil and cook for 1 to 2 minutes, or until thickened and reduced to ½ cup. Cut the chicken on the diagonal into ½"-thick slices. Spoon the sauce over the chicken and top with the orange segments. Serve with the vegetables.

• Makes 4 servings

PORK GYROS

Prep time: 45 minutes
Cook time: 25 minutes

2 tablespoons safflower or olive oil
2 tablespoons red wine vinegar
1 teaspoon dried oregano
4 cloves garlic, minced
1 pork tenderloin (1 ¼ pounds), trimmed
¼ teaspoon black pepper
½ teaspoon salt
⅓ cup fat-free plain Greek yogurt
2 tablespoons chopped fresh dill
4 whole wheat pitas, halved and toasted if desired
2 cups packed baby spinach
1 tomato, cut into thin wedges
Watermelon-Cucumber Salad (recipe follows)

• In a large resealable plastic bag, combine 1 tablespoon of the oil, 1 tablespoon of the vinegar, the oregano, and all but ¼ teaspoon of the garlic. Add the pork, seal the bag, and turn to coat the pork with the marinade. Let stand for 30 minutes.

• Preheat the oven to 425°F. Remove the pork from the bag and discard the marinade. Season the pork with the pepper and ¼ teaspoon of the salt. Heat the remaining 1 tablespoon oil in a large ovenproof skillet over medium-high heat. Add the pork and cook for 5 minutes, turning occasionally, until browned. Place the skillet in the oven and roast for 15 to 20 minutes, turning once, until a thermometer inserted in the thickest portion registers 155°F and the juices run clear. Remove the pork to a cutting board and let rest for 5 minutes.

• Meanwhile, in a small bowl, combine the yogurt, dill, the remaining 1 tablespoon vinegar, the remaining ¼ teaspoon garlic, and the remaining ¼ teaspoon salt.

• Thinly slice the pork. Stuff the pita halves with the pork, spinach, and tomato and drizzle with the yogurt sauce.

• Watermelon-Cucumber Salad: In a medium bowl, combine 2 cups diced seedless watermelon; ½ peeled, halved, and sliced cucumber; 3 tablespoons crumbled feta cheese; and 1 tablespoon red wine vinegar.

• Makes 4 servings

Abs-olutely Awesome Meals

ROAST SALMON WITH WHITE BEAN COMPOTE

Prep time: 15 minutes
Cook time: 20 minutes

1 pound wild salmon fillet (in one piece)
1 pint grape tomatoes
1 tablespoon olive oil
½ teaspoon salt
¼ teaspoon black pepper
1 can (15 ounces) reduced-sodium cannellini beans, rinsed and drained
½ cup roasted red and yellow bell peppers, chopped
¼ cup pitted kalamata olives, chopped
1 tablespoon lemon juice
¼ cup chopped fresh basil
1 teaspoon balsamic vinegar
Sauteed Escarole (recipe follows)

• Preheat the oven to 425°F. Coat a rimmed baking sheet with olive oil nonstick spray.

• Place the salmon on the prepared baking sheet. Arrange the tomatoes around the salmon. Drizzle the tomatoes with 1 teaspoon of the oil. Sprinkle the salmon and tomatoes with ¼ teaspoon of the salt and ⅛ teaspoon of the pepper. Roast for 12 to 15 minutes, or until the salmon is just opaque in the center and the tomatoes are soft.

• Meanwhile, in a medium bowl, combine the beans, bell peppers, olives, and lemon juice.

• Remove the tomatoes to a small bowl and stir in the basil, vinegar, and the remaining 2 teaspoons oil, ¼ teaspoon salt, and ⅛ teaspoon pepper. Cut the salmon into 4 pieces, discarding the skin. Serve over the bean compote with the tomato mixture spooned on top.

• Sauteed Escarole: In a large nonstick skillet, heat 1 tablespoon olive oil over medium heat. Add 2 cloves garlic, thinly sliced, and cook for 30 seconds. Add 1 bunch escarole, cut into 2" pieces. Cook for 4 to 5 minutes, stirring frequently, or until the escarole is wilted and tender. Stir in ⅛ teaspoon salt.

• Makes 4 servings

SMOOTHIES

MIXED FRUIT BREAKFAST SMOOTHIE

Prep time: 2 minutes
Cook time: 0 minute

¾ cup soy milk
¼ cup low-fat ricotta cheese
1 scoop vanilla whey protein
½ cup frozen cranberries
⅓ cup frozen mixed fruit

• In a blender or food processor, combine the soy milk, ricotta, whey protein, cranberries, and fruit. Blend or process for 1 minute, or until pureed and well blended.

HIGH-PROTEIN BLUEBERRY YOGURT SHAKE

Prep time: 5 minutes
Cook time: 0 minute

1 cup frozen wild blueberries
½ cup plain Greek yogurt
1 scoop plain or vanilla whey protein powder
1 banana
½ cup pomegranate juice
¼ cup walnut pieces
½ teaspoon vanilla extract

• In a blender, combine the blueberries, yogurt, protein powder, banana, pomegranate juice, walnuts, and vanilla extract. Process until smooth.

CHOCOLATE–PEANUT BUTTER SMOOTHIE

Prep time: 3 minutes
Cook time: 0 minute

1 scoop chocolate protein powder

1 tablespoon cacoa powder

1 tablespoon peanut butter

6 ounces almond milk

4 ice cubes

• In a blender, combine the protein powder, cacoa powder, peanut butter, almond milk, and ice cubes. Blend and serve.

STRAWBERRY-BANANA PROTEIN SMOOTHIE

Prep time: 3 minutes
Cook time: 0 minute

1 whole banana

½ cup strawberries

1 cup almond milk

1 ½ scoops vanilla whey protein powder

4 ice cubes

• In a blender, combine the banana, strawberries, almond milk, protein powder, and ice cubes. Blend and serve.

MINT CHOCOLATE CHIP SMOOTHIE

Prep time: 7 minutes
Cook time: 0 minute

6 ounces water

1 mint tea bag

6 ice cubes

1 scoop chocolate whey protein powder

½ cup unflavored Greek yogurt

1 tablespoon cacao powder

1 tablespoon cacao nibs or semisweet chocolate chips

• Boil the water and let the tea bag steep for 5 to 7 minutes. In a blender, combine the tea, ice cubes, protein powder, yogurt, cacao powder, and cacao nibs or chocolate chips. Blend and serve.

Chapter 7
Abs for Every Eater

Whether you're lactose intolerant, a vegetarian, or don't eat gluten, this is the solution for your special dietary needs.

Dieting can make

Dieting can make the weight loss process feel like high hurdles. Rather than simply running toward your goal, you're constantly forced to jump over obstacles that you can't avoid. Don't eat this. Limit that. The rules don't seem like they were made for a human, let alone a guy who knows what he wants, when he wants it. We understand that the worst part of your diet isn't necessarily what you can eat—it's what you can't. And we're not talking about cookies, cakes, or Denny's Grand Slam breakfast. Those are indulgences that have their place but can lead you astray. This is more about the hurdles you face as a result of personal health practices or health limitations.

In today's society, dietary restrictions have become a real burden for people who choose to eat a certain way or are forced

Abs for Every Eater

to avoid certain food groups. Whether you're a vegetarian, lactose intolerant, or practicing gluten-free eating, most diet plans don't account for the restrictive nature of your eating approach. And it doesn't matter if your "picky" habits are by choice or necessity. When you aren't given the options that work within the confines of the food you eat, it's hard to create an effective weight loss program.

Look no further than the eating plan suggested in this book. We've shown you that eating a high-protein diet is a great way to burn body fat and maintain muscle. But what happens if you're a vegetarian? Most high-protein food suggestions include some sort of animal protein. Does that mean you can't follow a high-protein approach? Of course not.

Vegetarians aren't the only ones frustrated by limited suggestions. Options like milk and cheese are commonly included as meals and snacks because calcium has been scientifically shown to shrink your gut and help fight against the aging process. However, if you're lactose intolerant, those foods could destroy your insides before making your outsides look better. The same can be said about those who follow a gluten-free diet.

There's no reason for your personal dietary preferences to stand in the way of any goal. Whether you're a calorie counter, a vegetarian, or lactose intolerant, or you just want to eat at a restaurant, you'll find suggestions to help tailor your eating to meet your specific needs. We turned to Mike Roussell, PhD, founder of Naked Nutrition, to ensure that your unique relationship with food isn't a hindrance to uncovering your abs. After all, the reason this diet works is because it complements your lifestyle. Dr. Roussell created this guide to help you navigate some of the most common and complicated diet scenarios and restrictions that make it seem impossible to follow a healthy plan. These tips and tricks offer a solution that will make your eating headaches a thing of the past.

THE HURDLE:
You're Lactose Intolerant

If no one suffered from lactose intolerance, odds are we'd all be a little healthier and trimmer. That's because research suggests that the calcium you consume from dairy is a stealthy way to eat more food and still lose weight—because the calories you eat from dairy are more likely to provide energy than be stored as body fat. More surprisingly, avoiding dairy makes you more likely to pack on the pounds. According to a study in the *American Journal of Clinical Nutrition*, reducing the amount of dairy you eat sends a signal in your body to make more fat cells.

The process might seem a bit magical, but it's nothing more than your body reacting to a primary need. When you don't have enough calcium in your body, you try to hold on to what you have. This triggers a reaction where your body releases a compound called calcitriol, which increases the production of fat cells. If you want fewer fat cells, eating extra calcium suppresses calcitriol, which breaks down fat and makes your fat cells leaner and your belly flatter.

Fortunately, having to avoid dairy because of lactose intolerance doesn't need to stand in the way of finding your abs. It is important to remember that if you're lactose intolerant, there are different levels of severity. Being lactose intolerant simply means that your body does not produce sufficient amounts of the enzyme lactase. Lactase is responsible for chopping the dairy sugar, lactose, in half so that your body can use it for energy. If lactose goes undigested, you're left feeling bloated and uncomfortable.

Some people can tolerate small amounts of lactose, while others cannot tolerate any. Figure out which one you are and then apply these tips accordingly, to help ignite more weight loss.

Add the Missing Ingredient
Sometimes the best approach is the simplest: Eat dairy. For those who don't have severe intolerance, taking a lactase supplement with a dairy-filled meal can help you experience all the benefits of milk and cheese. By supplementing with the enzyme, you're giving your body what it is missing. A diet high in dairy has been estimated to boost weight loss by as much as 70 percent, so using the supplement might be the extra kick you need, says Dr. Roussell.

Choose a "Better" Protein Powder
Whey is the most common protein used in protein powder, but there are different ways that whey is purified and processed in order to extract it from milk. Some of these processes leave small amounts of lactose that can cause you to bloat and cramp. If your protein powder is causing these symptoms, switch to a powder that only contains whey protein isolate, suggests Dr. Roussell. This is the purest form of whey, in which all the lactose is removed.

Eat More Probiotics
Dairy products such as kefir and certain brands of cottage cheese and yogurt contain good bacteria called probiotics. These cultured dairy products contain lower levels of lactose because the probiotics break down the lactose sugar for you, making it easier on your stomach, says Dr. Roussell. Oftentimes people who can tolerate low levels of lactose can eat these products without any problems. Cottage cheese and plain yogurt are both high in protein and serve as good snacks on a weight loss diet. Kefir is a great milk substitute for smoothies, and its high concentration of probiotics can help ease your intestinal discomfort.

Remove Dairy Entirely
If your lactose intolerance is severe, or if you have trouble achieving a sleek midsection, your best option might be to remove dairy entirely. While restrictive, this will eliminate the cause of your intestinal problems while also reducing the total amount of sugar that you consume in your diet. Though the sugar

81
Percent more body fat that dieters lost over 12 weeks when they ate 3 servings of yogurt a day compared to those who had no yogurt

Abs for Every Eater

CALCIUM CONTROL

Just because you're not eating dairy doesn't mean you can't have calcium in your diet. Remember, not enough calcium triggers the release of fat-friendly calcitriol. Because calcium-rich diets are essential in treating and managing many conditions, it's imperative that you maximize your opportunities to supplement calcium with other options. These include dark leafy greens (spinach, kale), almonds, sesame seeds, salmon, and fortified foods (orange juice).

from dairy is not a bad thing, it does serve as a hidden source that could put you over the edge and farther away from your hard body.

THE HURDLE:
You're a Vegetarian

Being a vegetarian poses dietary challenges that can hinder your weight loss. It's not that a plant-based diet is bad for you. After all, one of the foundational aspects of the eating plan in this book is eating more greens. Meals that are rich in vegetables provide nutrients that can help you fight off every disease from cancer to cardiovascular breakdown, as well as slow the aging process and help you supercharge your body with energy. But vegetarians have a tendency to eat less protein. And as you know, eating protein not only burns more calories during the digestion process, it also helps you build more muscle and improve your metabolism.

Another issue: Vegetarians eat a diet that tends to be excessively high in carbohydrates. While eating carbohydrates is part of a balanced eating plan, they are not as filling as protein. This means that in order to feel satisfied, vegetarians eat more and more carbs in order to satisfy their hunger. This unintentionally leads them to underestimate how much they eat, consume more calories than they should, and put on weight. With a few small adjustments, any vegetarian can maintain a green-based approach while accelerating fat loss.

Use Protein Powder

If you want to make sure that you lose fat and not muscle, you need to include more protein in your diet. For vegetarians, hitting daily protein goals without overeating carbohydrates can be difficult. That's because many of the best vegetarian protein sources such as beans, legumes, and higher protein grains contain more carbohydrates than protein (per serving). Your solution: protein powder. These powders are a convenient way to boost your protein intake without adding excess carbohydrates to your meals or snacks. Add a scoop to the foods you bake or to carb-based meals such as oatmeal, or blend as a smoothie.

Go Nuts

One of the best foods for vegetarians is also one of the most effective snacks for any diet. Nuts, such as almonds, cashews, and walnuts, are loaded with fat-fighting benefits. Adding 1 to $1\frac{1}{2}$ ounces (about a handful) of nuts each day is a great carbohydrate-controlled way to fuel your body while continuing to shed fat and eliminate hunger. Nuts contain fiber, protein, and fat, all of which will keep you fuller longer while also slowing digestion. What's more, nuts can help control rises in your blood sugar. This is essential for optimizing your fat loss hormones and age-proofing your body against weight gain. While nuts have many health benefits, they are packed with calories. Several handfuls can quickly set you back.

Take Strategic Supplements

While eating whole foods is always the foundation of any good eating plan, vegetarians should add a few supplements to fill gaps created on a plant-based diet. Creatine and docosahexaenoic acid (DHA) are two supplements that are essential for vegetarians concerned about weight loss and their general health, says Dr. Roussell. Creatine is typically viewed as a muscle-building formula, but it has many additional benefits for vegetarians. Supplementing with 5 grams of creatine following each of your workouts will help you maintain your lean muscle and improve brain function.

DHA is an omega-3 fat found in fish oil supplements that will potentially boost weight loss by stopping the growth of fat cells. If you don't eat fish, you can still add the vegetarian (or vegan) version of the supplement to your diet. DHA is produced by algae, and when fish consume the algae, they become a concentrated and potent source of the powerful, healthy fat. Vegetarians should take at least 1 gram of DHA per day from an algae-based supplement.

THE HURDLE:
You Follow a Gluten-Free Diet

A funny thing happened to the wheat industry thanks to the low-carb movement: People stopped eating breads and grains. And that wasn't all that happened. Lots of dieters who made the change lost weight and felt better than ever. But the reason wasn't what everyone assumed. While a lower-carb diet can help you lose weight, it's not that carbs are the enemy. In fact, they are a vital nutrient that will help you get lean fast and keep you energized for your workouts. The reason the diet changes made such a difference was because many people were overeating carbs, and the change in diet meant they were eating more protein and vegetables.

The shift also shed light on a growing medical problem: gluten intolerance. Turns out, thousands of people are sensitive to gluten, a compound that is found in most grains, breads, and wheat products. So when the foods were removed, people's digestive health improved, which aided in weight loss.

Even if you're not allergic to gluten, removing the by-product from your diet is one of the best ways to lose weight. That's because gluten-containing foods are packed with faster-acting carbohydrates, which can hinder your weight loss, says Dr. Roussell. Whether you're gluten free by choice or necessity, use these suggestions to make that approach work for you.

Don't Overdo Gluten-Free Foods

Gluten-free eating is very popular right now, but as a result there are myriad gluten-free food substitutes available in your local supermarket, such as gluten-free pretzels, bagels, and breads. Much like the low-fat craze of the 1980s and '90s, and the low-carb movement in the early 2000s, just because a food is low in

5 Tips to Staying Gluten Free

If you have a gluten allergy (i.e., celiac disease), then staying away from gluten is very important. Celiac disease is an inflammatory condition, and high levels of inflammation run counter to your weight loss efforts. If you are having trouble breaking through a weight loss plateau, make sure that you are truly gluten free. Foods like soy sauce, deli meats, marinade and sauces, meal replacement shakes, and oats (which don't contain gluten but a similar compound that many people with celiac disease don't respond well to) may secretly be adding gluten to your diet without you knowing, says Dr. Roussell.

TIP #1 Read foods labels carefully to make sure that gluten or wheat isn't being added as a binding or thickening agent to marinades or sauces that you are using.

TIP #2 Look for oat- and gluten-free hot cereal to replace your morning oatmeal.

TIP #3 Make sure you are buying soy sauce that is specifically labeled gluten free.

TIP #4 Skip the deli meats; instead, cook and slice your own. If you like using deli meats for convenience, choose a brand that doesn't contain additives or preservatives. This will limit your exposure to hidden sources of gluten.

TIP #5 Meal replacement shakes oftentimes contain oat and/or barley fiber to enhance the fiber content of the shakes. These are ingredients you should avoid if you are gluten free. Instead, make your own. In a blender, combine 1 ½ scoops vanilla protein powder, 3 tablespoons walnuts, 2 tablespoons ground flaxseed, ½ cup blueberries, 1 teaspoon powdered green tea, 1 ½ cups water, and 3 ice cubes for a gluten-free, carbohydrate-controlled, 400-calorie meal replacement shake.

gluten (or fat or carbs) doesn't mean it's a health food.

You should approach these foods as you would any other meal. Make sure that they fit in to your dietary needs, and buy accordingly. These foods—gluten free or not—will hinder your weight loss by adding unnecessary sugars and calories to your diet. Starchy (rice, potatoes) and grain-based (breads, pasta, bagels) foods should be limited while trying to get your abs to shine through. Eat them in smaller quantities first thing in the morning or directly after you exercise for the best return on your weight loss efforts.

Watch Out for So-Called High-Protein Foods

We've made it more than clear that you need to eat more protein to see your abs and maximize weight loss. But when you go gluten free, you must be wary of high-protein foods that aren't naturally loaded with protein. This includes foods like granola, cereal, and high-protein grains that have been engineered to boost your protein intake. While great in theory, the protein in these foods is usually fortified with pure gluten and can be a stealthy nightmare on your cleaner eating approach.

THE HURDLE:
You Always Eat Out

Making a home-cooked meal is the easiest way to ensure better nutrition. You buy the ingredients and know exactly what went into your meals.

Unfortunately, most people don't have the time or confidence to cook on a daily basis. In fact, the number of calories that Americans consume outside of their homes has doubled since the late 1970s—and that number is directly linked to our increase in weight gain. A study in Spain found that people who ate at restaurants two or more times per week were 33 percent more likely to become overweight or obese.

Control Your Environment

When you eat out, no one is going to control calories for you, and you shouldn't be expected to count calories for yourself. But these are the facts: You are likely to eat 36 percent more calories when you eat out than when you're at home. So you need to take steps that help limit overindulgence.

Calorie Saver #1: Ask your server to remove the bread basket from the table.

Calorie Saver #2: Tell your server what you would like on your plate. If your meal comes with french fries or chips, ask for those to be left off your plate.

Calorie Saver #3: Ask for sauces or salad dressing to be brought on the side. This way, you can add them in the amounts you need (not in the excess amounts that most restaurants provide).

Calorie Saver #4: It's very hard to overeat vegetables, but rice, potatoes, pastas, and breads are carbohydrate- and calorie-dense foods that can sabotage your weight loss.

ABOUT THE EXPERT

Mike Roussell holds a doctorate in nutrition from Penn State University. He is a sought-after nutritional consultant known for his evidence-based approach that transforms complex nutritional concepts into practical nutritional habits and strategies for his clients. "Dr. Mike" works with a range of clientele that includes professional athletes, executives, food companies, and top-rated fitness facilities. He is a widely published author, and his work can be seen regularly on newsstands, on leading fitness Web sites, and at your local bookstore. To learn more, check out Facebook.com/nutritionphd.

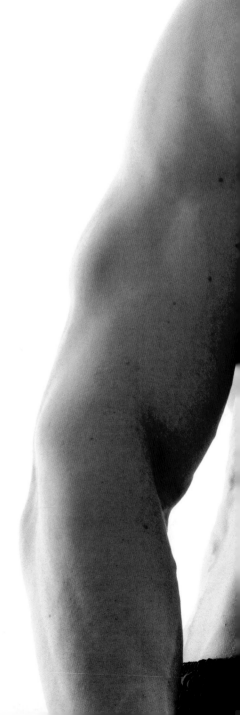

Chapter 8
The Abs Workout

Build your best body ever with this
butt-kicking total-body workout.

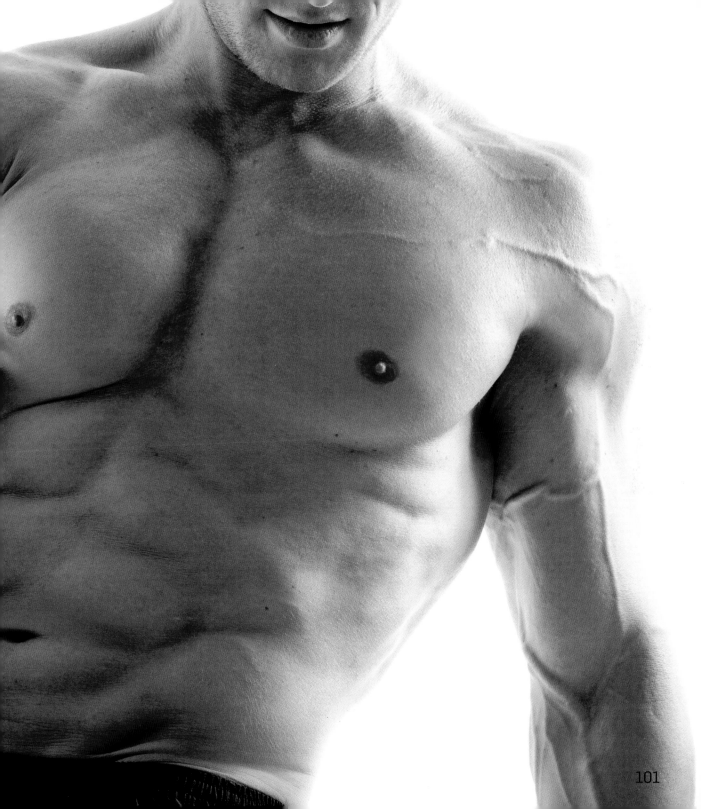

The Abs Workout

When you visit the gym, you probably have your routine. Maybe it includes some cardio, a few machines, and the inevitable subtle flexing in the mirror. Yeah, we've seen you do it. And while you may burn a few calories or be sore the next day, your training probably falls short of your expectations. In fact, if you're like most men, the lack of results might be the reason why you quit the gym altogether or choose to use other activities as your primary form of fitness. In a world where time is your most valuable asset, you need an exercise plan that guarantees every second of your workouts will lead to visible results.

That's why we created The Abs Workout. It doesn't matter if you've been exercising for 10 years or never set foot in the gym—you've never experienced a workout like this. We created a fat-scorching plan designed specifically to build your abs and incinerate the fat around your entire body to show off a lean, more muscular you. It's the perfect combination of time-tested exercises that challenge your muscles, and innovative movements that build your core and keep your workouts fun and engaging. The program is so effective, you'll only lift weights 3 days a week. That's because the exercises will exhaustively work all the muscles in your body, and you'll need the rest of the week to recover so you can continually improve. This leaves you with plenty of leisure time to be moderately active in the park, yard, court, or pool.

The Fall of Machines

This workout offers everything you'll ever need to transform your body as efficiently as possible. But as you check out your new workout, you might think you notice a flaw: There are no machines. That's not a mistake. If you want some insight into why so many people struggle to lose weight, just step into any cookie-cutter gym. There, in the big open space, you have a template for obesity: lots of cardio equipment lined up in front of televisions. Rows and rows of beautiful exercise machines, strategically organized to help you work every single muscle in your body.

The gym owners aren't stupid. They built these facilities to make you feel at home and comfortable. Machines are welcoming, convenient, and enjoyable. But there's nothing worse than spending hundreds of dollars on a membership, and hours and hours in a gym, and still not see results from your hard work. While there might be several reasons for your struggles, the machines deserve some blame. After all, machines—for all their convenience—are less effective at making changes to your body, say Canadian researchers.

In fact, both dumbbells and body-weight resistance are better alternatives and can help you burn more calories, say researchers from Columbia University. They found that free weights activate more muscle fibers, which results in more calories burned. While you won't notice a difference, your body will. That's because the non-mechanical approach allows you to perform your entire workout in fewer exercises. Think about it: Machines target each body part specifically and hold you in one restrictive range of motion, whereas it's much more efficient to select exercises that work multiple muscles at the same time. So instead of doing leg curls, leg extensions, and calf raises, you could just do squats—and see better results in a fraction of the time.

Faster results are one thing, but aren't machines safer? That's the general feeling among most people who train at a gym. After all, you're much more likely to drop a dumbbell than experience a machine falling apart while you're using it. However, a review of physical therapists discovered that machines are actually more likely to cause injuries than dumbbell and barbell exercises. That's why we've outlined a new plan that removes machines from the equation and, at times, removes all equipment entirely so you can do your entire workout at home. Your bodyweight can help you score the ultimate body.

We reached out to the top fitness experts, and they insisted that a machine-free approach is not only cheaper, but also better at helping you bust out of a slump and putting you on the fast track to shed sizes and shrink your belly.

Your Abs—Revealed

By now you might feel that you have a pretty good idea of what it takes to flip the switch on the ultimate body makeover. So let's try a little pop quiz.

Which of the following is true?
- **(a) Your abs are the key to a flatter belly.**
- **(b) Gimmick devices and supplements will help you eliminate your beer belly.**
- **(c) Crunches are the worst exercise for your abs.**

So what'd you pick? Hopefully, you were waiting for **(d) None of the above.**

You see, the lessons of the lean are not what they used to be, which means the methods of changing your body are not what you commonly see in the gym. So let's start with the basics: The terms core and abs are not interchangeable. Crunches work your abs. But for the biggest benefits, you need to work your entire core, which is made up of the four layers of the abs (rectus abdominis, external and internal obliques, and the transverse abdominis), hip flexors, spine extensors, hip adductors (inner thigh muscles), hip abductors (including gluteus medius), and multifidus (a series of muscles that connect and support your spine; they are activated first to protect your spine from injury).

That's the real purpose of your core: to prevent movement. So when you are focusing on doing crunches—or creating movement—you're doing the opposite of what was intended for your body. While crunches feel like they're doing something, they're actually one of the last exercises you want to include in an ab-revealing routine. Not only do they

The Abs Workout

put your back at risk for injury, they also work your muscles significantly less than other alternatives. In fact, a study published in the *Journal of Strength and Conditioning Research* found that crunches create a 64 percent activation of your six-pack muscles. That sounds great until you realize that Canadian researchers found that a variation of the basic plank achieves 100 percent activation of the same muscles.

The message is simple: The more you train your abs for stability—with planks, side planks, and other exercises that activate your entire core—the better you'll look. The best part: You'll barely have to move, which should eliminate your strains and pains. Just beware: The exercises in this program are deceptively difficult but surprisingly effective at finally uncovering your abs.

Your Program

To create a workout that has to deliver the impossible, you need to consult with the best. That's why we turned to strength coach John Romaniello, an expert known for transforming clients into the best shape of their life. That's what you'd expect from a man whose reputation is based on the ability to make fat disappear permanently. His programs present a unique combination of heavy lifting, explosive movements, dynamic exercises, and bodyweight training so that you can strip off pounds of fat while adding muscle mass and developing your abs. If it seems like that's too much to accomplish with one

program, you have yet to experience the benefits of a carefully crafted, scientifically designed regimen.

On this program, you will train 3 days per week to optimize your results and recovery, with each workout coming from one of three specific training protocols.

Training Methods

In order to achieve multiple physical goals during the same time frame, you can't follow your typical training plan, which usually builds in phases such as adding strength, packing on muscle, and then focusing on metabolic training to melt away fat. Instead, Romaniello has combined these elements in a unique fashion. It's not as simple as changing rep ranges. This is muscle science, with each workout being designed to allow you to improve on the goals simultaneously—without taking forever to see results.

The interplay between these three protocols is unique: They will have an additive effect, meaning that the results will stack on each other nicely; but they'll also have a synergistic effect, meaning that simply doing one makes the others more effective and increases your results. Allowing for both additive and synergistic effects is the only way to achieve simultaneous fat loss and muscle growth—what we call body re-composition—and the only way to do that is by utilizing multiple training methods. Your abs workouts will include:

A Positive Pyramid Scheme

Pyramid training is a method that has been used for decades by some of the world's most successful athletes. The idea of pyramids is pretty simple: Do short sets with descending numbers of reps, allowing you to perform a good deal of work in minimal time, all while having built-in rest periods.

Let's say you can lift 25 pounds for an exercise. If you perform a normal set of 10 reps, you are lifting a total of 250 pounds (10 reps x 25 pounds = 250 pounds lifted). Not too bad. Now let's say you use that same weight for a descending pyramid.

You lift that same 25 pounds, but for a total of 15 reps split into multiple sets with short rest periods (for instance: 5 + 4 + 3 + 2 + 1 = 15). You never reach complete fatigue on any set. But this way, you are able to lift your 10-rep max (10 RM)—25 pounds in this example—for 5 more reps than is normally possible. Why? Because of strategic rest periods that are built in to the protocol, so you are able to recover and keep working. In the end, you will have lifted a total of 375 pounds, or 125 pounds more. That's the type of increase in work capacity that will help you build muscle and lose fat fast.

With descending pyramids, you are doing more reps with a weight you normally could not lift that number of times, all for more total weight lifted. That's one way you'll achieve significant muscle growth and fat loss.

The Abs Workout

Heavy Metal

Lifting heavy weight is an integral part of training for muscle growth. Although lifting heavy necessitates utilizing lower reps, by keeping the volume (relatively) high with a greater number of total sets, we allow for enough microtrauma—the physical act of breaking down your muscle tissue so that it can build back bigger—to induce muscle growth.

Training with heavy loads also increases both myogenic and neurogenic muscle tone. Myogenic muscle tone is residual tension in a muscle at rest. That is, once you are lean enough, having a high level of myogenic muscle tone will give you a harder, leaner, more impressive physique—the lithe, fit look that you want. Neurogenic muscle tone is the temporary size that most guys enjoy in the gym. This refers to the look of your muscles when you're training; the pumped look that always seems to fade too soon once you leave the gym. This type of training will make your muscles look harder and bigger during your workouts.

Bodyweight Work

Before the inception of weights, machines, genetic engineering, or the Internet, people who wanted to get big and strong had to train using only their bodyweight. This training method continues to be used because of its efficacy.

Bodyweight exercises are fundamentally different from most weight-bearing exercises—even when the same muscles or movement patterns are involved.

Bodyweight exercises like pullups, pushups, squats, and lunges belong to a group of movements known as closed kinetic chain exercises (CKCE). These are exercises performed where the hand or foot is fixed or in constant contact with a surface, and does not move relative to the body. Speaking generally, you are moving your body toward or away from an object.

Compare these with exercises like the pulldown, bench press, leg press, or leg curls, which are known as open kinetic chain exercises (OKCE). In contrast to CKCEs, open kinetic chain exercises are performed without the hand or foot being fixed, and instead allow movement relative to body position. In this case, you are moving something either toward or away from your body.

From a neurological standpoint, there is a tremendous difference between pulling yourself toward a fixed object and pulling an object toward your body in a fixed position. Incorporating bodyweight CKCEs into training programs stimulates your nervous system in a way that is completely different from OKCEs. This different type of stimulus challenges your muscles and plays an important role in promoting new muscle growth, increasing how many calories you burn, and targeting fat loss.

Cardio, of Course

You'll be doing one high-intensity interval training (HIIT) cardio workout per week and one moderate-intensity cardio session per week.

The Schedule

Below is a complete layout of how you will be spending the next 4 weeks. Follow the guidelines as closely as possible to experience the full benefits of The Abs Workout.

WEEK 1	WEEK 2	WEEK 3	WEEK 4
Monday: Workout 1 (page 108)	**Monday:** Workout 4 (page 114)	**Monday:** Workout 5 (page 116)	**Monday:** Workout 2 (page 110)
Tuesday: HIIT cardio (page 120)	**Tuesday:** Off	**Tuesday:** HIIT cardio (page 120)	**Tuesday:** 20-minute moderate-intensity cardio workout (page 121)
Wednesday: Workout 2 (page 110)	**Wednesday:** Workout 5 (page 116)	**Wednesday:** Workout 4 (page 114)	**Wednesday:** Workout 1 (page 108)
Thursday: Off	**Thursday:** HIIT cardio (page 120)	**Thursday:** 20-minute moderate-intensity cardio workout (page 121)	**Thursday:** Off
Friday: Workout 3 (page 112)	**Friday:** Workout 6 (page 118)	**Friday:** Workout 3 (page 112)	**Friday:** Workout 2 (page 110)
Saturday: 20-minute moderate-intensity cardio workout (page 121)	**Saturday:** Off	**Saturday:** Off	**Saturday:** HIIT cardio (page 120)
Sunday: Light physical activity (walk, jog) during the day	**Sunday:** 20-minute moderate-intensity cardio workout (page 121)	**Sunday:** Off	**Sunday:** Light physical activity

BONUS WEEKS

By now, you should have seen some amazing results. But don't stop here. If you want to take on a new challenge, try any of the workouts in Chapter 11. Or, to keep progressing, continue with these two additional weeks to get in the best shape of your life.

WEEK 5	WEEK 6
Monday: Workout 2 (page 110)	**Monday:** Workout 5 (page 116)
Tuesday: HIIT cardio (page 120)	**Tuesday:** HIIT cardio (page 120)
Wednesday: Workout 3 (page 112)	**Wednesday:** Workout 6 (page 118)
Thursday: Off	**Thursday:** 20-minute moderate-intensity cardio workout (page 121)
Friday: Workout 4 (page 114)	**Friday:** Light physical activity
Saturday: Light physical activity	**Saturday:** Workout 1 (page 108)
Sunday: 20-minute moderate-intensity cardio workout (page 121)	**Sunday:** 20-minute moderate-intensity cardio workout (page 121)

The Abs Workout

BEFORE YOU BEGIN

Start each workout with a 10-minute warmup, like the one found on page 340. Make sure you push yourself hard enough during your warmup. Your heart rate should be elevated, and you should have light perspiration before you begin. For more on why your warmup is one of the most important components of your workouts, see "The Total Body Jump Start" on page 340.

Workout 1 / HEAVY TRAINING

CIRCUIT 1

Alternate between 1A and 1B for 6 sets of each. There is no need to time rest periods. Just don't waste time hanging out by the cardio area trying to catch the attention of that chick on the elliptical—she has a boyfriend. Trust me, I asked. After your last set of deadlifts, perform mountain climbers for 120 seconds. If you can't perform for the 120 seconds, set a timer and rest as necessary until the time is up.

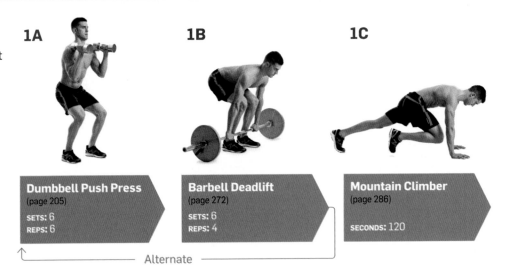

1A

Dumbbell Push Press
(page 205)

SETS: 6
REPS: 6

1B

Barbell Deadlift
(page 272)

SETS: 6
REPS: 4

1C

Mountain Climber
(page 286)

SECONDS: 120

——— Alternate ———

CIRCUIT 2

Perform 2A, 2B, and 2C sequentially, resting 60 seconds between exercises and 180 seconds between circuits. Perform this circuit five times, for a total of 5 sets of each exercise.

2A

2B

2C

Hold the top portion of the plank on your hands, instead of on your elbows

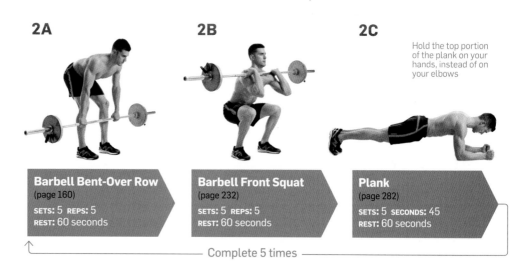

Barbell Bent-Over Row
(page 160)
SETS: 5 REPS: 5
REST: 60 seconds

Barbell Front Squat
(page 232)
SETS: 5 REPS: 5
REST: 60 seconds

Plank
(page 282)
SETS: 5 SECONDS: 45
REST: 60 seconds

↑———————— Complete 5 times ————————

CIRCUIT 3

Alternate between exercises, resting 30 seconds between each. Perform this circuit twice, then proceed to jumping rope. NOTE: AMAP means "as many as possible."

3A

3B

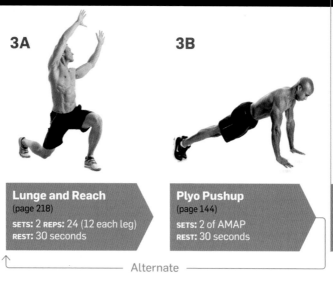

Lunge and Reach
(page 218)
SETS: 2 REPS: 24 (12 each leg)
REST: 30 seconds

Plyo Pushup
(page 144)
SETS: 2 of AMAP
REST: 30 seconds

↑———————— Alternate ————————

FINISH

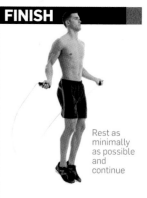

Rest as minimally as possible and continue

Jump Rope
5 to 10 minutes of jump rope work, performed as quickly and efficiently as you can.

The Abs Workout

Workout 2 / DESCENDING PYRAMIDS

CIRCUIT 1

Setup: Using your 10-rep max, perform 5 forward lunges with your left leg, then 5 with your right leg. Then 4 with your left leg and 4 with your right leg. Continue in a descending fashion until you reach 1 rep with each leg. This circuit is to be performed twice, with 60 seconds of rest between them. After the second run through, proceed immediately to circuit 2.

1A

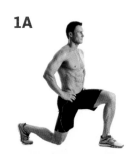

Bodyweight Lunge
(page 246)
SETS: 5 (non-alternating)
REPS: 5, 4, 3, 2, 1

CIRCUIT 2

Setup: Perform a plank for 30 seconds, then do 20 pushups. Without rest, transition back to the plank and hold for 25 seconds, followed by 15 pushups. Perform a plank for 20 seconds, followed by 10 pushups. Perform a plank for 15 seconds, followed by 5 pushups. Perform a plank for 10 seconds, followed by as many pushups as possible. Perform this circuit only once. Rest 120 seconds and proceed to circuit 3.

2A

2B

Plank
(page 282)
SETS: 5
SECONDS: 30, 25, 20, 15, 10

Pushup
(page 132)
SETS: 5
REPS: 20, 15, 10, 5, AMAP

Rest

SECONDS: 120

⌐— Complete 5 times with descending reps —

CIRCUIT 3

Perform 6 bicep curls. Then perform 6 front squats. At the apex of your last squat, press the dumbbells overhead for 6 reps. Lower the dumbbells back down to your sides, and perform 5 biceps curls, 5 squats, and 5 presses. Continue until you do 1 rep of each. That is 1 set. Rest and repeat.

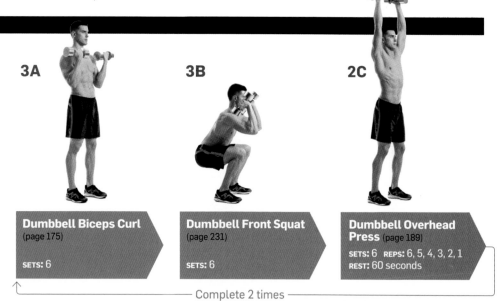

3A

Dumbbell Biceps Curl (page 175)

SETS: 6

3B

Dumbbell Front Squat (page 231)

SETS: 6

2C

Dumbbell Overhead Press (page 189)

SETS: 6 REPS: 6, 5, 4, 3, 2, 1
REST: 60 seconds

— Complete 2 times —

CIRCUIT 4

This circuit is to be performed four times, resting 30 seconds between each circuit. Perform 4 reps of split squats, followed immediately by 4 reps of front raises. Rest 30 seconds, then do 3 reps of each. Continue this pattern until you complete 1 rep of each exercise, then proceed to jumping rope.

FINISH

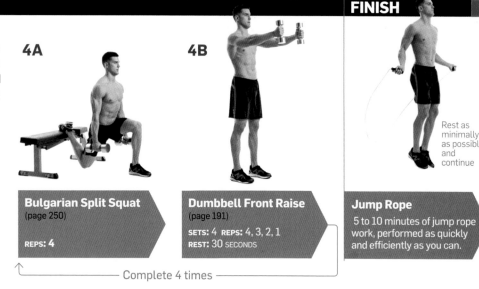

4A

Bulgarian Split Squat (page 250)

REPS: 4

4B

Dumbbell Front Raise (page 191)

SETS: 4 REPS: 4, 3, 2, 1
REST: 30 SECONDS

Rest as minimally as possible and continue

Jump Rope

5 to 10 minutes of jump rope work, performed as quickly and efficiently as you can.

— Complete 4 times —

111

The Abs Workout

Workout 3 / BODYWEIGHT TRAINING

In this phase, you'll be experimenting with pulse reps. This is a simple way to make your traditional bodyweight exercises more difficult. When pulse reps are indicated, pause 1 second at the bottom of each movement and 2 seconds at the top. This will result in more time under tension, which will make your muscles work a little harder without adding any weight.

CIRCUIT 1

Perform 1A to 1E sequentially (only do 1F if you failed the pushup test on page 126), without resting between exercises. Rest 60 seconds and move on to circuit 2.

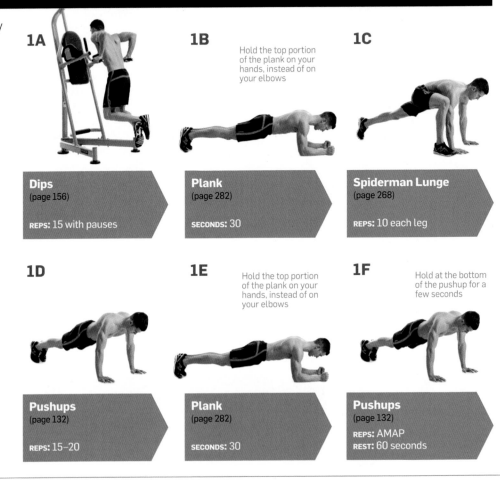

1A

Dips
(page 156)

REPS: 15 with pauses

1B
Hold the top portion of the plank on your hands, instead of on your elbows

Plank
(page 282)

SECONDS: 30

1C

Spiderman Lunge
(page 268)

REPS: 10 each leg

1D

Pushups
(page 132)

REPS: 15–20

1E
Hold the top portion of the plank on your hands, instead of on your elbows

Plank
(page 282)

SECONDS: 30

1F
Hold at the bottom of the pushup for a few seconds

Pushups
(page 132)

REPS: AMAP
REST: 60 seconds

CIRCUIT 2

Perform this circuit twice, resting 60 seconds between each. Rest 120 seconds and proceed to circuit 3.

2A

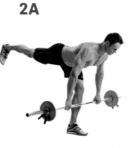

2B

2C

2D

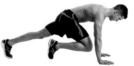

Single-Leg Barbell Romanian Deadlift (page 254)
REPS: 20 per leg **REST:** 60 seconds

Dumbbell Reverse Lunge (page 274)
REPS: 10/leg with pulses
REST: 60 seconds

Plank (page 282)
SECONDS: 60
REST: 60 SECONDS

Mountain Climber (page 286)
SECONDS: 60
REST: 120 SECONDS

―――― Complete 2 times ――――

CIRCUIT 3

Perform this circuit twice, resting 180 seconds between each. During this rest period, perform the abdominal exercise of your choice.

3A

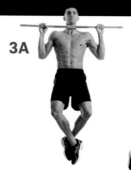

3B

Hold the top portion of the plank on your hands, instead of on your elbows

3C

3D

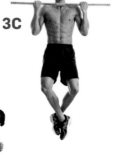

Pullup (page 171)
REPS: AMAP
REST: 180 seconds

Plank (page 282)
SECONDS: 30
REST: 180 seconds

Chinup (page 334)
REPS: AMAP
REST: 180 seconds

Inverted Row (page 161)
PULSE REPS ONLY: 25
REST: 180 seconds

―――― Complete 2 times ――――

The Abs Workout

Workout 4 / HEAVY TRAINING

CIRCUIT 1

Setup: Alternate between 1A and 1B eight times. There is no need to time your rest periods, but if more than half a song on your iPod has gone by, you're probably taking too long. Pick it up. After your last set, proceed to the Jumping Jacks.

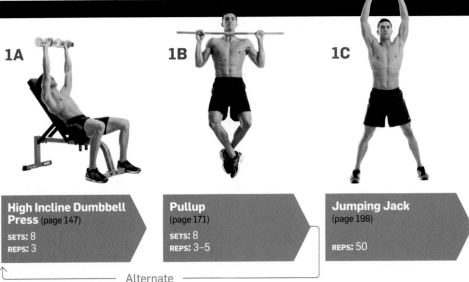

1A

1B

1C

High Incline Dumbbell Press (page 147)
SETS: 8
REPS: 3

Pullup (page 171)
SETS: 8
REPS: 3–5

Jumping Jack (page 198)
REPS: 50

Alternate

CIRCUIT 2

Perform 5 sets of the hack squat, resting about 60 to 90 seconds in between each. If you find you need longer rest periods, utilize the time by performing 1 set of 10 to 15 reps of the abdominal exercise of your choice. Immediately after your last set, perform the jump for 2 minutes. After your jumps, rest 60 seconds and perform 5 more sets of the hack squats.

2A

2B

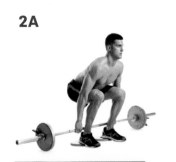

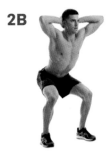

Barbell Hack Squat (page 271)
SETS: 5 REPS: 5
REST: 60–90 seconds

Squat Jump (page 234)
MINUTES: 2 REPS: AMAP
REST: 60 seconds

CIRCUIT 3

Alternate between exercises, resting 30 seconds between each. Perform this circuit twice, then proceed to jumping rope.

FINISH

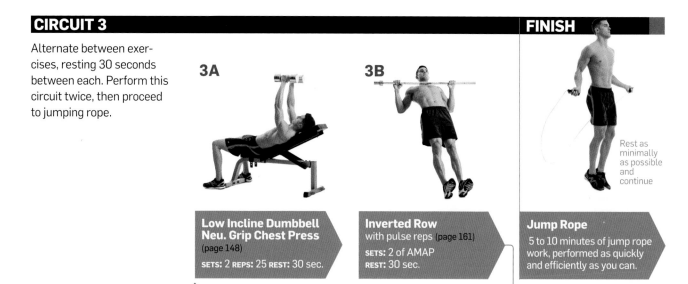

3A

3B

Rest as minimally as possible and continue

Low Incline Dumbbell Neu. Grip Chest Press (page 148)
SETS: 2 **REPS:** 25 **REST:** 30 sec.

Inverted Row with pulse reps (page 161)
SETS: 2 of AMAP
REST: 30 sec.

Jump Rope
5 to 10 minutes of jump rope work, performed as quickly and efficiently as you can.

Alternate

ABOUT THE EXPERT

The Abs Workout was created by **John "Roman" Romaniello**, a fat loss specialist and creator of the Final Phase Fat Loss training program. He is the founder of Roman Fitness Systems and a New York City–based trainer, coach, writer, and model. He works with clients of every stripe—from overweight teenagers to professional athletes to media and literary sensation Gary Vaynerchuk. Romaniello has been featured in *Men's Health*, *Men's Fitness*, and *SHAPE* magazine, and has appeared on *Good Morning America*. You can find out more about him at www.romanfitnesssystems.com.

The Abs Workout

Workout 5 / DESCENDING PYRAMIDS

CIRCUIT 1

Using your 12-rep max, perform 6 split squats with your left leg, then 6 with your right leg, then 5 with your left leg, and so forth until you do 1 rep on each leg. That is one set. Perform this circuit twice, with 60 seconds of rest between them. After the second circuit, proceed immediately to circuit 2.

1A

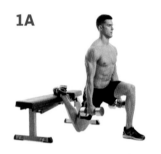

Bulgarian Split Squat
(page 250)
SETS: 2
REPS: 6, 5, 4, 3, 2, 1

Rest

SECONDS: 60

↑ ——————— Complete 2 times ———————

CIRCUIT 2

Perform 8 Inchworms, moving back and forth as quickly as you can. At the end of your last rep, stand up, and perform 8 Squat Jumps. Immediately proceed back to Inchworms for 7 reps, followed by 7 jumps. Follow this method until you have completed all reps for all sets. Perform this circuit only once. Rest 90 to 120 seconds and proceed to circuit 3.

2A

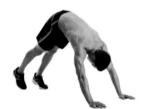

Inchworm
(page 224)
SETS: 8
REPS: 8, 7, 6, 5, 4, 3, 2, 1

2B

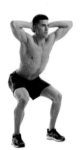

Squat Jump
(page 234)
SETS: 8
REPS: 8, 7, 6, 5, 4, 3, 2, 1

Rest

SECONDS: 60

CIRCUIT 3

Perform 4 pushups (on dumbbells), then 4 pushup rows with your right arm. Perform 4 more pushups, then 4 pushup rows with your left arm. Perform 3 pushups, then 3 pushup rows with your right arm. Continue this pattern until you have completed all sets. This circuit is to be performed three times, with 60 seconds of rest between each. Then proceed immediately to Circuit 4.

3A

3B

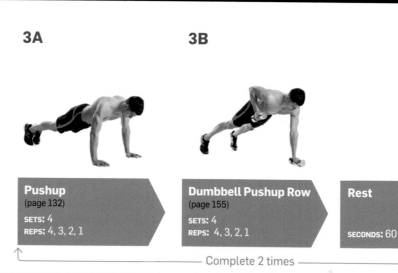

Pushup (page 132)
SETS: 4
REPS: 4, 3, 2, 1

Dumbbell Pushup Row (page 155)
SETS: 4
REPS: 4, 3, 2, 1

Rest
SECONDS: 60

Complete 2 times

CIRCUIT 4

Perform 6 Squat to Overhead Presses, then put the dumbbells down and get into a plank. Hold this for 30 seconds. Pick up the dumbbells and perform 5 more of the presses, then hold a plank for 25 seconds. Repeat this pattern until all sets are completed. Perform this circuit twice, resting 120 seconds between each circuit.

4A

4B

FINISH

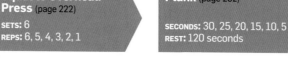

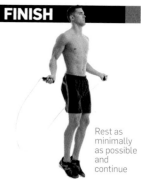

Squat to Overhead Press (page 222)
SETS: 6
REPS: 6, 5, 4, 3, 2, 1

Plank (page 282)
SECONDS: 30, 25, 20, 15, 10, 5
REST: 120 seconds

Rest as minimally as possible and continue

Jump Rope
5 to 10 minutes of jump rope work, performed as quickly and efficiently as you can.

Complete 2 times

The Abs Workout

Workout 6 / BODYWEIGHT TRAINING

CIRCUIT 1

Perform 1A to 1D sequentially. Do not rest between exercises. Perform this circuit three times, resting 60 seconds between each. After your last circuit, rest 90 seconds and move on to circuit 2.

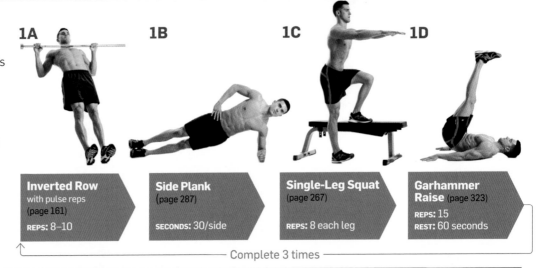

1A **1B** **1C** **1D**

Inverted Row
with pulse reps
(page 161)
REPS: 8–10

Side Plank
(page 287)
SECONDS: 30/side

Single-Leg Squat
(page 267)
REPS: 8 each leg

Garhammer Raise (page 323)
REPS: 15
REST: 60 seconds

—— Complete 3 times ——

CIRCUIT 2

Perform 2A to 2D sequentially. Do not rest between exercises, but rather transition smoothly from one to the next. Perform this circuit two times, resting 120 seconds between rounds. Rest 60 seconds and move to circuit 3.

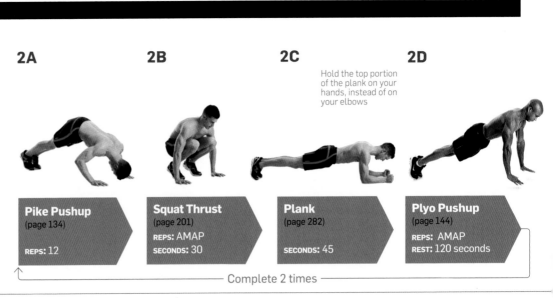

2A **2B** **2C** **2D**

Hold the top portion of the plank on your hands, instead of on your elbows

Pike Pushup
(page 134)
REPS: 12

Squat Thrust
(page 201)
REPS: AMAP
SECONDS: 30

Plank
(page 282)
SECONDS: 45

Plyo Pushup
(page 144)
REPS: AMAP
REST: 120 seconds

—— Complete 2 times ——

CIRCUIT 3

Perform 3A to 3D sequentially. Rest minimally between exercises. Perform this circuit twice, resting 120 seconds between each.

3A   **3B**   **3C**   **3D**

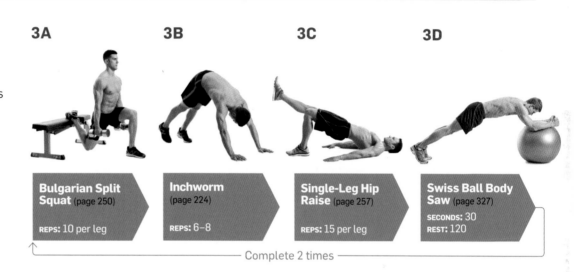

Bulgarian Split Squat (page 250)

REPS: 10 per leg

Inchworm (page 224)

REPS: 6–8

Single-Leg Hip Raise (page 257)

REPS: 15 per leg

Swiss Ball Body Saw (page 327)

SECONDS: 30
REST: 120

Complete 2 times

The Abs Workout

Cardio Workout / HIGH-INTENSITY INTERVAL TRAINING (HIIT)

WARM UP: 4-MINUTE JOG

Use this chart to guide you through the HIIT cardio workout. The number on the left represents your work time—that is, the amount of seconds you sprint. The number on the right is the amount of time you rest.

Start on a track or treadmill and sprint for the prescribed number of seconds, and when time is up, "rest" by slowing down your pace to a walk or very slow jog. When the rest time runs out, kick it back into a sprint. Complete all of the work and rest segments, and finish up with a full sprint for 30 seconds. After that, cool down.

NOTE: Don't think you're locked into only running. This workout can also be done on an elliptical, rowing machine, jump rope, or any piece of cardio equipment. Alternatively, you could use kettlebells and perform things like swings or snatches.

WORK	REST
30	10
20	10
20	20
10	30
10	10
10	10
10	50
10	60
20	60
10	40
30	

COOLDOWN: 2-MINUTE JOG, FOLLOWED BY 1 MORE MINUTE OF WALKING.

CardioWorkout / 20-MINUTE MODERATE-INTENSITY

The following routine is your 20-minute moderate-intensity cardio workout. This is to be performed on a scale of subjective intensity, using the Rate of Perceived Exertion. The warmup is just a walk, which on a scale of 1 to 10 should be 3 to 4. Toward the end of the workout, you'll do an all-out sprint, which after 16 minutes of fluctuating difficulty, should hit a 10 on anyone's scale.

MINUTE	DIFFICULTY	RATE OF PERCEIVED EXERTION
1	Warmup	3 out of 10
2	Warmup	4 out of 10
3	Warmup	4 out of 10
4	Moderate	6 out of 10
5	Moderate	6 out of 10
6	Hard	8 out of 10
7	Moderate	5 out of 10
8	Hard	7 out of 10
9	Moderate	4 out of 10
10	Hard	8 out of 10
11	Easy	3 out of 10
12	Hard	7 out of 10
13	Moderate	5 out of 10
14	Moderate	5 out of 10
15	Easy	4 out of 10
16	Moderate	6 out of 10
17	Crazy!	10 out of 10
18	Dying	2 out of 10
19	Less dead	4 out of 10
20	That wasn't so bad	3 out of 10

ARE YOUR ABS WEAK?

You've probably heard the old saying, "Everyone has abs— there's just a layer of fat covering them." While this is technically true, stripping away excess weight won't give you a rock-solid core. For that, you need a combination of exercises that target your weakness and build up your strength. So it serves you well to build up those muscles so you can look great on the beach and in the gym.

As you become leaner and start to see your abs, it's not always easy to determine what areas need the most work. Abs are abs, right? That's why we turned to strength coach and fitness expert Mike Robertson, CSCS. He identified six ways to test your core strength and the plan you need to make sure there are no flaws in your newly chiseled body.

Test yourself, see how you stack up, and then follow the tips to take your body to the next level.

Breathing

While the breathing assessment may seem silly at first glance, it should not be disregarded, says Robertson. Proper diaphragmatic breathing and function is a key component of proper core stability. Quite simply, without proper function of the diaphragm, your body will be forced to rely on "outer core" muscles such as the rectus abdominis, obliques, and the spinal erectors to create stability.

The Test

Lie on your back with your legs straight. Place your right hand on your belly and your left hand on your chest.

From this position take three full, deep breaths. Notice which hand rises faster, as well as which one moves higher.

The Results

Your right hand (the one on your belly) should rise higher and faster than your left. You might have a faulty breathing pattern if the left hand rises higher and/or faster (chest breathing) or if your right hand actually moves down when inhaling (paradoxical breathing). If your breathing is normal, your stomach should rise when you inhale and come back down when you exhale. If your breathing is off, that means other muscles are working unnecessarily and impacting your core.

The Fix

Lie on your back with your hips and knees flexed 90 degrees and your feet flat against a wall. Take 10 deep breaths, with a focus on filling the belly and not the chest. Think about breathing low into your belly button. Repeat one to two times per day.

Plank

The plank tests your core stability—that is, your ability to stabilize your spine, hips, and pelvis and hold it for periods of time. Oftentimes your core is imbalanced due to poor posture and poor core training programs.

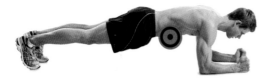

The Test

Start in plank position and have a friend lay a broomstick or PVC pipe lengthwise on your back. The back of your head, your upper back, and your buttocks should all be in contact with the pipe. Your elbows should be directly underneath your shoulders, your body in a straight line and up on your toes. Your friend should be able to slide his fingertips underneath the pipe at your lower back up to his knuckles. Time yourself. Do not break form.

The Results

You should be able to hold the three-points-of-contact position for a minimum of 2 minutes. If you can't achieve this position or can't hold it for the 2-minute time period, you failed the test.

The Fix

Perform the plank for shorter periods of time to build up your core stability. If necessary, you can even start on your knees instead of on your toes, to decrease the load and intensity.

Instead of holding for 40 seconds, try eight 5-second holds. Make sure to get into ideal alignment. Robertson tends to start his clients with 3 sets of 6 to 8 repetitions, holding each rep for 5 seconds.

Side Plank

The side plank tests lateral core stability. Often, the lateral core is very weak and dominated by big muscles such as the spinal erectors.

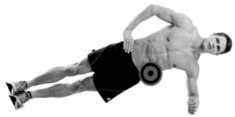

The Test

You'll need a friend or a trainer at your gym to help you with this one. Set up in a side plank position and have your friend hold a broomstick or PVC pipe on your back. The back of your head, your upper back, and your buttocks should all be in contact with the pipe. Furthermore, you should be in a straight line from your feet, through your hips, and up through your head.

Your elbow should be directly underneath your shoulder, your top hand should be placed on the opposite shoulder, and your feet can be either stacked on top of or placed slightly in front of each other.

The Abs Workout

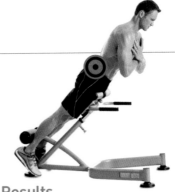

Finally, your friend or trainer should be able to slide his fingertips in between the pipe and your lower back up to his knuckles.

The Results

This test has three components:

Qualitative—You should be able to achieve the three-points-of-contact position and not break form.

Quantitative—You should be able to hold the three-points-of-contact position for a minimum of 90 seconds.

Symmetry—Your times between sides should have no greater than a 10 percent discrepancy.

If you can't achieve the three-points position, can't hold for the 90-second time period, or have asymmetries greater than 10 percent in hold time, you've failed the test.

The Fix

Perform the side plank for shorter periods of time. You can even start on your knees instead of on your toes, to decrease the load and intensity.

Instead of holding for 30 seconds, try six 5-second holds. Make sure to get into ideal alignment. Start with 3 sets of 4 to 6 repetitions, holding each "rep" for 5 seconds.

Static Back Extension

The static back extension tests posterior core stability. Often, your posterior core is dominated by the bigger muscles located on your lower back.

The Test

Set up in a static back extension machine with a broomstick or PVC pipe on your back. The back of your head, your upper back, and your buttocks should all be in contact with the pipe.

The Results

This test has two components:

Qualititative—You should be able to achieve the three-points-of-contact position and not break form.

Quantitative—You should be able to hold the three-points-of-contact position for a minimum of 2 minutes.

Failure to either achieve the three-points position or hold for the 2-minute time period should be considered a failing test.

The Fix

Perform the static back extension for shorter periods of time. Instead of holding for 40 seconds, try eight 5-second holds. Make sure to get into ideal alignment, and start with 3 sets of 6 to 8 repetitions, holding each "rep" for 5 seconds.

The Pushup

The pushup tests your core while your upper and lower body are both working. While most think of the pushup as an upper body pressing exercise, its role as a core stabilization drill is equally important.

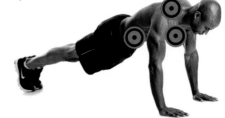

The Test

Start in pushup position on the floor with your hands just outside your torso and elbows tucked to approximately a 45-degree angle. Your entire body should be resting and relaxed on the ground, with the exception of your toes. Have a friend place a broomstick or PVC pipe on your back. The back of your head, your upper back, and your buttocks should all be in contact with the pipe.

The Results

When pressing up, your body should move as a seamless, integrated unit. At no point should you lose your three-points-of-contact position. Failure to either achieve the three-points position or maintain that position throughout the test should be considered a failing test. Make sure your friend is not holding the broomstick in place. If the pipe rolls off your body, it's a sign that you need to improve your core strength in order to do pushups correctly.

The Fix

If you can't plank properly, don't bother doing pushups yet. If you can plank properly, try performing your pushups in a power rack or with your torso elevated in some fashion (such as putting your hands on a bench). The goal here isn't to maximally load your upper body; instead, you want to unify your upper and lower body so your body stays in a straight line throughout. As your core stability improves, work to decrease the incline of your torso.

The Squat

The squat examines relative stiffness between your core and your lower body. In terms of your squat, "stiffness" is really the flexibility between

your core and your body. For most people who squat, the muscles that surround your hips are less flexible than those around your lower back. So when you squat, you are forced to round your back, which is not a good thing.

The Test

Start with your feet approximately hip- or shoulder-width apart, with your toes pointing forward. Extend your arms straight out in front of your body. Squat down as low as possible, preferably while standing next to a mirror.

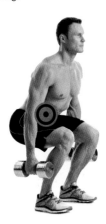

The Results

You should be able to squat down with your thighs below parallel (the crease of your hip below your knees) without losing the normal arch of your lower back. If your lower back tucks under—or begins to round—it means that your hips have less flexibility than your core. With a perfect squat, your hips push back first and then you bend your knees and sit down. All the while, the shape of your spine should not change at all. So if you round your upper or lower back, then you need to strengthen your core.

The Fix

All of the exercises listed above should help as will Goblet Squats. This variation helps keep your spine in perfect alignment and teaches you a more natural way to squat without any weight on your back that might force the rounding of your spine.

Chapter 9
The Best Abs Exercises Ever Created

These cutting-edge moves will work every muscle
in your body and help you strip away fat faster than ever.

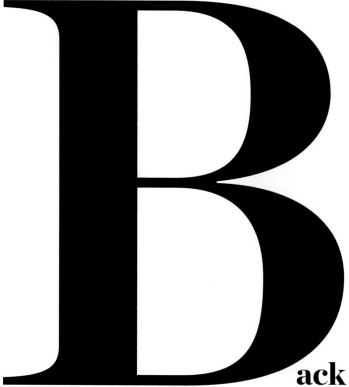

Back when you first started exercising (or restarted, or restarted after that), you probably had a workout that seemed like it provided all the right ingredients you needed to lose weight, pack on slabs of new muscle, and have more energy. A few reps here, a couple of sets there, and you were done. Still, as time went on, the magic of exercise disappeared. While your muscles felt like they were working, and sweat dripped from your brow and covered your shirt, the movements you did rarely took off the pounds or came close to creating a new you.

So what did you do wrong? Technically, nothing. You did the exercises and worked hard. That should be enough to lose weight—but it's not. The secret to a lean body isn't wrapped in just any random mix of exercise. You need variety, but that

The Best Abs Exercises Ever Created

doesn't mean simply trying every machine in the gym. If you want to see your abs, the movements you perform must challenge your entire body and not individual muscles like your arms and shoulders. When that's achieved, you activate more muscle fibers, burn more calories, and—boom!—start to see your abs.

In order to put an end to your frustrating workouts, we had some of the best fitness minds handpick their favorite exercises. Some exercises may look familiar, like pushups, squats, and lunges. These are staples of any great routine. But where most workouts stop is where these workouts actually begin. Our experts created a list of hundreds of moves that will work every muscle in your body, including your abs. We call these the best abs exercises ever created because they work you harder and faster for guaranteed results.

Not only will these exercises keep you from straying from your workout, they'll actually have you looking forward to your next gym day. And while a great workout doesn't require much equipment, these exercises will provide enough variety that you can do them in your own home or with the expensive machines at your local training facility. The big difference: These moves are so original that you'll be excited by the challenge of something new. And they'll work all of the regions that make up your core: upper abs, lower abs, obliques, transverse abdominis, and lower back muscles. Even if you've never lifted a weight before, you'll find that these exercises are more fun than you'd have imagined. But even better—they'll do more than make you sweat. They'll actually produce changes you can see and appreciate.

Hard Abs Made Easy

The Abs Exercise Rating System makes it easy to figure out which exercises are right for you on any given day. Just look for the key: Easy, Moderate, or Hard Core. So if you're looking to upgrade your workout, or want to create your own, use our guide to find the right level of difficulty for your expertise.

EASY

MODERATE

HARD CORE

The Abs Advantage

Creating your own flat belly plan requires a healthy dose of core exercises. But the best workouts include exercises that challenge every muscle in your midsection without you even knowing it.

We've included dozens of these exercises for you to use in your workouts. They have been specially designed to work more muscles, shrink your belly, and leave you with a toned, tight body in a fraction of the time.

The Big Six

If there was one goal we kept in mind for this book it's that we wanted it to be for everyone. Big guys, small guys, skinny guys, fat guys, and even muscle-up guys who are still searching for that get-lean secret to reveal their hard body. In order to work for everyone, you need a special blend of exercises, and the right experts to design programs that work.

But before you can begin to see the benefits of diverse rep ranges and advanced training techniques, each program needs a foundation. That foundation is compound exercises. These are the multi-muscle movements that will be the key to all of your results. They require the most focus, the most intensity, and your success improving on these exercises will ultimately determine just how much you transform your body. Here are the six exercises (and their variations) that will be—with exception to your mirror—the best assessment and measure of your success.

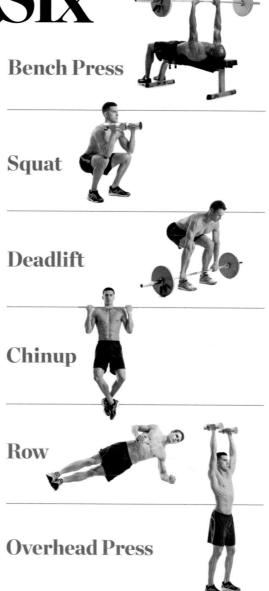

Bench Press

Squat

Deadlift

Chinup

Row

Overhead Press

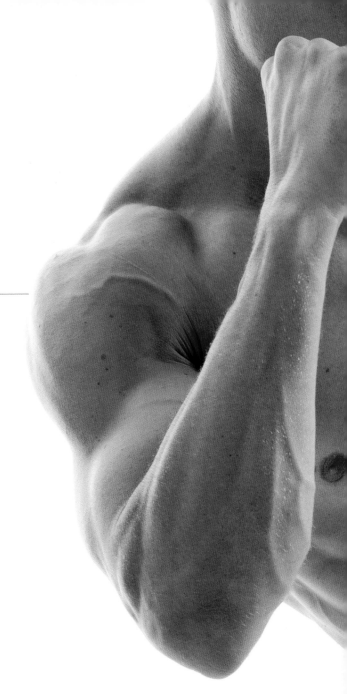

Upper Body Exercise
CHEST

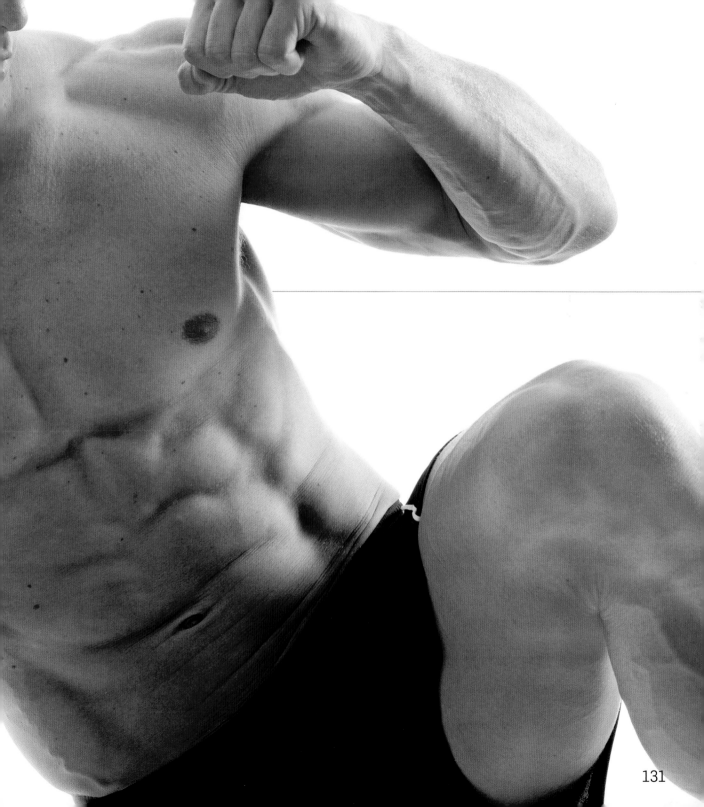

Upper Body Exercise: Chest

▌Pushup

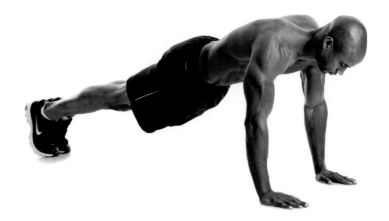

- Get on all fours and place your hands on the floor slightly wider than and in line with your shoulders. Your body should form a straight line from your ankles to your shoulders.
- Squeeze your abs as tight as possible and keep them contracted for the entire exercise.

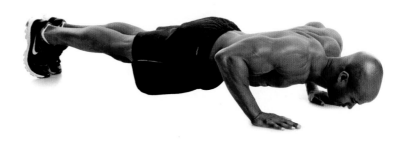

B

- Lower your body until your chest nearly touches the floor, making sure that you tuck your elbows close to the sides of your torso.
- Pause, then push yourself back to the starting position.

▌**PUSHUPS—SIMPLIFIED!**
If you struggle with normal pushups, bend your knees and cross your ankles behind you. Your body should still form a straight line from your ankles to your shoulders. Then, lower your body until your chest nearly touches the floor and press back up to the starting position.

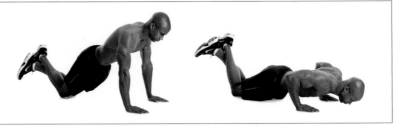

▮Pushup Plus

- Get on all fours and place your hands on the floor slightly wider than and in line with your shoulders. Your body should form a straight line from your ankles to your shoulders.
- Squeeze your abs as tight as possible and keep them contracted for the entire exercise.

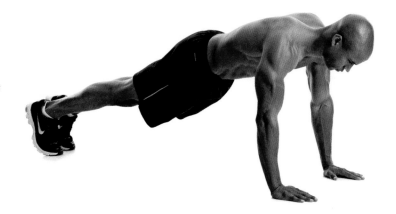

- Lower your body until your chest nearly touches the floor, making sure that you tuck your elbows close to the sides of your torso.
- Pause, then push yourself back to the starting position.

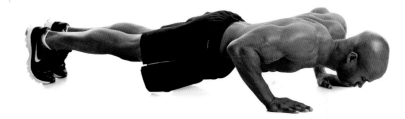

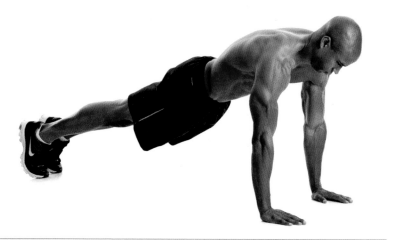

- Once your arms are straight, push your upper back toward the ceiling. It's a subtle move, but it should feel like your shoulder blades are flaring out.
- Pause, then repeat the entire movement.

Upper Body Exercise: Chest

Pike Pushup

A

- Start in a traditional pushup position, but walk your feet toward your hands and raise your hips into the air. Your body should look like an inverted V.

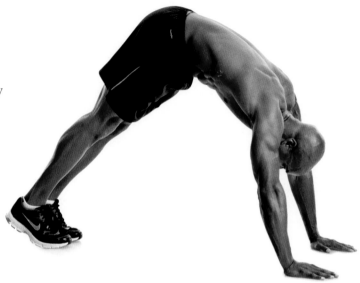

B

- Keeping your hips raised, lower your body until your chin nearly touches the floor.
- Pause, then press back up to the starting position.

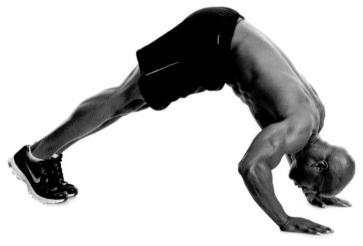

Dumbbell T-Pushup

- Place a pair of dumbbells (preferably hex) on the floor about shoulder-width apart. Important note: Use hex dumbbells as a base. Round dumbbells will roll out from under you.
- Start in a pushup position and grab the dumbbells.

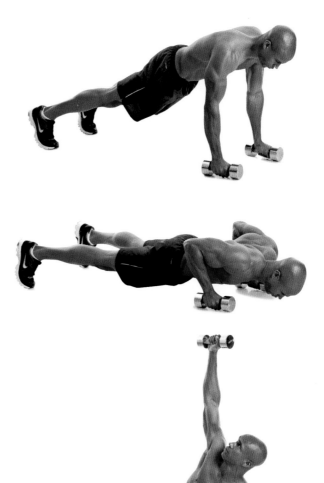

B

- Perform a pushup while holding the dumbbells.

C

- As you press back up, rotate your body to the right and pull the dumbbell in your right hand up and above your shoulder. In the top position, your right arm should be straight and your body turned to the side so that you form the letter T.
- Lower the dumbbell back to the starting position, perform another pushup, and repeat—this time turning to the left.

T-PUSHUPS—SIMPLIFIED! If the Dumbbell T-Pushup is too difficult, simply perform the exercise without the dumbbells. The movement will be identical, but you won't have the added resistance.

Upper Body Exercise: Chest

Pushup and Step Out

A

- Begin in the standard pushup position.

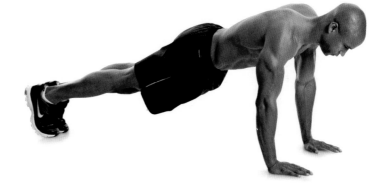

B

- Perform a pushup.

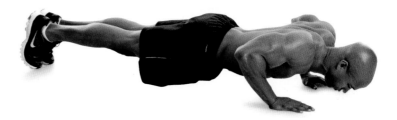

C

- Then "walk" your hands forward so your body is extended.
- Walk your feet forward so your hands are once again underneath.

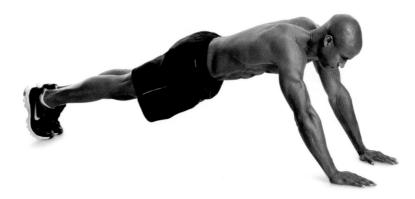

Single-Leg Pushup

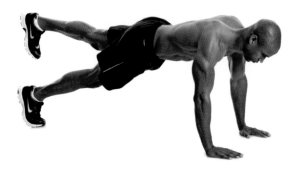

 A

- Begin in the standard pushup position with your body forming a straight line from your ankles to your shoulders.
- Raise one foot off the floor.

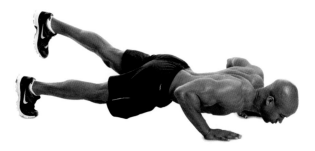

B

- Lower your body toward the floor and then press back up, all the while keeping your leg off the floor.
- Try to perform all reps without lowering your leg.

Pushup Jack

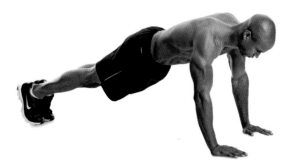

A

- Begin in the standard pushup position with your body forming a straight line from your ankles to your shoulders.

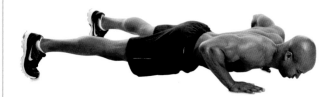

B

- As you lower your body to the floor, jump your feet outward so that your feet end up shoulder-width apart at the bottom of the movement.
- As you press your body back up, jump your legs back together and return to the starting position.

Upper Body Exercise: Chest

▌Pushup with Hand Raise

A

- Begin in the standard pushup position with your body forming a straight line from your ankles to your shoulders.

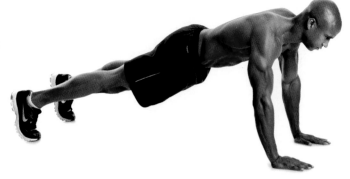

B

- Lower your body to the floor and then press back up.

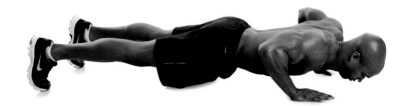

C

- As you return to the starting position, raise your right hand so it's in line with your body.
- Hold for 2 seconds, then return your hand to the starting position.
- Do another pushup and repeat, this time raising your left hand.

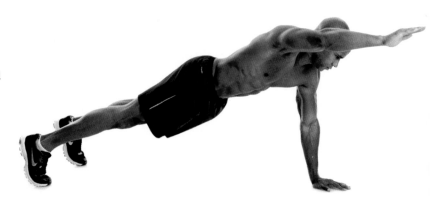

■Single-Leg Pushup with Shoulder Touch

- Begin in the standard pushup position with your body forming a straight line from your ankles to your shoulders.

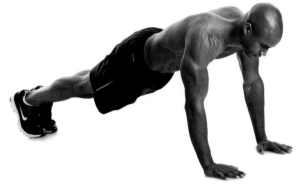

- Raise your right foot off the floor, hold it, and perform a pushup.

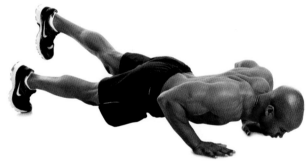

- As you press back up, take your left hand and touch your right shoulder.
- Return your hand to the starting position and perform another pushup. This time, raise your left foot for the pushup, and take your right hand and touch your left shoulder.
- Continue alternating legs and arms on each rep.

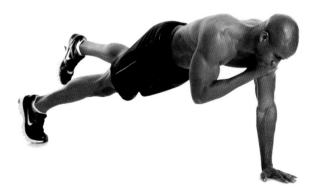

Upper Body Exercise: Chest

▌Grasshopper Pushup

A

- Begin in the standard pushup position with your body forming a straight line from your ankles to your shoulders.

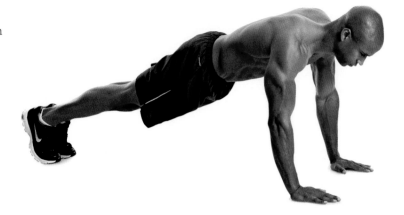

B

- Bend your right knee and slide your leg underneath your body.
- Perform a pushup, trying to prevent your right leg from touching the floor.

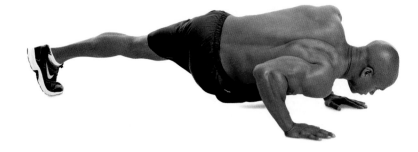

C

- Press back up, return your right leg to the starting position, and then repeat with your left leg.

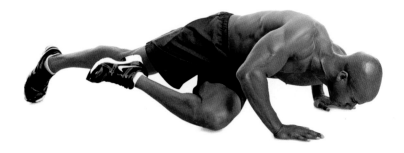

▮Knee to Elbow Pushup

A

- Begin in the standard pushup position with your body forming a straight line from your ankles to your shoulders.

B

- Bring your right knee to your left elbow, and pause before returning your leg to the starting position.

C

- Now lower your body as you would for a standard pushup.

D

- Push back to the starting position and repeat, this time bringing your left knee to your right elbow.

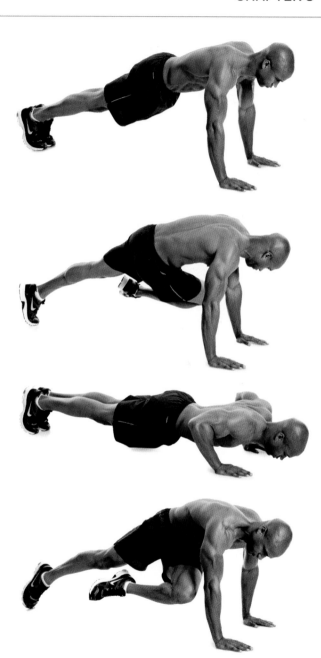

Upper Body Exercise: Chest

Divebomber Pushup

- Begin in the standard pushup position, but move your feet forward and raise your hips so your body almost forms an inverted V.

- Keeping your hips elevated, lower your body until your chin nearly touches the floor.

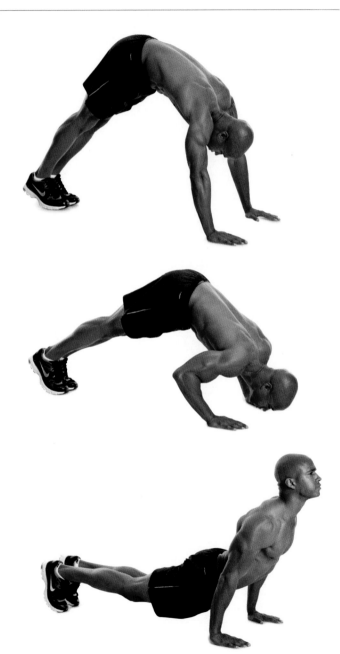

C

- Lower your hips until they almost touch the floor, as you simultaneously raise your head and shoulders toward the ceiling. Reverse the movement back to the starting position and repeat.

▮Side-to-Side Pushup

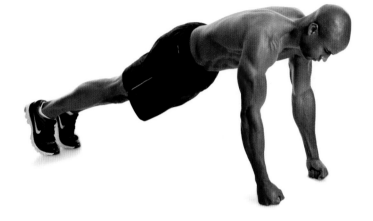

A

- Assume a pushup position, but form fists with your hands so your knuckles are flat against the floor.

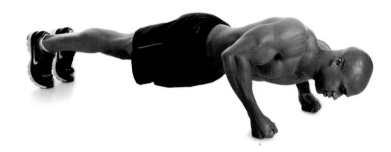

B

- Keeping your right arm straight, lower your chest to your left hand, pause, and push back up.

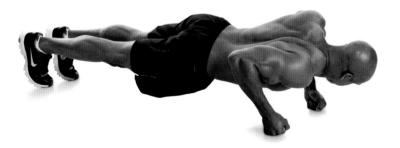

C

- Repeat, this time keeping your left arm straight and lowering your chest to your right hand. Alternate sides each rep.

Upper Body Exercise: Chest

█ Plyo Pushup

- Assume a pushup position.

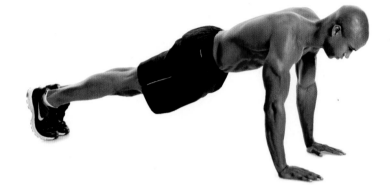

- Then lower your body until your chest nearly touches the floor.

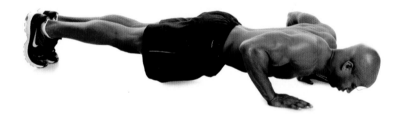

- Press yourself up so that your hands leave the floor. "Land" back in the start position, lower your body, and repeat.

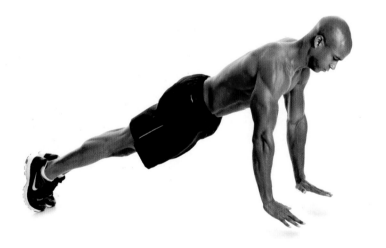

Dumbbell Chest Press

- Grab a pair of dumbbells and lie faceup on a flat bench.
- Hold the dumbbells above your chest with your arms straight. The dumbbells should be nearly touching, and your palms should be facing your feet.

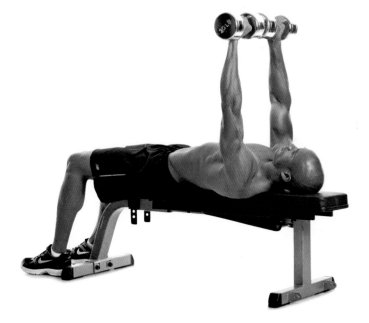

B

- Keeping your elbows tucked close to your body, lower the weights to the sides of your chest.
- Pause, then press the dumbbells back above your chest.

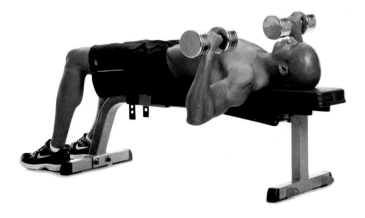

Upper Body Exercise: Chest

▮Incline Dumbbell Press

A

- Set an adjustable bench to an incline of 30 to 45 degrees.
- Grab a pair of dumbbells and lie faceup on the bench. Hold the dumbbells directly above your shoulders with your arms straight and your palms facing each other.

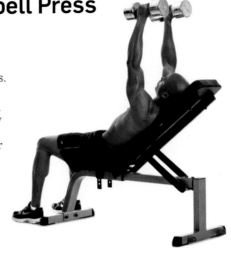

B

- Lower the dumbbells to the sides of your chest, pause,

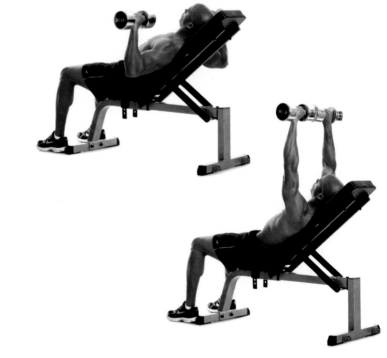

C

- Then press the weights back above your chest.

▮High Incline Dumbbell Press

A

- Set an adjustable bench to an incline of 45 to 60 degrees.
- Grab a pair of dumbbells and lie faceup on the bench. Hold the dumbbells directly above your shoulders with your arms straight and your palms facing each other.

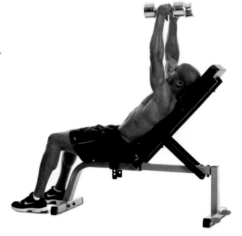

B

- Lower the dumbbells to the sides of your chest and pause.

C

- Press the weights back above your chest.

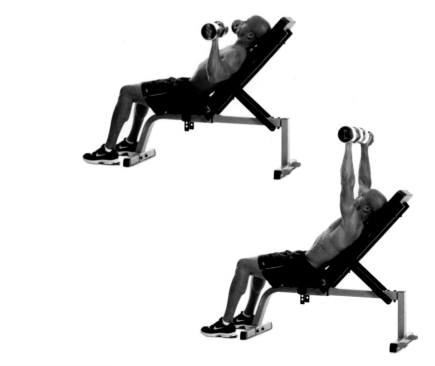

Upper Body Exercise: Chest

Low Incline Dumbbell Neutral Grip Chest Press

A

- Set an adjustable bench to an incline of 15 to 30 degrees.
- Grab a pair of dumbbells and lie faceup on the bench. Hold the dumbbells directly above your shoulders with your arms straight and your palms facing each other.

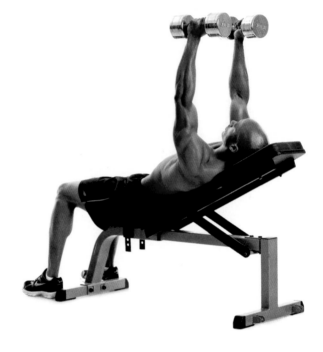

B

- Lower the dumbbells to the sides of your chest, pause, and then press the weights back above your chest.

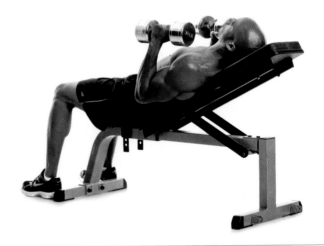

Single-Arm Dumbbell Chest Press

A

- Grab a dumbbell in one hand and lie on your back on a flat bench, holding the dumbbell over your chest.

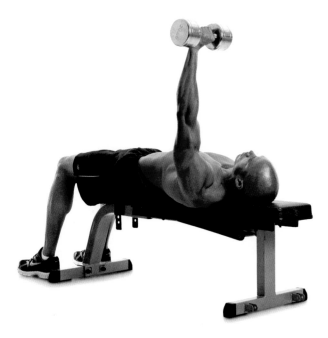

B

- Lower the dumbbell to the side of your chest, pause, and then press the weight back up to the starting position as quickly as you can.
- Do all reps on one arm, move the weight to your other arm, and repeat.

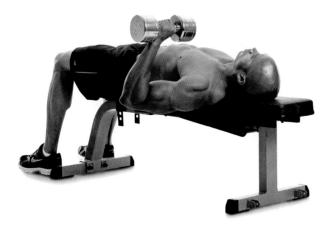

Upper Body Exercise: Chest

█ Close-Grip Bench Press

A

- Grab a barbell with an overhand grip that's closer than shoulder width and hold it above your sternum with your arms straight.

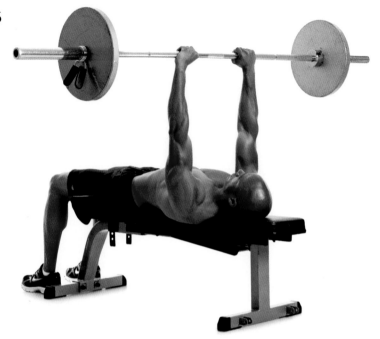

B

- Lower the bar straight down, pause, then press the bar in a straight line back up to the starting position.
- Make sure you keep your elbows tucked in, so that your upper arms form a 45-degree angle with your body in the "down" position.

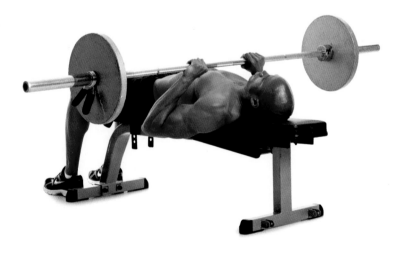

Barbell Chest Press

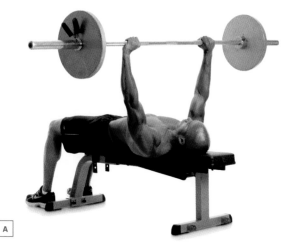

A

- Grab a barbell with an overhand grip that's just wider than shoulder width and hold it above your sternum with your arms straight.

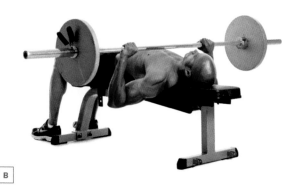

B

- Lower the bar straight down, pause, then press the bar in a straight line back up to the starting position.
- Make sure you keep your elbows tucked in, so that your upper arms form a 45-degree angle with your body in the "down" position.

Incline Barbell Chest Press

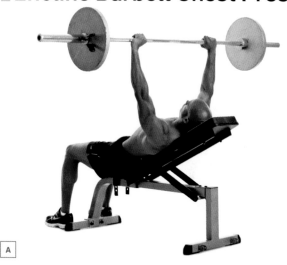

A

- Set an adjustable bench to an incline of 30 degrees.
- Grab a barbell and lie faceup on the bench. Hold the barbell directly above your shoulders with your arms straight.

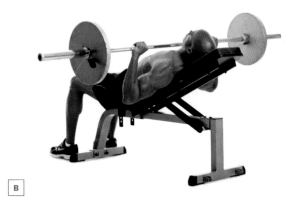

B

- Lower the barbell to the top of your chest, pause, and then press the weights back above your chest.

Upper Body Exercise: Chest

Cable Punch

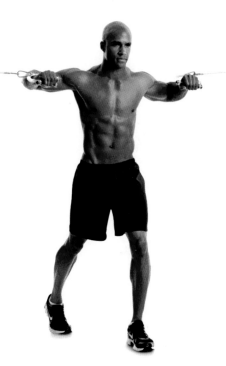

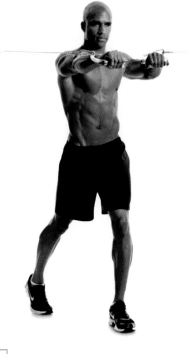

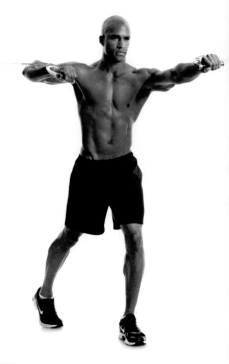

A

- Attach two D-handles to a cable station and adjust the pulley so the handles are at chest height.
- Grab the handles and face away from the weight stack.
- Stagger your feet and make sure the handles are positioned in front of your shoulders. Your arms should be parallel to the floor.

B

- Push one handle forward and straighten your arm in front of you.

C

- Pause and return to the starting position. Immediately repeat with your other arm. Continue alternating.

■ Spiderman Pushup

A

- Begin in the standard pushup position with your body forming a straight line from your ankles to your shoulders.

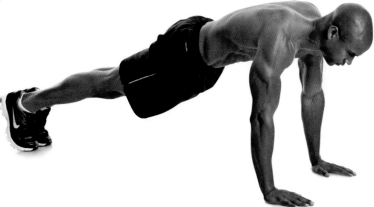

B

- As you lower your body toward the floor, lift your right foot off the floor. Bring your right leg out to the side and try to touch your knee to your right elbow.
- Reverse the movement, then push your body back up to the starting position.
- Perform another pushup, but try to touch your left knee to your left elbow. Alternate sides on each repetition.

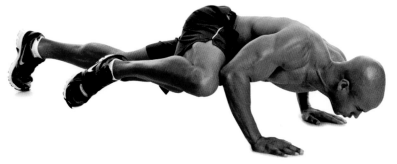

Upper Body Exercise: Chest

▌Valslide Spiderman Pushup

A

- Position your feet on a pair of Valslides and begin in the standard pushup position with your body forming a straight line from your ankles to your shoulders.

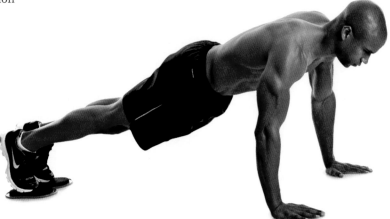

B

- As you lower your body toward the floor, bring your right leg out to the side and try to touch your knee to your right elbow, while keeping both feet on the Valslides.
- Reverse the movement, then push your body back up to the starting position.
- Perform another pushup, but try to touch your left knee to your left elbow. Alternate sides on each repetition.

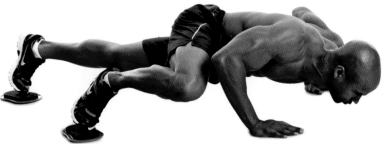

Dumbbell Pushup Row

A

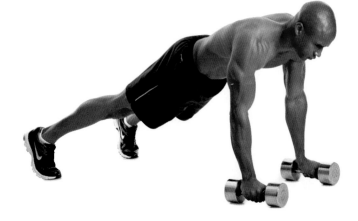

- Place a pair of dumbbells (preferably hex) about shoulder-width apart on the floor. Grab the dumbbell handles and position yourself in a pushup position.

B

- Lower your body to the floor and then press back up.

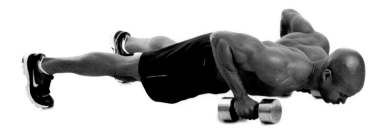

C

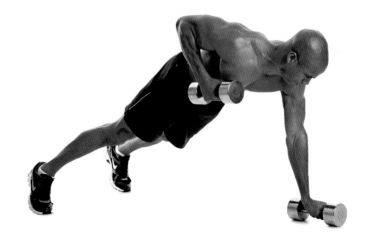

- Once you're back in the starting position, pull the dumbbell in your right hand up toward the side of your chest.
- Pause, then return the dumbbell back to the floor and repeat with your left hand. That's 1 rep. Try to prevent your torso from rotating each time you row the weight.

IMPORTANT NOTE: Use hex dumbbells as a base. Round dumbbells will roll out from under you.

Upper Body Exercise: Chest

▍Dips

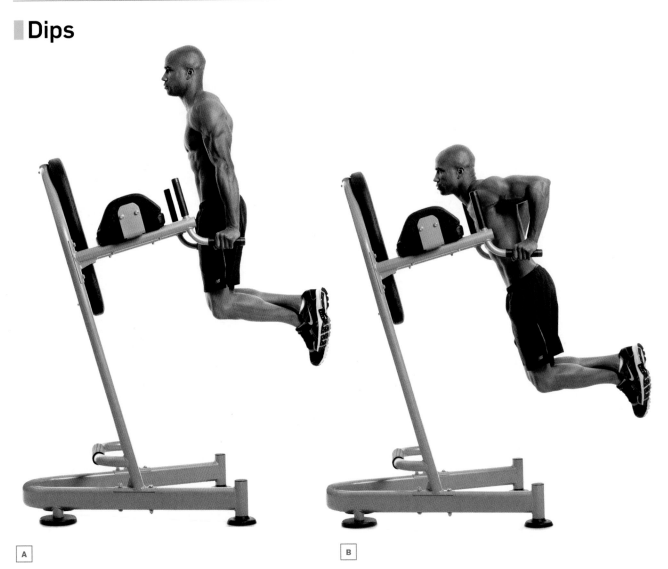

A

- Hoist yourself up on parallel bars with your torso perpendicular to the floor. You'll maintain this posture throughout the exercise.
- Bend your knees and cross your ankles.

B

- Slowly lower your body until your shoulder joints are below your elbows.
- Push back up until your elbows are nearly straight but not locked.

Side-Lying Windmill

A

- Lie on your left side with both arms extended out in front of your chest.
- Bring your right knee up toward your body so that your right hip is flexed 90 degrees.

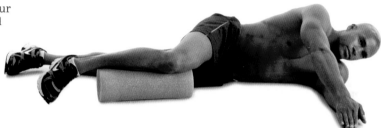

B

- In one motion, bring your right hand up and over your head in a sweeping counter-clockwise motion. Make sure your head follows your hand at all times.

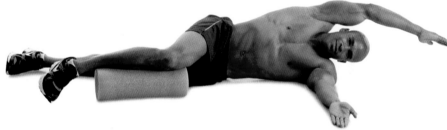

C

- Make a full revolution (like a windmill) until your hand is back at the start.
- Perform all reps, then switch to your right side and repeat with your left arm.

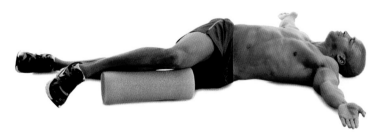

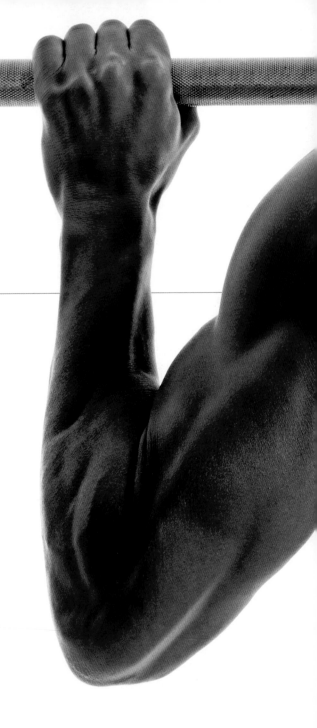

Upper Body Exercise
BACK

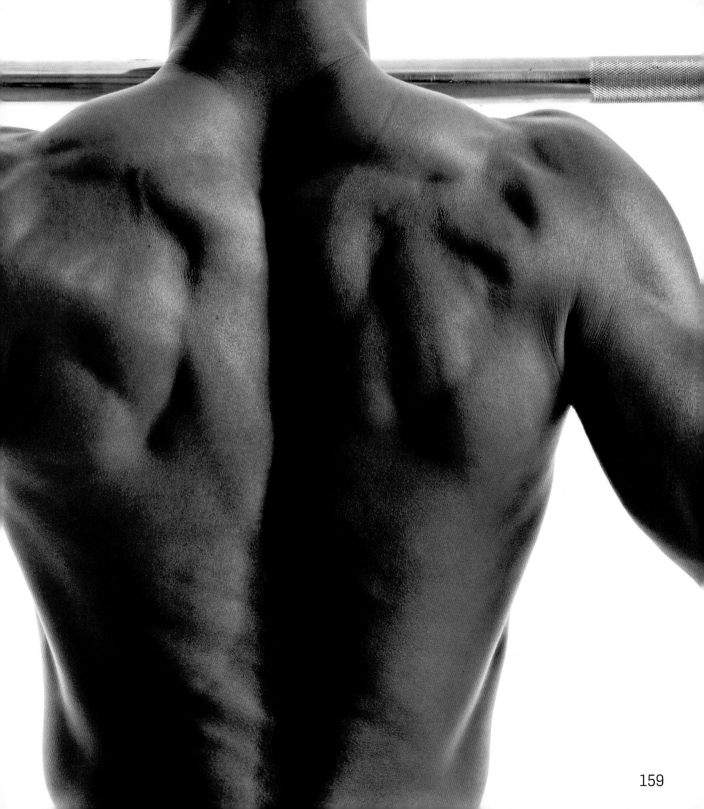

159

Upper Body Exercise: Back

Barbell Bent-Over Row

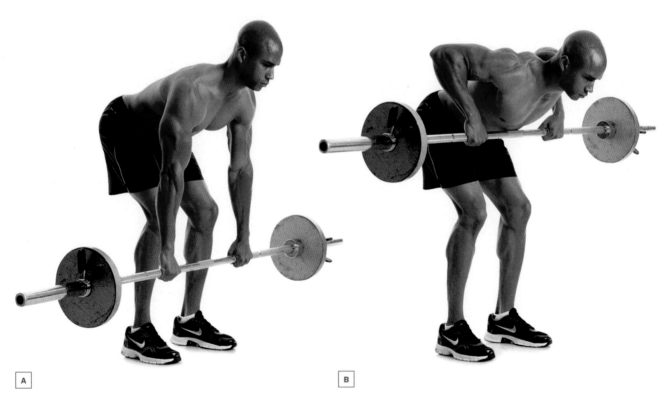

A

- Grab a barbell with an overhand grip with your hands about shoulder-width apart.
- Hold the bar at arm's length, and then bend at your hips and lower your torso until it's almost parallel to the floor. Your knees should be slightly bent and your lower back naturally arched.

B

- Squeeze your shoulder blades together and pull the bar up to your upper abs.
- Pause, then return the bar back to the starting position.

Inverted Row

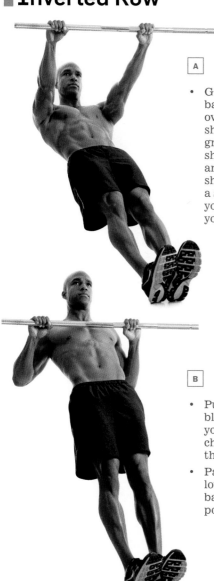

A

- Grab a stationary bar with an overhand, shoulder-width grip. Your arms should be straight and your body should form a straight line from your shoulders to your ankles.

B

- Pull your shoulder blades back and lift your body until your chest touches the bar.
- Pause, then slowly lower your body back to the starting position.

Dumbbell Bent-Over Row

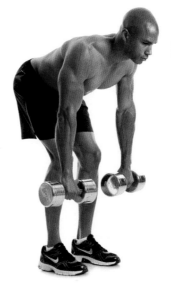

A

- Grab a pair of dumbbells with an overhand grip with your hands about shoulder-width apart.
- Hold the dumbbells at arm's length, and then bend at your hips and lower your torso until it's almost parallel to the floor. Your knees should be slightly bent and your lower back naturally arched.

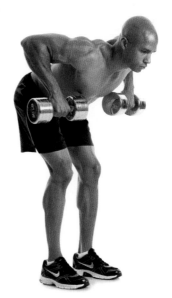

B

- Squeeze your shoulder blades together and pull the dumbbells up to the sides of your torso.
- Pause, then return to the starting position.

Upper Body Exercise: Back

Dumbbell Bent-Over Row (Neutral Grip)

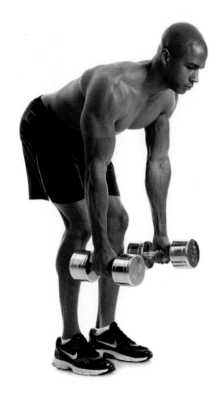

- Grab a dumbbell in each hand with your palms facing each other.
- Push your hips back and bend over until your torso is almost parallel to the floor. Your arms should hang at arm's length.

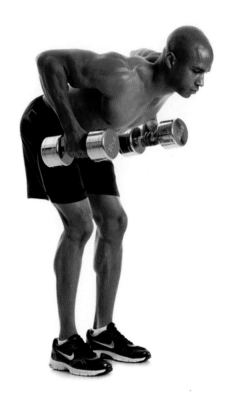

- Keeping your elbows close to your body, pull the dumbbells up to your chest by squeezing your shoulder blades back.
- Pause, then lower back to the starting position.

Underhand Barbell Bent-Over Row

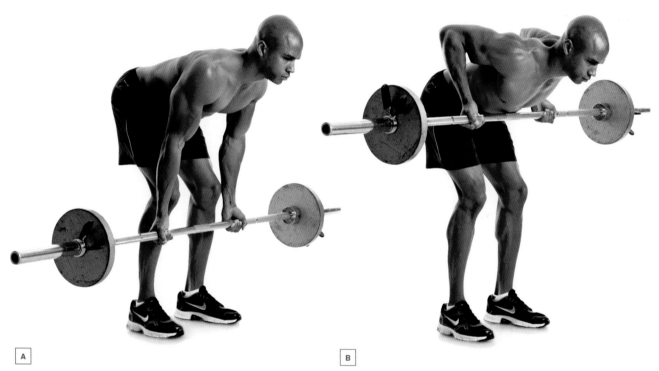

A

B

- Grab a barbell with an underhand grip with your hands about shoulder-width apart.

- Hold the bar at arm's length, and then bend at your hips and lower your torso until it's almost parallel to the floor. Your knees should be slightly bent and your lower back naturally arched.

- Squeeze your shoulder blades together and pull the bar up to your upper abs.

- Pause, then return the bar back to the starting position.

Upper Body Exercise: Back

█ Band Pull-Apart

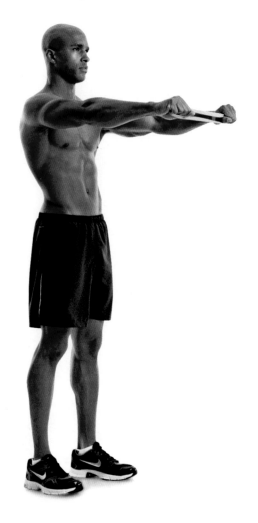

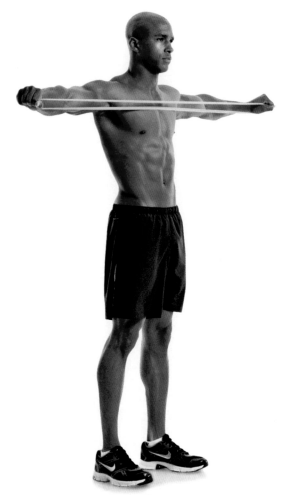

A

- Grab a resistance band in both hands and hold the ends a little more than shoulder-width apart.
- Raise your arms so that the band is at arm's length in front of your chest.

B

- Pull each end of the band and squeeze your shoulder blades together. (Try to snap the band in half.)
- Pause, then return your hands to the starting position.

Assisted Chinup

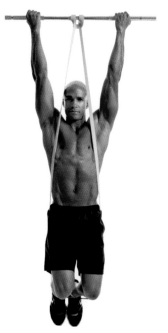

A

- Loop one end of a large resistance band around a chinup bar and then pull it through the other end of the band.
- Grab the bar with a shoulder-width, underhand grip.
- Place your knees in the loop of the band and hang at arm's length.

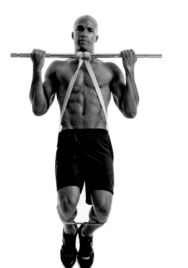

B

- Perform a chinup by pulling your chest up to the bar.
- Once your chest touches the bar, pause, then lower your body back to the starting position.

Split Stance Single-Arm Cable Row

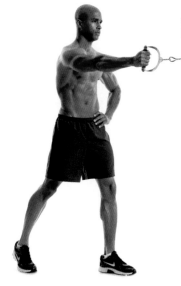

A

- Attach a D-handle to the pulley on a cable station and set the cable to about chest height.
- Grab the handle in your right hand, step away from the cable tower, and stand in a staggered stance.

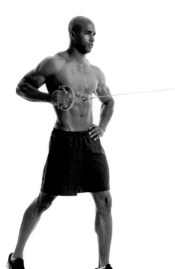

B

- Pull the handle toward your right side by squeezing your shoulder blade back.
- Pause, then return to the starting position.
- Perform all reps, switch hands, and repeat.

Upper Body Exercise: Back

Face Pulls

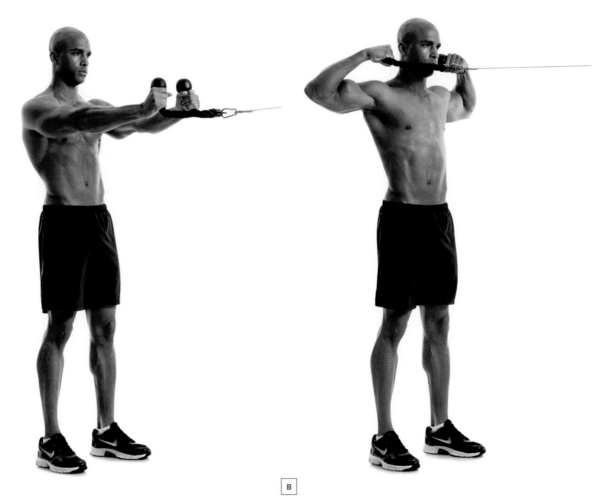

A

- Attach a rope to the high pulley of a cable station and grab an end with each hand so your palms face each other, thumbs toward you.
- Back a few steps away from the weight stack until your arms are straight in front of you and you feel tension in the cable.

B

- Pull the rope toward your eyes so your hands end up just outside your ears. You should be positioned in the classic bodybuilder's "double-biceps pose."
- Allow your arms to straighten out slowly in front of you and return to the start.

▮Three-Point Dumbbell Row

- Grab a dumbbell in your right hand.
- Push your hips back and bend over until your torso is almost parallel to the floor. Place your left hand on a bench in front of your body. Your right arm should hang at arm's length with your palm facing your other arm.

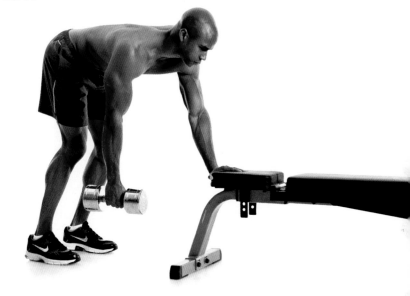

B

- Keeping your elbow close to your body, pull the dumbbell up to your chest by squeezing your shoulder blade back.
- Pause, then lower back to the starting position.
- Complete all prescribed reps, then switch arms and repeat.

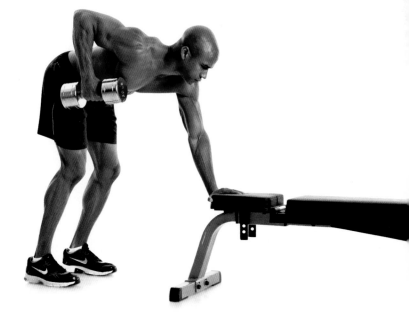

Upper Body Exercise: Back

Seated Lat Pulldown

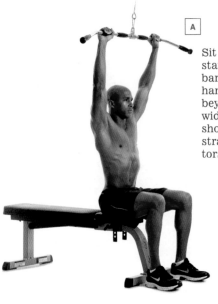

A

Sit at a lat pulldown station and grab the bar with an overhand grip that's just beyond shoulder width. Your arms should be completely straight and your torso upright.

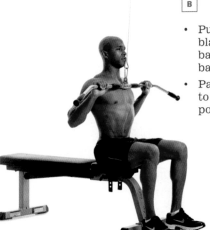

B

- Pull your shoulder blades down and back, and bring the bar to your chest.
- Pause, then return to the starting position.

Dumbbell Row with Rotation

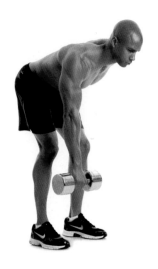

A

- Grab a dumbbell with an overhand grip in your right hand.
- Hold the dumbbell at arm's length, and then bend at your hips and lower your torso until it's almost parallel to the floor. Your knees should be slightly bent, your lower back naturally arched, and your other hand on your hip.

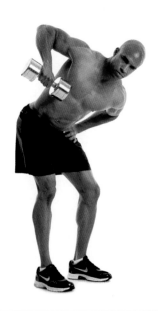

B

- Squeeze your shoulder blades back, then pull the dumbbell up to the side of your torso and rotate your torso upward.
- Pause, then return to the starting position.
- Complete all prescribed reps, switch arms, and repeat.

Weighted Wide Grip Pullup

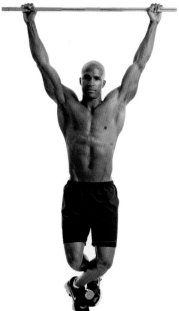

A

- Hold a dumbbell with your feet by crossing your ankles around the "head" of the weight. Grab a chinup bar with an overhand grip that's about 1.5 times shoulder-width apart.
- Hang at arm's length and pull your shoulder blades down and back so that your shoulders are as far from your ears as possible.

B

- Pull your chest to the bar as you squeeze your shoulder blades together.
- Pause, then lower your body back to a dead hang.

Kneeling Mixed-Grip Pulldown

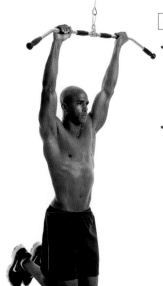

A

- Attach a bar to a lat pulldown station and grab the bar with a mixed grip—one hand over the other.
- Kneel on the floor so that your body forms a straight line from your shoulders to your knees.

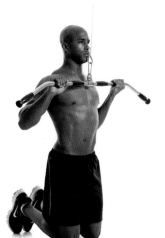

B

- Squeeze your shoulder blades down and back, then bring the bar to your chest.

Upper Body Exercise: Back

45-Degree Cable Row

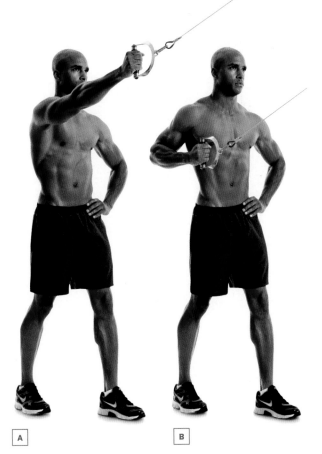

A

- Attach a D-handle to the pulley on a cable station and set the cable to the highest setting.
- Grab the handle in your right hand, step away from the cable tower, and stand in a staggered stance.

B

- Pull the handle down and toward your right side by squeezing your shoulder blade back.
- Pause, then return to the starting position.
- Perform all reps, switch hands, and repeat.

Resistance Band Pulldown

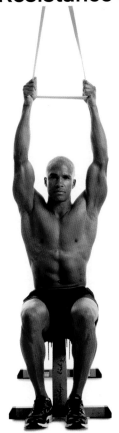
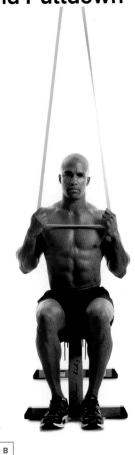
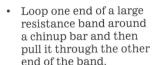

A

- Loop one end of a large resistance band around a chinup bar and then pull it through the other end of the band.
- Grab the band with both hands about shoulder-width apart and your arms straight.

B

- Squeeze your shoulder blades down and back, and pull your hands to the sides of your chest.
- Pause, then return to the starting position.

Pullup

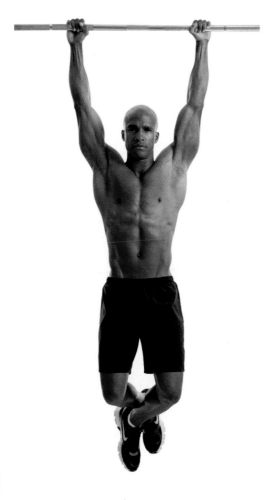

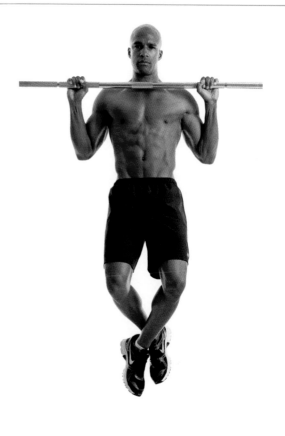

A

B

- Grab a chinup bar with a shoulder-width overhand grip.
- Hang at arm's length and pull your shoulder blades down and back so that your shoulders are as far from your ears as possible.

- Pull your chest to the bar as you squeeze your shoulder blades together.
- Pause, then lower your body back to a dead hang.

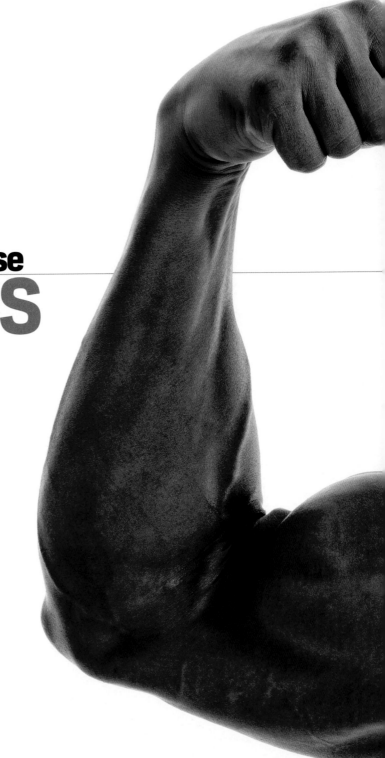

Upper Body Exercise
ARMS

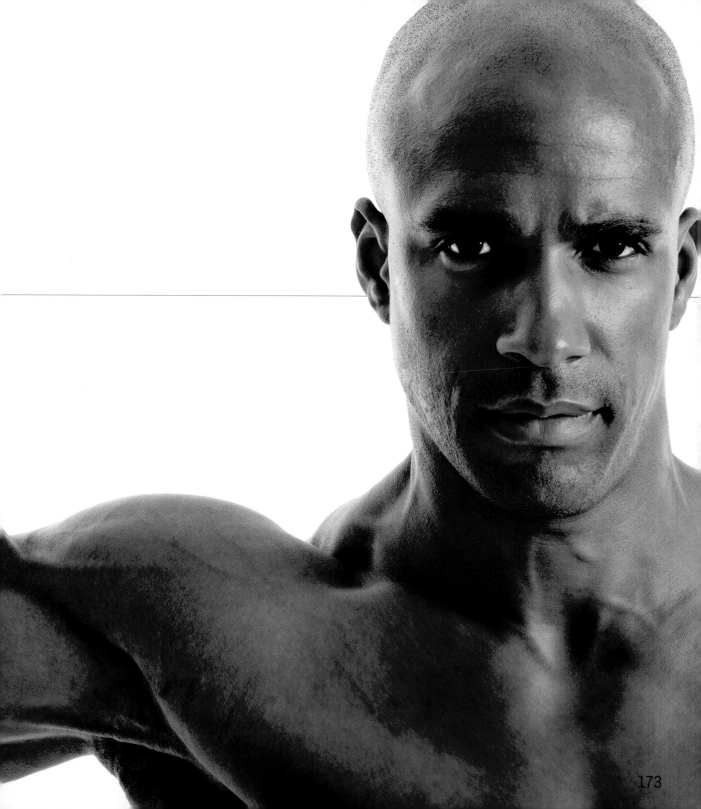

173

Upper Body Exercise: Arms

█ Triceps Rope Extension

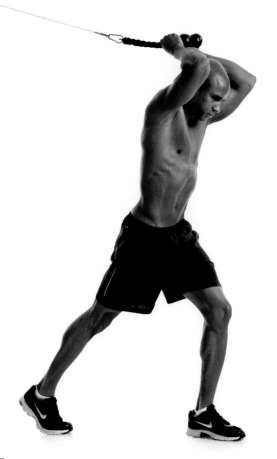
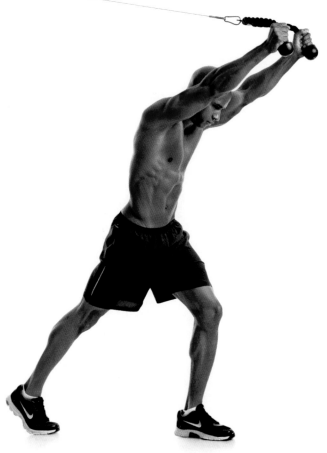

 A

- Attach a rope to a cable station and set it at a height above your head.
- Grab the rope with each hand and stand with your back to the cable station.
- Stand in a staggered stance, bend at your torso, and hold the rope behind your head with your elbows bent 90 degrees.

B

- Without moving your upper arms, pull the rope forward until your arms are straight.
- Pause, then return to the starting position.

▌Dumbbell Biceps Curl

▌Seated Dumbbell Biceps Curl

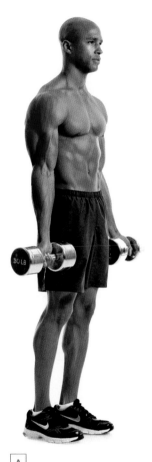
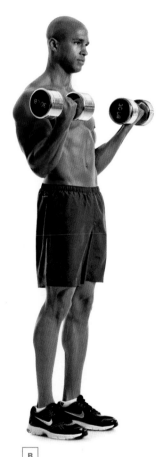

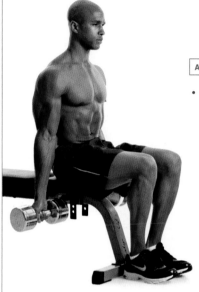

A

- Sit on a bench and grab a pair of dumbbells. Let them hang at arm's length next to your sides with your palms facing forward.

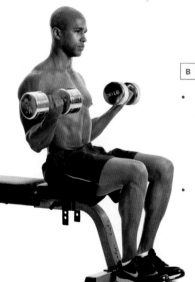

B

- Without moving your upper arms, bend your elbows and curl the dumbbells as close to your shoulders as you can.
- Pause, then lower the weights back to the starting position.

A

- Grab a pair of dumbbells and let them hang at arm's length next to your sides with your palms facing forward.

B

- Without moving your upper arms, bend your elbows and curl the dumbbells as close to your shoulders as you can.
- Pause, then lower the weights back to the starting position.

Upper Body Exercise: Arms

▊Resistance Band Overhead Triceps Press

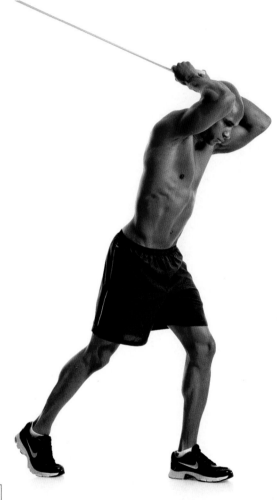

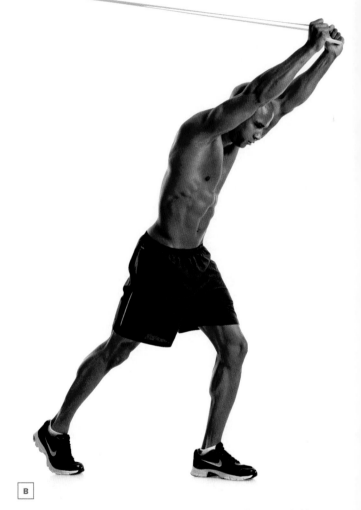

A

- Loop one end of a large resistance band around a chinup bar (or a secure object) and then pull it through the other end of the band.
- Grab the band with each hand. Stand in a staggered stance, one foot in front of the other, with your back to the anchor point.

B

- Hold the band behind your head, your elbows pointing forward and bent 90 degrees.
- Without moving your upper arms, push your forearms forward until your arms are straight.
- Pause, then return to the starting position.

▮Resistance Band Biceps Curl

▮Standing Overhead Dumbbell Triceps Press

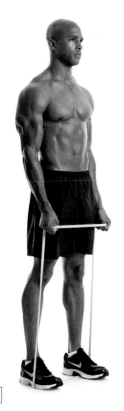 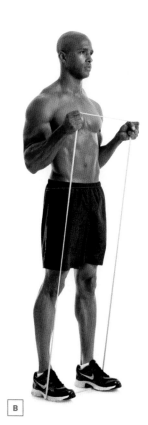 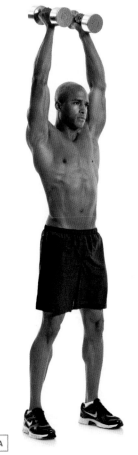 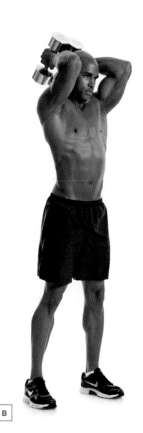

A

B

A

B

- Stand on one end of a resistance band with both feet about shoulder-width apart.
- Grab the other end of the band with your hands about shoulder-width apart and your arms at your sides.

- Without moving your upper arms, bend your arms and pull the band as close to your shoulders as you can.
- Pause, then lower the band to the starting position.

- Grab a pair of dumbbells and stand tall with your feet shoulder-width apart. Hold the dumbbells at arm's length above your head, your palms facing each other.

- Without moving your upper arms, lower the dumbbells behind your head.
- Pause, then straighten your arms to return the dumbbells to the starting position.

Upper Body Exercise: Arms

Dumbbell Zottoman Curl

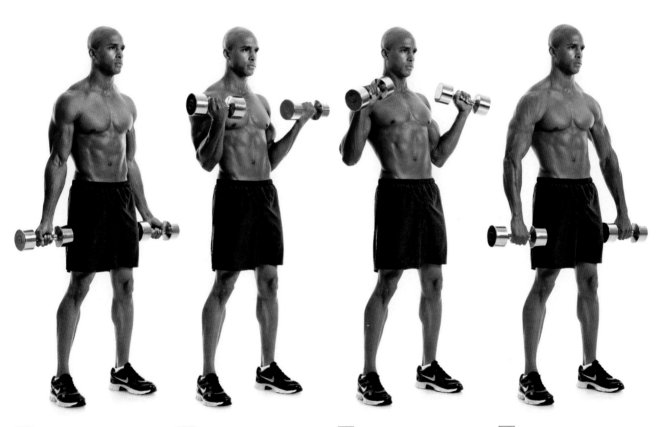

A
- Grab a pair of dumbbells and hold them at arm's length with your palms facing forward.

B
- Without moving your upper arms, curl the weights toward your shoulders.

C
- At the top of the curl, rotate your wrists outward so your palms face forward. Then, lower them from there back to the starting position.

D
- Rotate your wrists and the dumbbells back to the initial position and repeat.

EZ Bar Curl

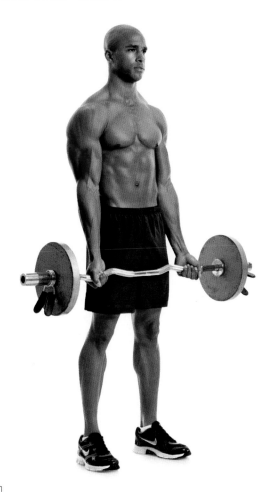

- Grab an EZ curl bar with an underhand, shoulder-width grip so that your palms are angled slightly inward.
- The bar should hang at arm's length in front of your waist.

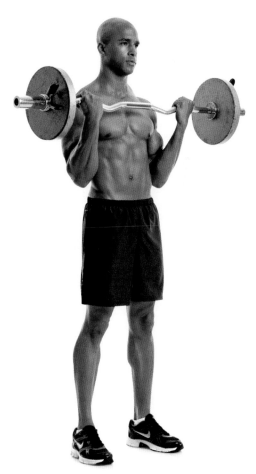

- Without moving your upper arms, bend your elbows and curl the bar as close to your shoulders as you can.
- Pause, then lower the weight back to the starting position.

Upper Body Exercise: Arms

Reverse Grip EZ Bar Curl

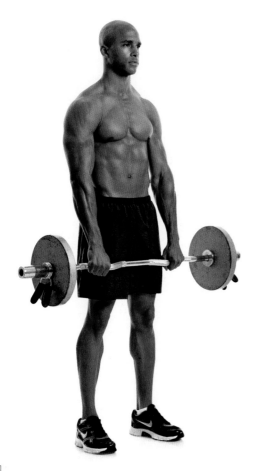

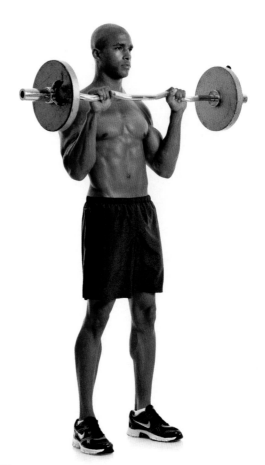

 A

- Grab an EZ curl bar with an overhand, shoulder-width grip so that your palms are angled slightly inward.
- The bar should hang at arm's length in front of your waist.

B

- Without moving your upper arms, bend your elbows and curl the bar as close to your shoulders as you can.
- Pause, then lower the weight back to the starting position.

Dumbbell Skull Crusher

A

- Grab a pair of dumbbells and lie faceup on a flat bench. Hold the dumbbells over your head with your arms straight and palms facing each other. Your arms should be angled slightly back.

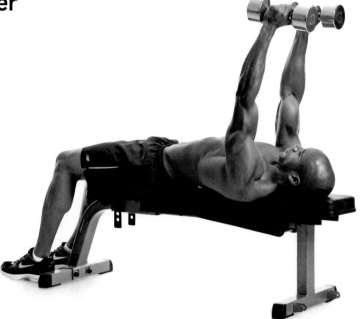

B

- Without moving your upper arms, bend your elbows to lower the dumbbells until your forearms are beyond parallel to the floor.
- Pause, then lift the weights back to the starting position by straightening your arms.

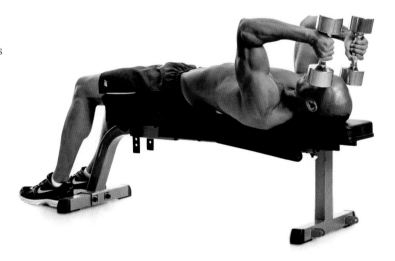

SHOULDERS

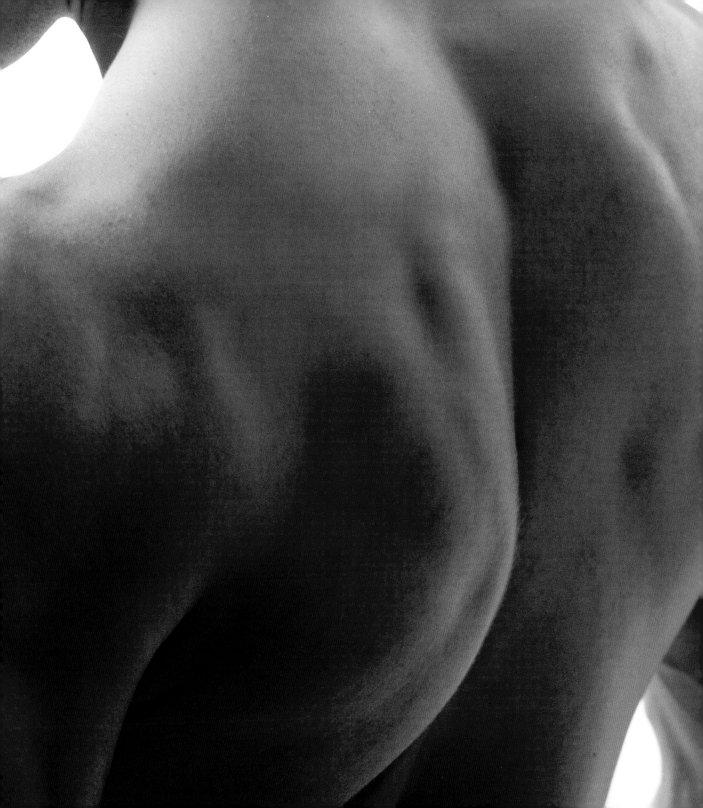

Upper Body Exercises: Shoulders

Barbell Shoulder Press

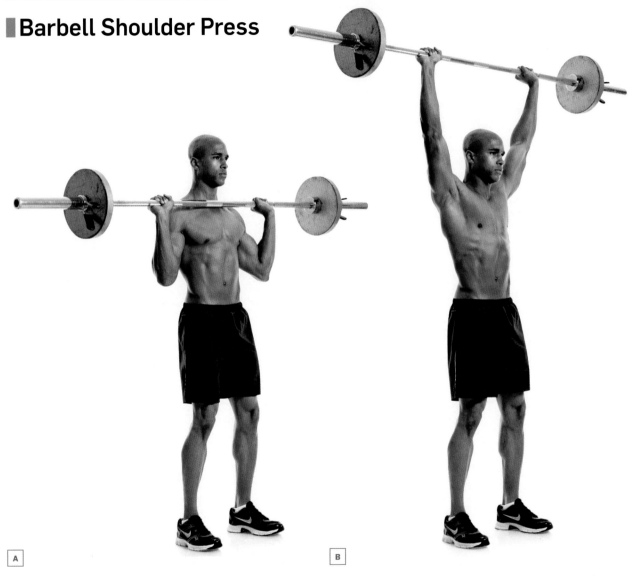

A

- Grab a barbell with an overhand grip that's just beyond shoulder width and hold it at shoulder level in front of your body. Stand with your feet shoulder-width apart and your knees slightly bent.

B

- Push the barbell straight overhead, while keeping your torso upright.
- Pause, then lower the bar back to the starting position.

Dumbbell Lateral Shoulder Raise

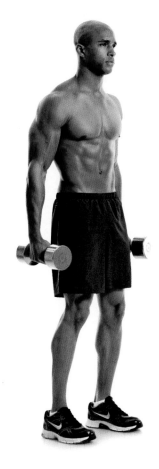

A

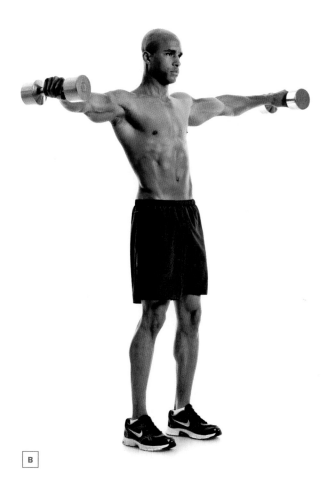

B

- Grab a pair of dumbbells and let them hang at arm's length next to your sides. Stand tall and make sure your palms are facing your body.

- Keeping your elbows slightly bent, raise your arms straight out to the sides until they're at shoulder level.

- Pause, then lower the weights back to the starting position.

Upper Body Exercises: Shoulders

█ Dumbbell Rear Lateral Raise

A

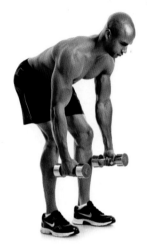

- Grab a pair of dumbbells and bend forward at your hips until your back is nearly parallel to the floor. Your arms should hang straight down from your shoulders with your elbows slightly bent.

B

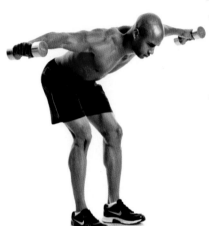

- Hold your body still and raise your arms out to the sides until your hands are in line with your shoulders.
- Pause, then return to the starting position.

█ T Raise (dumbbells optional)

A

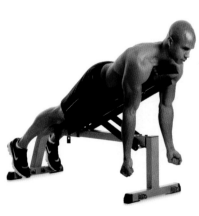

- Lie chest down on an adjustable bench set to a low incline (holding dumbbells optional). Your arms should hang straight down from your shoulders, and your palms should be facing each other.

B

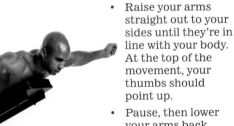

- Raise your arms straight out to your sides until they're in line with your body. At the top of the movement, your thumbs should point up.
- Pause, then lower your arms back to the starting position.

Y Raise (dumbbells optional)

A

- Lie chest down on an adjustable bench set to a low incline (holding dumbbells optional). Your arms should hang straight down from your shoulders, and your palms should be facing each other.

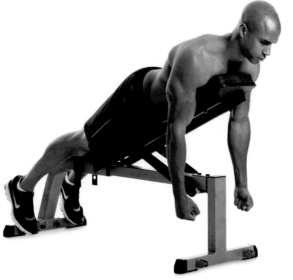

B

- Raise your arms at a 30-degree angle to your body until they are in line with your body. At the top of the movement, your arms and torso should form a Y.
- Pause, then lower back to the starting position.

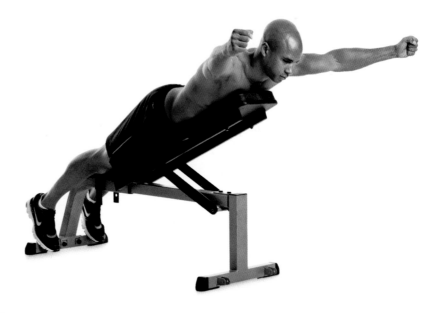

Upper Body Exercises: Shoulders

█ I Raise (dumbbells optional)

A

- Lie chest down on an adjustable bench set to a low incline (holding dumbbells optional). Your arms should hang straight down from your shoulders, and your palms should be facing each other.

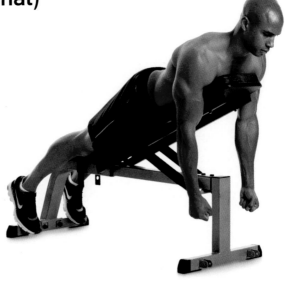

B

- Raise your arms straight up until they're in line with your body. Your arms and torso should form the letter I.
- Pause, then lower back to the starting position.

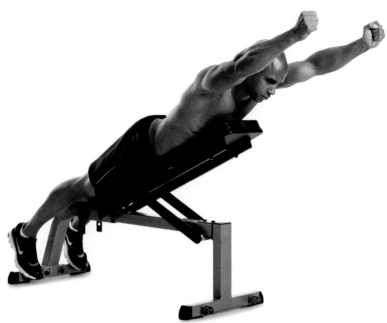

▮Dumbbell Overhead Press

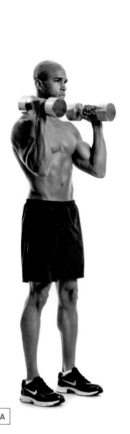 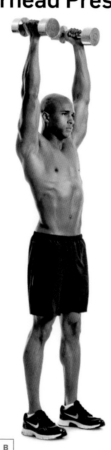

A

- Grab a pair of dumbbells and hold them just outside your shoulders with your palms facing each other.

B

- Press the weight overhead until your arms are completely straight.
- Pause, then slowly lower the dumbbells back to the starting position.

▮One-Arm Overhead Press

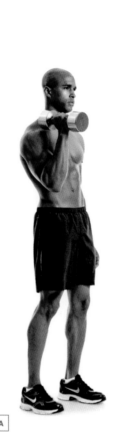 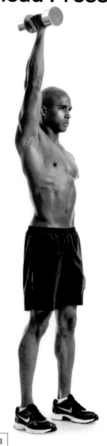

A

- Grab one dumbbell with one hand and hold it just outside your shoulder with your palm facing your head.

B

- Press the weight overhead until your arm is completely straight.
- Pause, then slowly lower the dumbbell back to the starting position.
- Complete all reps, then grab the dumbbell with your other hand and repeat.

Upper Body Exercises: Shoulders

Dumbbell Shrug

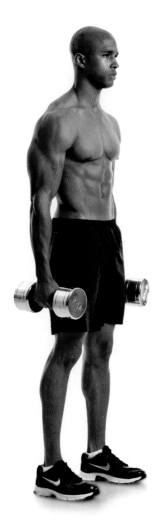

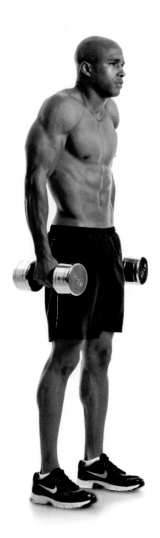

A

- Grab a pair of dumbbells and let them hang at arm's length with your palms facing each other.

B

- In one movement, explode upward and shrug your shoulders as high as you can, while keeping your arms straight.

Dumbbell Front Raise

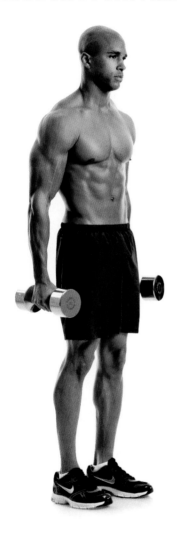

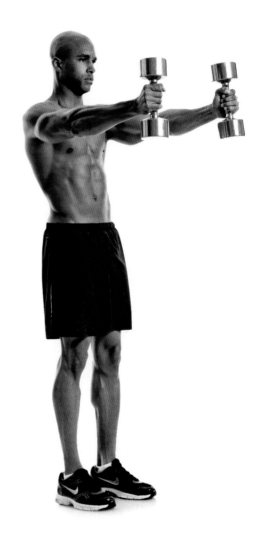

- Grab a pair of dumbbells and let them hang at arm's length next to your sides. Stand tall and make sure your palms are facing your body.

- Keeping your elbows slightly bent, raise your arms in front of your body until they're at shoulder level.
- Pause, then lower the weights back to the starting position.

Upper Body Exercises: Shoulders

Wall Slide

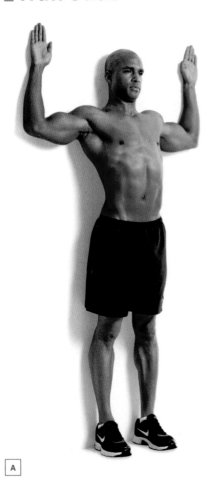

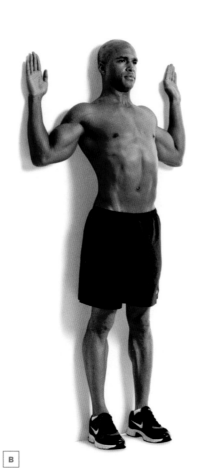

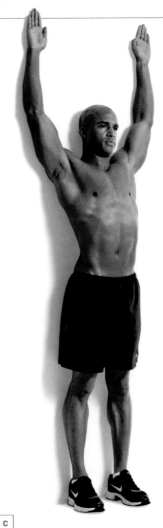

A

- Lean your head, upper back, and butt against the wall.
- Place your hands and arms against the wall in the "high-five" position, your elbows bent 90 degrees and your upper arms at shoulder height. Hold for 1 second. Don't allow your head, upper back, or butt to lose contact with the wall.

B

- Keeping your elbows, wrists, and hands pressed into the wall, slide your elbows down toward your sides as far as you can. Squeeze your shoulder blades together.

C

- Slide your arms back up the wall as high as you can while keeping your hands in contact with the wall.
- Lower and repeat.

■ Dumbbell Uppercut

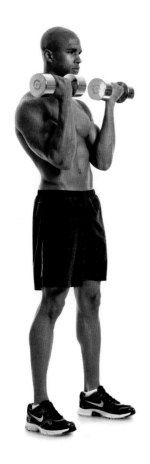
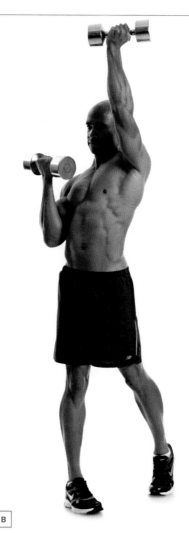
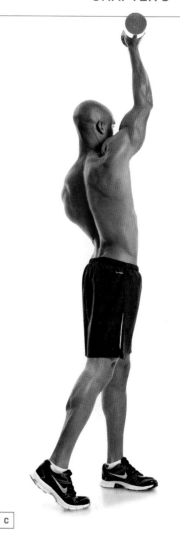

A

- Hold a pair of dumbbells at arm's length at your sides with your palms facing forward.
- Curl the weights up so that the dumbbells are at shoulder height with your palms facing your shoulders.

B

- Rotate your torso to the right and press the dumbbell in your left hand overhead.

C

- Then rotate all the way to the left and press the dumbbell in your right hand overhead. Continue alternating back and forth.

Upper Body Exercises: Shoulders

Standing Hips Flexed Ts and Ws

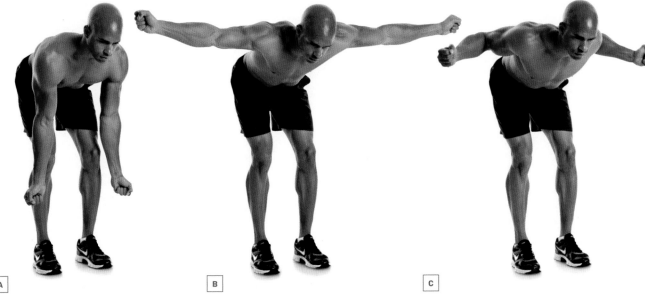

A

- Stand with your feet shoulder-width apart, your hips bent so your back is just above parallel to the floor, keeping your spine in a neutral position.
- With your arms hanging down straight and perpendicular to the floor, rotate your arms so that your palms are facing forward.

B

- Squeeze your shoulder blades together and lift your arms up as high as they go to form a T with your torso. Pause for a second.

C

- Keeping your thumbs up toward the ceiling, squeeze your shoulder blades back and down, and pull your elbows into your side to form a W.
- Pause for a second before returning to the T position and then back down.

Wall Snow Angel

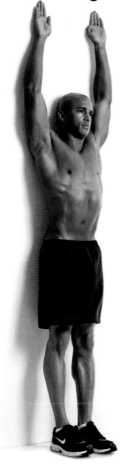

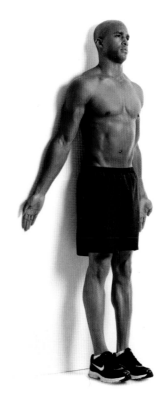

B

- Stand with your back against a smooth wall and your feet about 6 to 8 inches away from the wall.
- Put your arms into an overhead position so that the back of your hands and forearms are resting on the wall.

- While putting light pressure on the wall with your forearms, slide your arms in a big arc all the way down to your sides, squeezing your shoulder blades back and down during the movement.
- Pause for a second to feel the muscles on the insides of your shoulder blades engage, then return to the starting position.

TOTAL BODY
Exercises

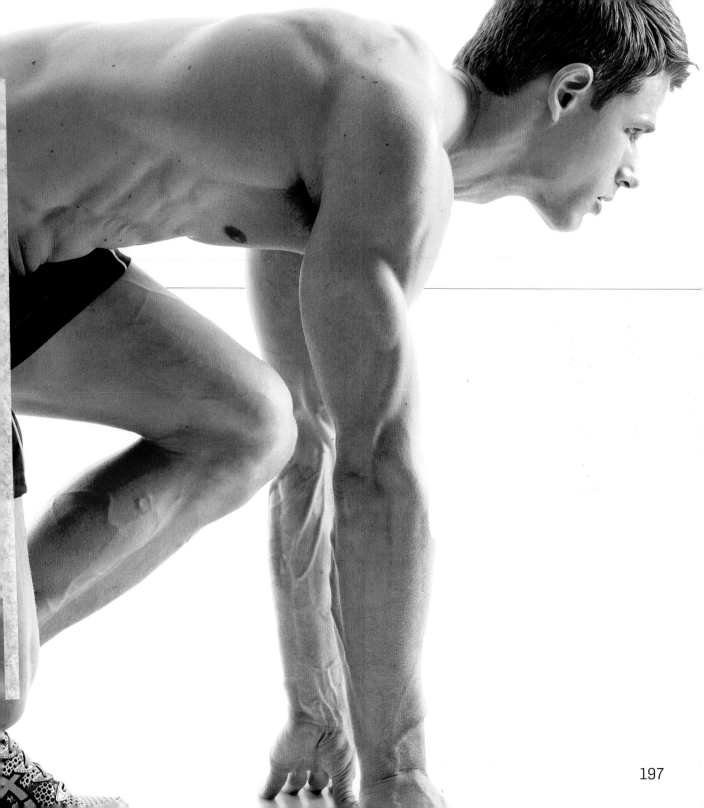

Total Body Exercises

Jumping Jack

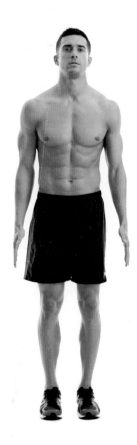

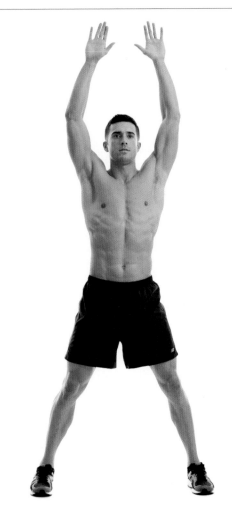

A

- Stand with your feet together and your hands at your sides.

B

- Simultaneously raise your arms above your head and jump your feet out to the sides.
- Immediately reverse the movement and jump back to the starting position.
- Repeat for all reps.

■ Squat to Press

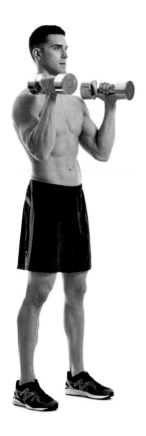

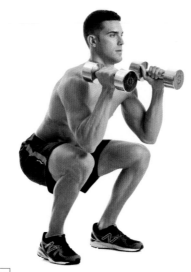

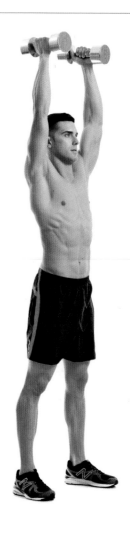

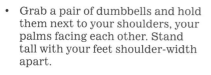

A

- Grab a pair of dumbbells and hold them next to your shoulders, your palms facing each other. Stand tall with your feet shoulder-width apart.

B

- Lower your body until the tops of your thighs are at least parallel to the floor.

C

- Push your body back to a standing position as you press the dumbbells directly over your shoulders.
- Lower the dumbbells back to the starting position.

Total Body Exercises

Dumbbell Curl to Squat to Press

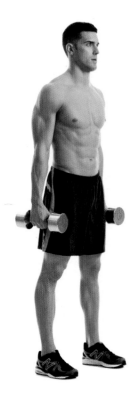

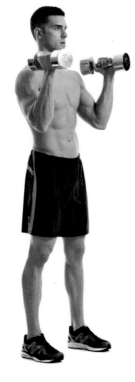

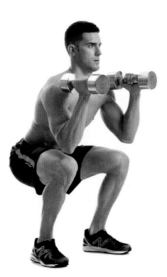

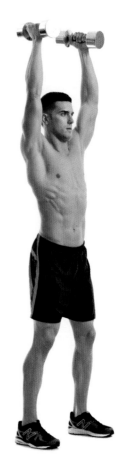

A

- Hold a pair of dumb-bells about shoulder-width apart and your arms at your sides with your palms facing forward.

B

- Without moving your upper arms, bend your arms and lift the weights as close to your shoulders as you can.

C

- Then, push your hips back and squat down until your upper thighs are at least parallel to the floor. Immediately explode upward and stand up.

D

- As you rise up, press the weights overhead.

▮Squat Thrust

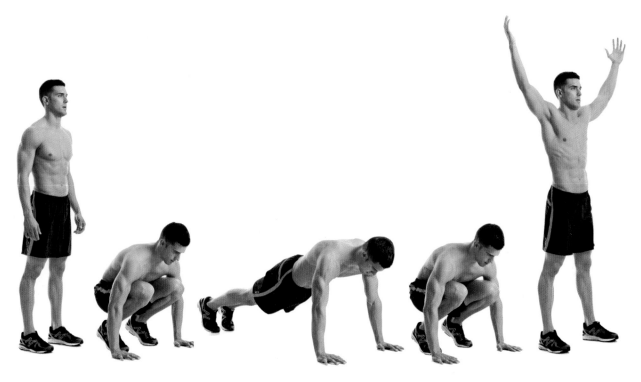

A
- Stand with your feet shoulder-width apart and your arms at your sides.

B
- Push your hips back, bend your knees, and lower your body as deep as you can into a squat.

C
- Place your hands on the floor and kick your legs backward into a pushup position.

D
- Kick your legs back to the squat position.

E
- Stand up and jump. That's 1 rep.

Total Body Exercises

▍Squat to Stand

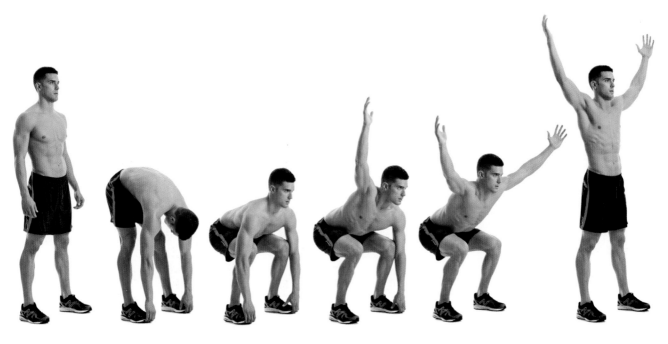

A
- Stand tall with your legs straight and your feet shoulder-width apart.

B
- Keeping your legs straight, bend over and grab your toes. (If you need to bend your knees, you can, but bend them only as much as necessary.)

C
- Without letting go of your toes, lower your body into a squat as you raise your chest and shoulders up.

D
- Staying in the squat position, raise your right arm up high and wide.

E
- Then raise your left arm.

F
- Now stand up.

Goblet Squat to Press

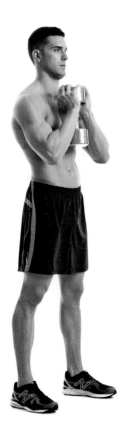
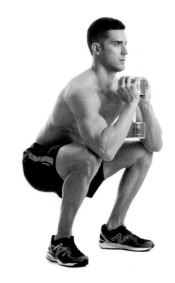
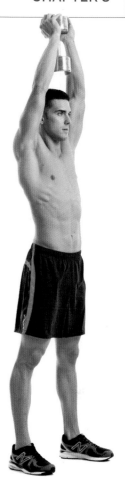

 A

- Hold a dumbbell vertically next to your chest, with both hands cupping the dumbbell head.

 B

- Push your hips back and lower your body into a squat until your upper thighs are at least parallel to the floor. Your elbows should brush the insides of your knees in the bottom position.

C

- Pause, then press your body back up and press the dumbbell overhead.
- Lower the dumbbell back to the starting position.

Total Body Exercises

Dumbbell Squat Thrust

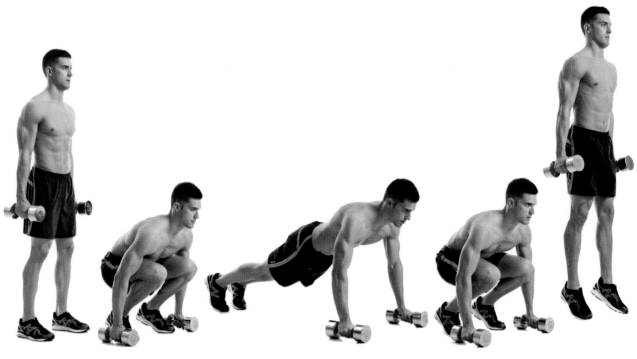

A
- Stand with your feet shoulder-width apart and your arms at your sides holding a pair of dumbbells (preferably hex).

B
- Push your hips back, bend your knees, and lower your body as deep as you can into a squat.

C
- Holding on to the dumbbells, place them on the floor, then kick your legs backward into a pushup position.

D
- Kick your legs back to the squat position.

E
- Stand up and jump. That's 1 rep.

Dumbbell Push Press

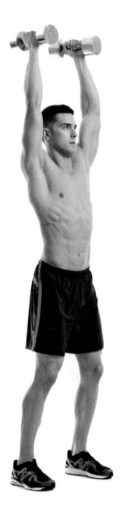

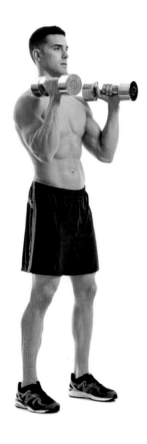

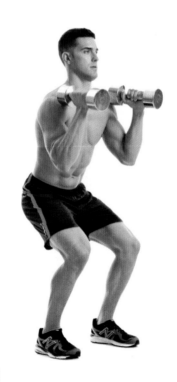

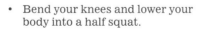

 A

- Grab a pair of dumbbells and hold them just outside your shoulders with your palms facing each other.

B

- Bend your knees and lower your body into a half squat.

C

- Press the weight overhead as you stand up tall and explode upward, pressing through your heels.
- Pause, then slowly lower the dumbbells back to the starting position.

Total Body Exercises

Single-Arm Dumbbell Push Press

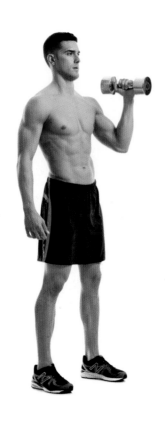

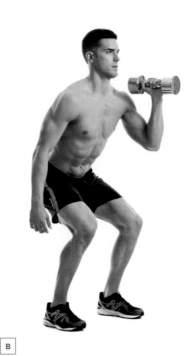

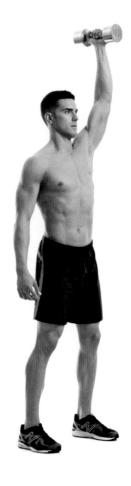

A

- Grab a single dumbbell and hold it just outside your shoulders with your thumb facing your body.

B

- Bend your knees and lower your body into a half squat.

C

- Press the weight overhead as you stand up tall and explode upward, pressing through your heels.
- Pause, then slowly lower the dumbbell back to the starting position. Do all reps, switch sides, and repeat.

■Push Jerks

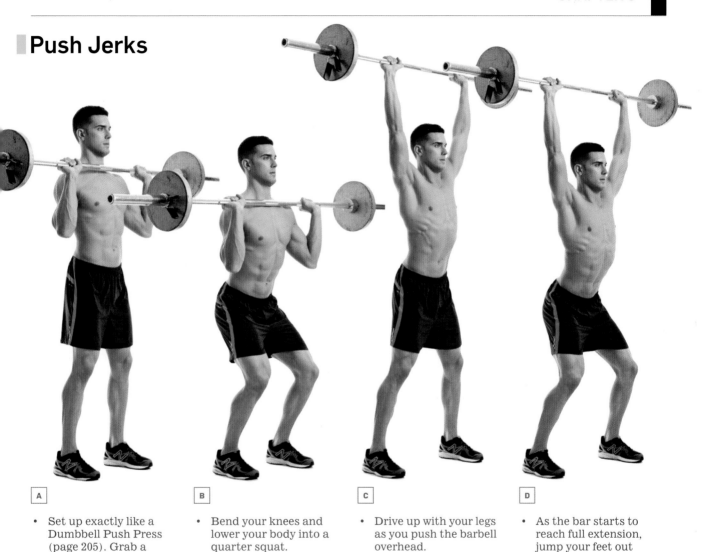

A

- Set up exactly like a Dumbbell Push Press (page 205). Grab a barbell and hold it just outside your shoulders.

B

- Bend your knees and lower your body into a quarter squat.

C

- Drive up with your legs as you push the barbell overhead.

D

- As the bar starts to reach full extension, jump your feet out slightly wider than your starting base and bend your knees to drop slightly under the bar. This portion is known as "the catch."
- Return to the starting position and repeat.

Total Body Exercises

Overhead Waiter's Carry

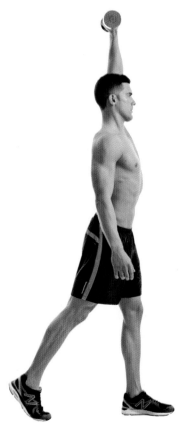

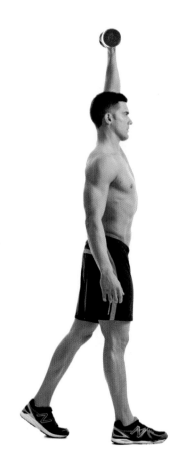

A

- Stand up tall and press one dumbbell overhead, locking your arm at the top.

B

- Keep your eyes straight ahead, chin tucked back, chest up, and shoulders blades packed back and down as you walk in a straight line for 25 yards.
- Switch arms, turn around, and walk back for a total of 50 yards.
- You should feel your grip and shoulders working. Avoid letting your lower back arch and prevent side bending throughout the exercise.

▮ Dumbbell Snatch

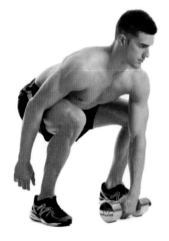
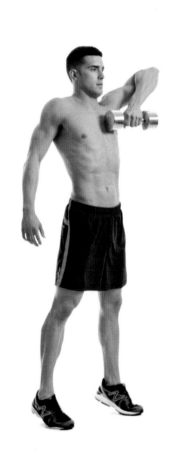
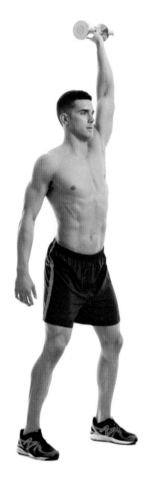

A

- Place a dumbbell on the floor and stand over it with your feet wider than shoulder-width apart.
- Bend at your hips and knees, and squat down until you can grab the dumbbell with one hand, in an overhand grip, without rounding your upper back.

B

- Keeping the dumbbell close to your body, pull it upward and try to throw it at the ceiling without letting go.

C

- As you raise the dumbbell, your forearm should rotate up and back, until your arm is straight and your palm is facing forward.
- Pause and then lower the weight back to the starting position.

Total Body Exercises

Dumbbell or Kettlebell Swing

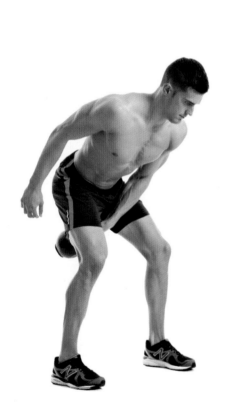

A

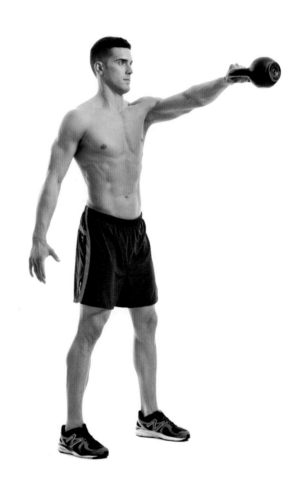
B

- Grab a dumbbell (or kettlebell) with an overhand grip and hold it with one hand in front of your waist at arm's length. Set your feet slightly wider than shoulder-width apart.

- Keeping your lower back slightly arched, bend at your hips and knees, and lower your torso until it forms a 45-degree angle to the floor.

- Now swing the dumbbell between your legs. Keeping your arm straight, thrust your hips forward, straighten your knees, and swing the dumbbell up to chest level as you rise to the standing position.

- Reverse the movement and swing the dumbbell back between your legs again. That's 1 rep.

- Do all reps, then switch arms and repeat.

█ Dumbbell Clean

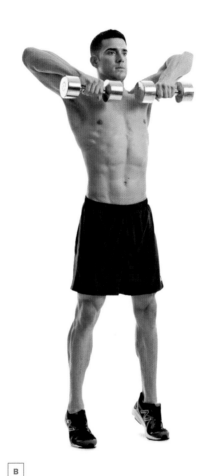

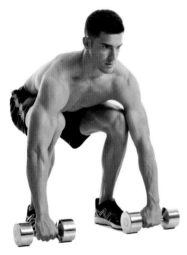

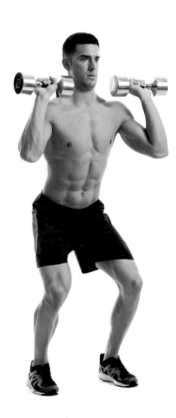

A
- Squat over a pair of dumbbells and grab them with an overhand grip.

B
- Stand and lift both weights up to chest height.

C
- Quickly drop underneath the weights and "catch" them on your shoulders, with your elbows high.
- Drop your elbows, keeping the dumbbells at shoulder level.

Total Body Exercises

Barbell High Pull

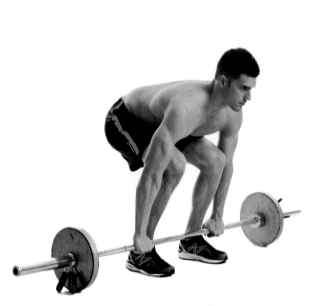

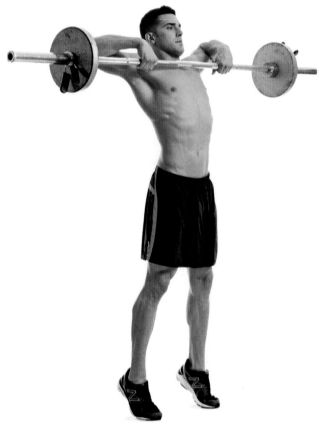

A

- Load the barbell and roll it against your shins.
- Grab the bar with an overhand grip that's just beyond shoulder width.
- Bend at your hips and knees to squat down.
- Raise your chest and hips until your arms are straight. Your lower back should be slightly arched.

B

- Pull the bar as high as you can by explosively standing up as you bend your elbows, raise your upper arms, thrust your hips forward, and rise up on your toes.
- Reverse the movement to return to the starting position.

▮ Barbell Clean and Press

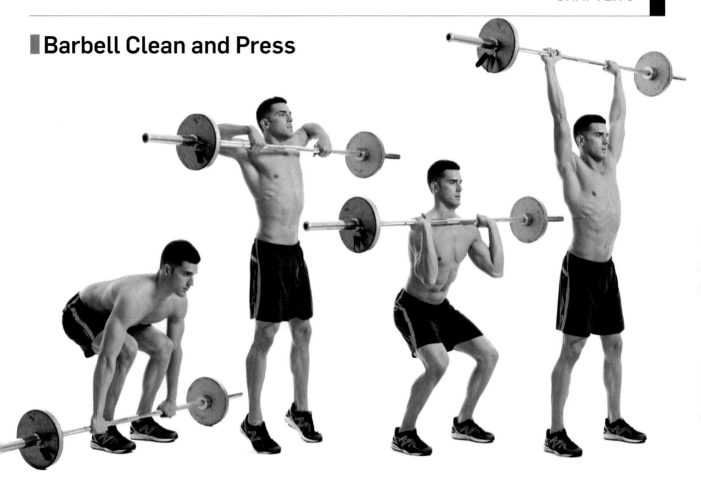

A

- Load a barbell with the appropriate weight and roll it against your shins.

B

- Grab the barbell with an overhand grip that's just beyond shoulder-width apart. Bend at your hips and knees to squat down. Pull the bar as high as you can by explosively standing up as you bend your elbows and raise your upper arms.

C

- "Catch" the weight as you let the barbell rotate around your wrist. Squat down.

D

- Then press the weight overhead.

Total Body Exercises

Dumbbell High Pull

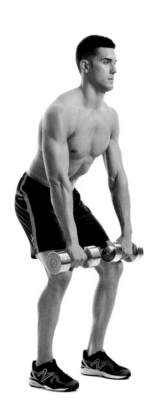

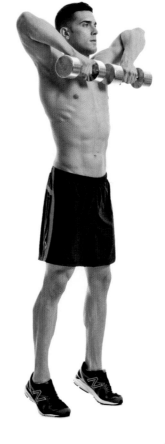

- Grab a pair of dumbbells with an overhand grip and hold them just below knee height.

B

- Explosively pull the dumbbells upward, rise onto your toes, and bend your elbows as you bring the weights up to shoulder height. Return to the starting position.

Rope High Pull

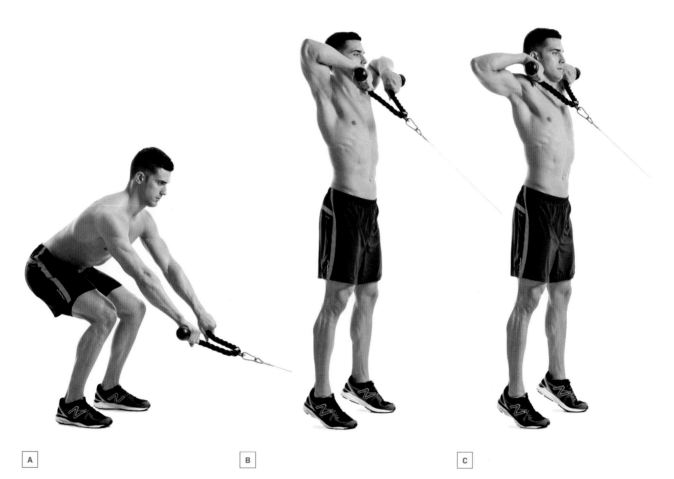

A

- Attach a rope to a low cable pulley. Grab the rope attachment in each hand with an overhand grip, just below knee height.

B

- Explosively pull the rope upward, rise onto your toes.

C

- Bend your elbows as you bring the rope up to shoulder height. Return to the starting position.

Total Body Exercises

Reverse Lunge and SA Cable Row

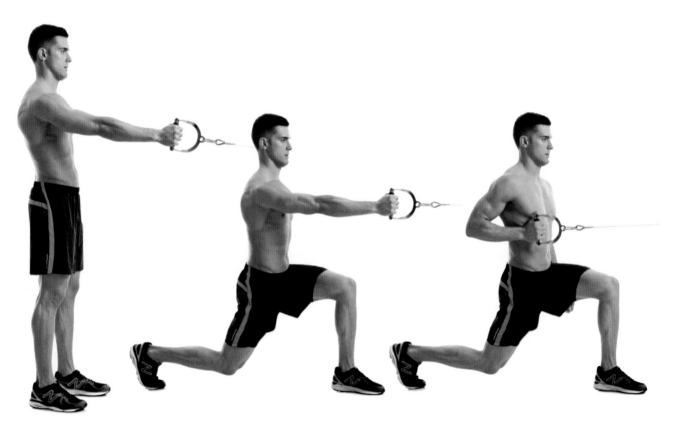

A

- Attach a D-handle at hip height to a cable station.
- Grab the handle with the right hand and step away from the tower until your arm is extended in front of your body.

B

- Step backward with your right leg into a lunge and lower your body until your front knee is bent 90 degrees.

C

- Pause, row the cable to the side of your chest, and then return to the starting position.
- Perform all reps, and then switch arms and repeat the process, stepping back with your left leg.

Dumbbell Hang Jump Shrug

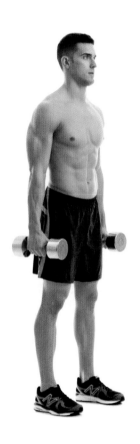
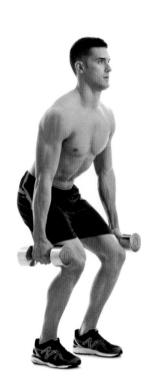
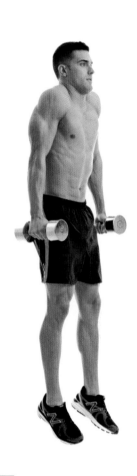

 A

- Grab a pair of dumbbells and let them hang at arm's length with your palms facing each other.

 B

- Push your hips back, slightly bend your knees, and lower the dumbbells until they are just below your knees.

C

- In one movement, explode upward and shrug your shoulders as high as you can, while keeping your arms straight.
- Land softly on the floor, dip your knees, and repeat.

Total Body Exercises

Lunge and Reach

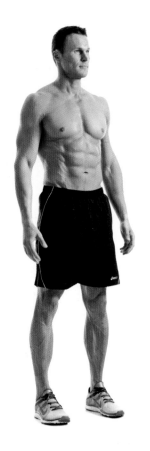

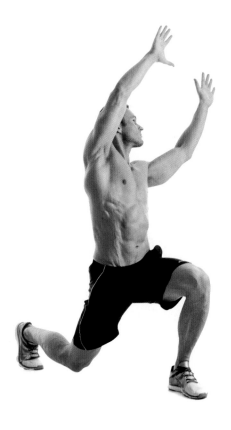

A

- Stand tall with your arms hanging at your sides. Brace your core and hold it that way.

B

- Lunge back with your right leg, lowering your body until your left knee is bent at least 90 degrees.
- As you lunge, reach back with both hands over your left shoulder.
- Reverse the movement back to the starting position.
- Complete the prescribed number of repetitions with your left leg, then step back with your left leg and reach over your right shoulder for the same number of reps. Keep your torso upright for the entire movement.

Dumbbell Renegade Crawl

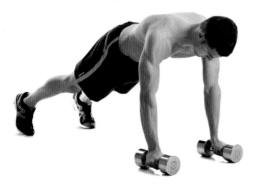

- Place a pair of dumbbells (preferably hex) at the spots where you position your hands for a pushup.

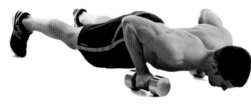

B

- Grasp a dumbbell with each hand and get into the pushup position.
- Lower your body to the floor, pause, then push yourself back up.

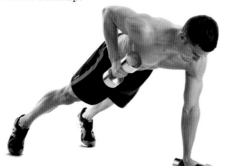

C

- Once you're back in the starting position, lift the dumbbell in your right hand to the right side of your chest.

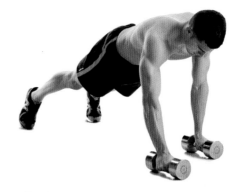

D

- Lower the dumbbell and repeat with your left hand.

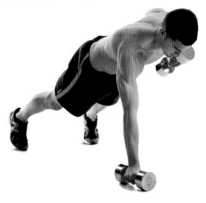

E

- "Walk" each hand one step forward, still holding the dumbbells, and follow with your feet so you're back in the starting position. That's 1 rep.

Total Body Exercises

▮ Squat and Cable Row

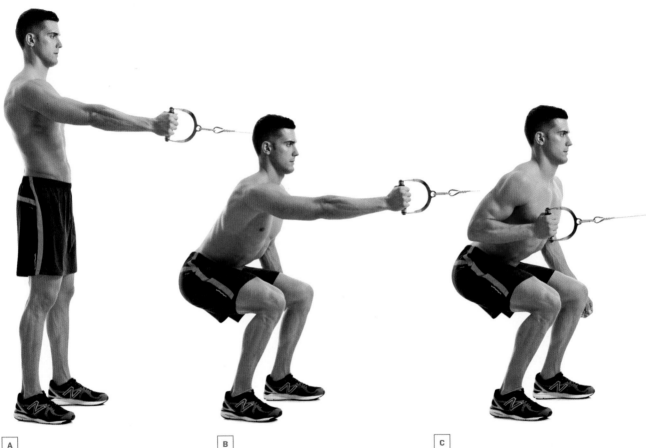

A

- Attach a D-handle at hip height to a cable station.
- Grab the handle with one hand and step away from the tower until your arm is extended in front of your body.

B

- Push your hips back and lower your body into a squat until your thighs are at least parallel to the floor.

C

- Pause, row the cable to the side of your chest, and then return to the starting position.
- Perform all reps, then switch arms and repeat the process.

Split Squat and Overhead Press

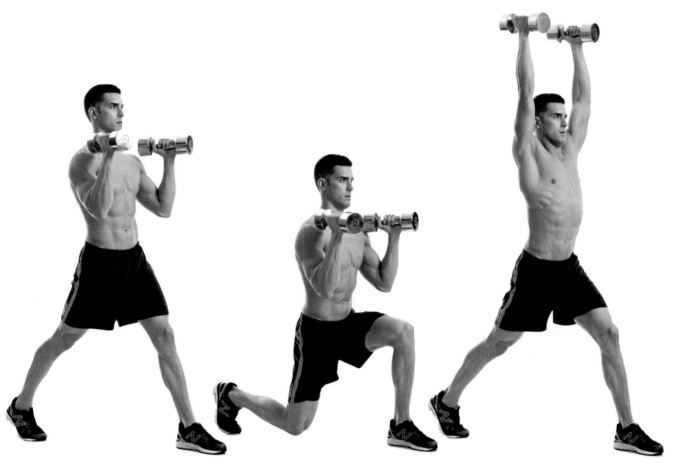

A

- Grab a pair of dumbbells and hold them next to your shoulders, your palms facing each other.
- Stand in a staggered stance with your left foot in front of your right and your front knee slightly bent.

B

- Lower your body as far as you can, or until your back knee nearly touches the floor.

C

- Push yourself back up to the starting position. As you stand up, press the dumbbells directly over your shoulder.
- Return to the starting position and repeat.

Total Body Exercises

▍Dumbbell Getup

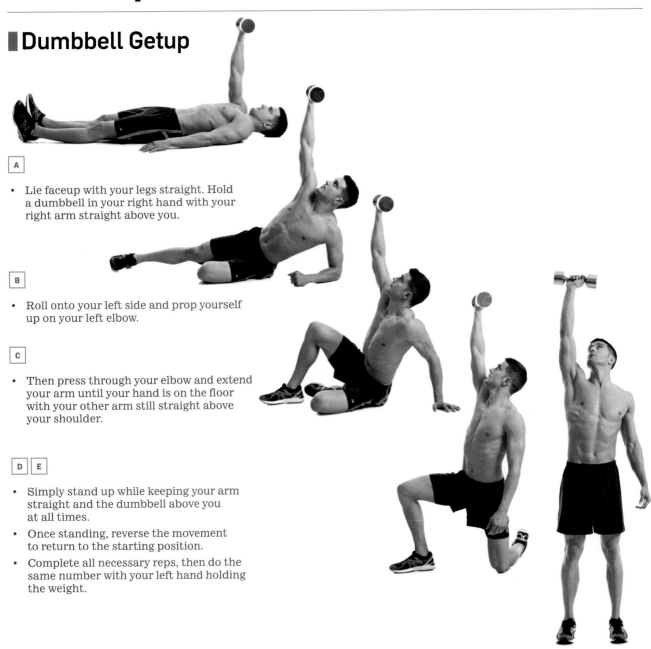

A

- Lie faceup with your legs straight. Hold a dumbbell in your right hand with your right arm straight above you.

B

- Roll onto your left side and prop yourself up on your left elbow.

C

- Then press through your elbow and extend your arm until your hand is on the floor with your other arm still straight above your shoulder.

D **E**

- Simply stand up while keeping your arm straight and the dumbbell above you at all times.
- Once standing, reverse the movement to return to the starting position.
- Complete all necessary reps, then do the same number with your left hand holding the weight.

Kettlebell Windmill

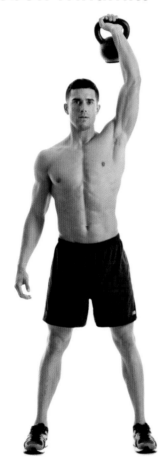

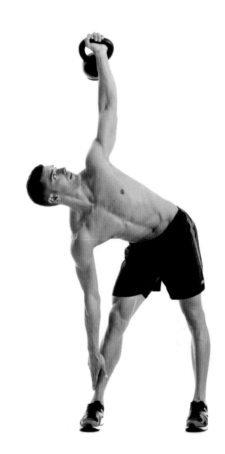

 A

- Stand with your feet wider than hip-width apart, and hold the kettlebell in your left hand.
- Raise it next to your left shoulder, then press it overhead.

 B

- Rotate your chest to the left and look up at the kettlebell as you try to touch your right hand to your right foot.
- Pause, then return to the starting position, keeping your left arm extended.
- Do the prescribed number of reps before lowering the weight, then repeat on the other side.

Total Body Exercises

Inchworm

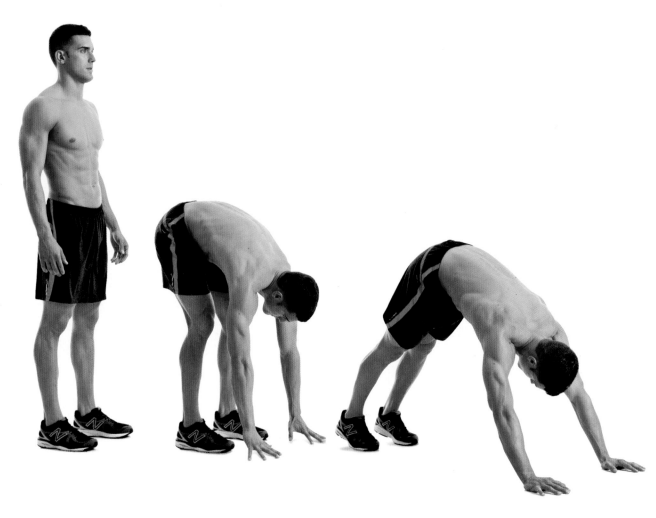

A
- Stand tall with your legs straight.

B
- Bend over and touch the floor.

C
- Keeping your legs straight, walk forward with your hands.

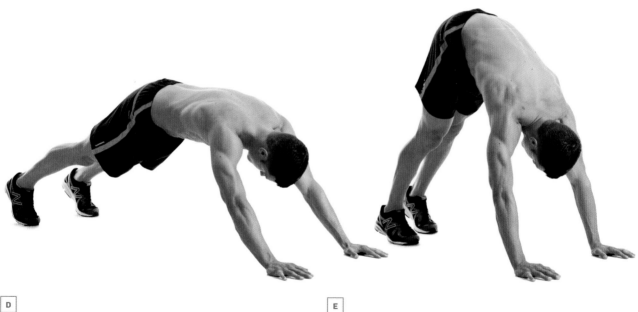

D

- Walk forward as far as you can without allowing your hips to sag.

E

- Walk your feet toward your hands. That's 1 rep.

Total Body Exercises

Kettlebell or Dumbbell Suitcase Carry

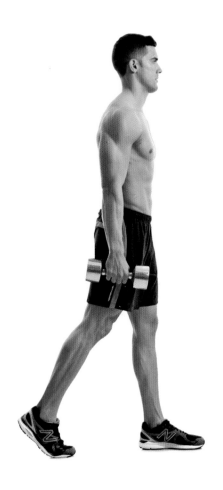

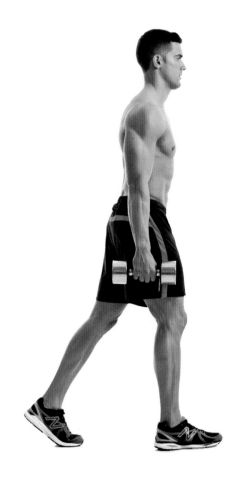

A

- Grab a heavy dumbbell or kettlebell and hold it at your side at arm's length.

B

- Now walk forward (or in a circle) for the prescribed time or distance. Make sure that you stand tall and don't allow the weight to "pull" you down. If you feel like you could have gone longer, grab heavier weights on your next set.

Dumbbell Farmer's Walk

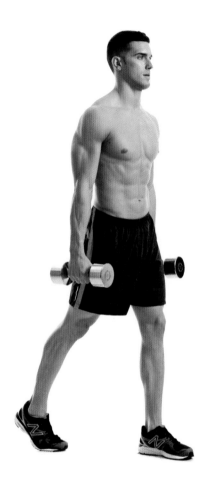

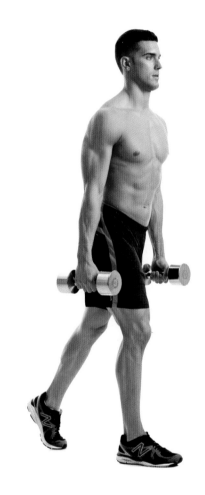

 A

- Grab a pair of heavy dumbbells and hold them at your sides at arm's length.

 B

- Now walk forward (or in a circle) for the prescribed time or distance. If you feel like you could have gone longer, grab heavier weights on your next set.

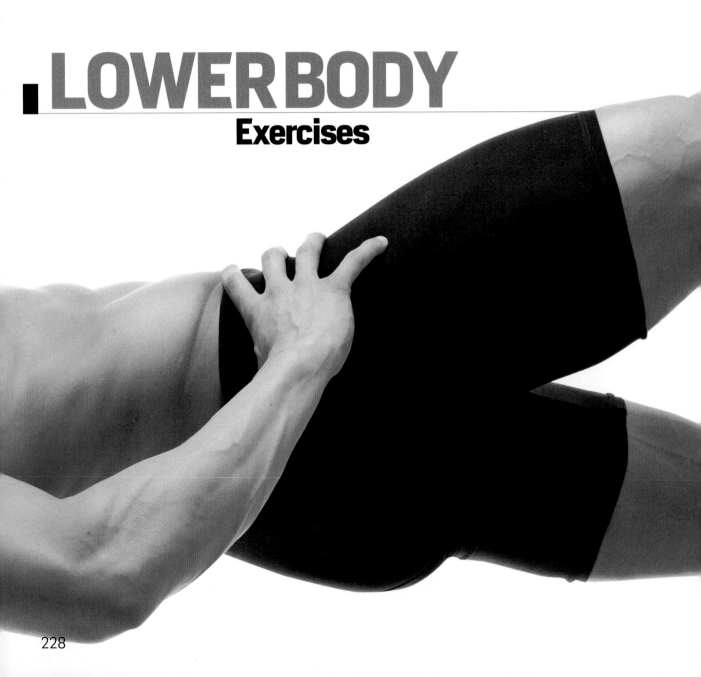

LOWER BODY
Exercises

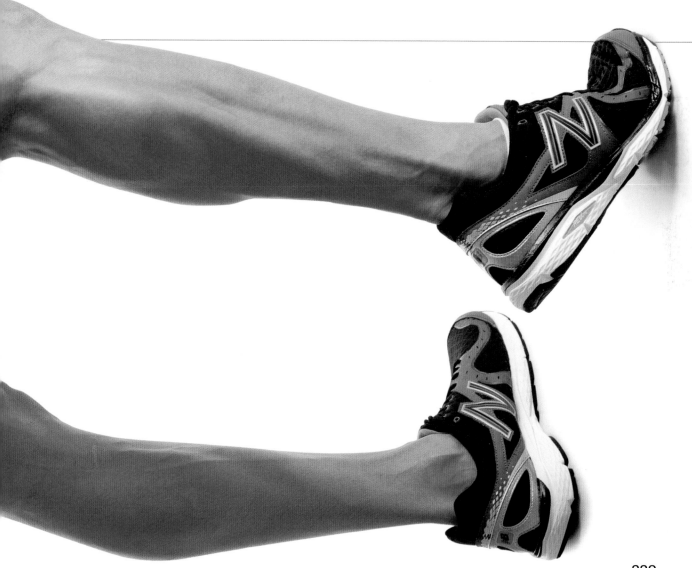

Lower Body Exercises

▍Barbell Squat

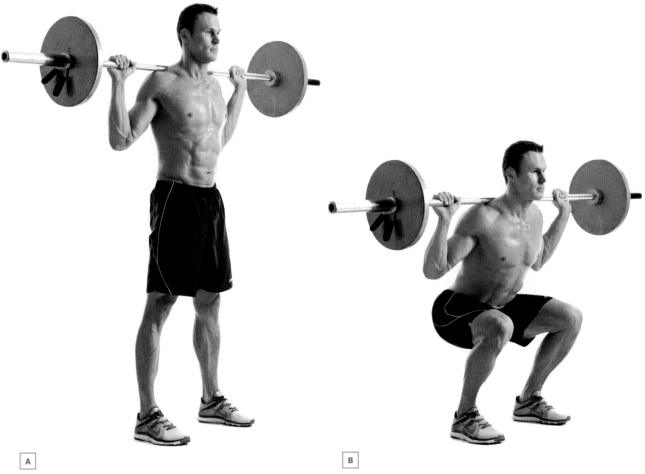

A

B

- Hold a barbell across your upper back with an overhand grip and your feet shoulder-width apart.

- Keeping your lower back arched, lower your body as deep as you can by pushing your hips back and bending your knees.
- Pause, then reverse the movement back to the starting position.

█ Bodyweight Squat

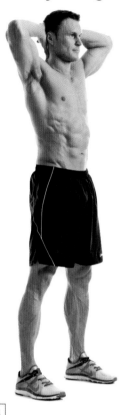
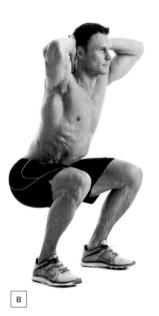

A

B

- Stand tall with your feet shoulder-width apart and place your fingers on the back of your head.

- Pull your shoulders and elbows back, and lower your body as far as you can by pushing your hips back and bending your knees.

- Pause, then push yourself back to the starting position.

█ Dumbbell Front Squat

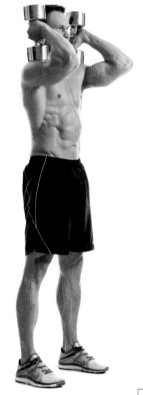
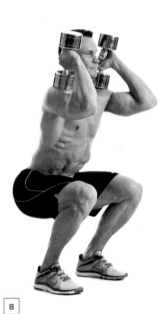

A

B

- Stand with your feet shoulder-width apart. Hold a pair of dumbbells so that your palms are facing each other, and rest one of the dumbbell heads on the meatiest part of each shoulder.

- Keep your body as upright as you can at all times, as your upper arms remain parallel to the floor.

- Brace your abs and lower your body as far as you can by pushing your hips back and bending your knees.

- Pause, then push yourself back to the starting position.

Lower Body Exercises

Barbell Front Squat

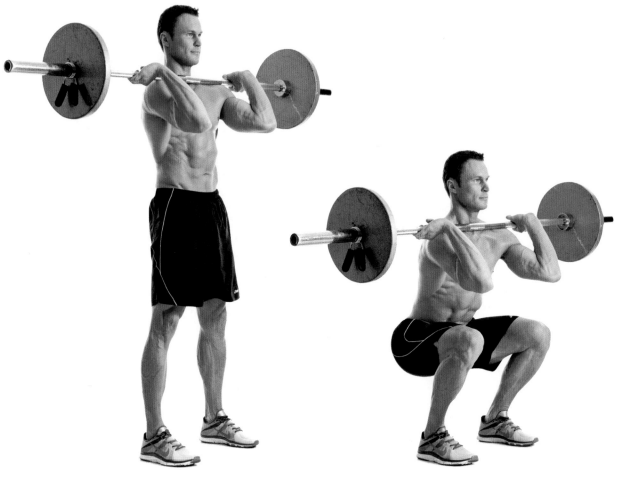

A

- Hold a barbell with an overhand grip that's just beyond shoulder width.
- Raise your upper arms until they're parallel to the floor.
- Allow the bar to roll back so that it's resting on the front of your shoulders.

B

- Lower your body until the tops of your thighs are at least parallel to the floor.
- Pause, then push your body back to the starting position.

Skater Jump

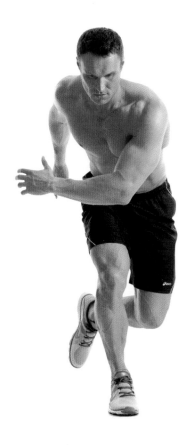

A

- Stand on your right foot with your right knee slightly bent, and place your left foot just behind your right ankle.
- Bend your right knee and lower your body into a partial squat.

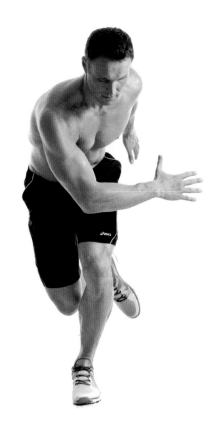

B

- Bound to the left by jumping off your right foot.
- Land on your left foot and bring your right foot behind your left as you reach toward the floor with your right hand.
- Repeat the move back toward the right, landing on your right foot and reaching with your left hand.

Lower Body Exercises

Squat Jump

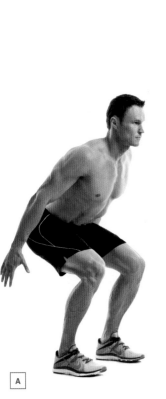

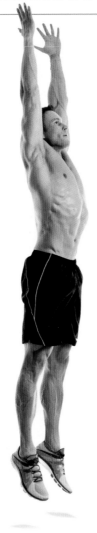

A

- Place your fingers on the back of your head and pull your elbows back so that they're in line with your body.
- Dip your knees in preparation to leap.

B

- Explosively jump as high as you can, raising your arms up in the air as you jump.
- When you land, immediately squat down and jump again.

Dumbbell Squat

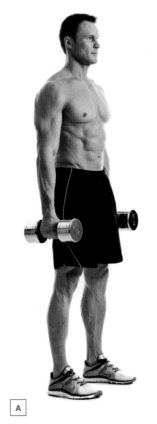

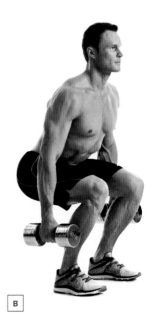

A

- Hold a pair of dumbbells at arm's length next to your sides, your palms facing each other.

B

- Brace your abs, and lower your body as far as you can by pushing your hips back and bending your knees.
- Pause, then push back up to the starting position.

■Dumbbell Split Squat

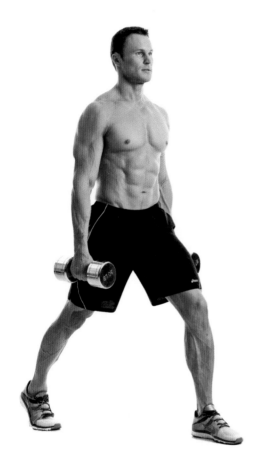

- Hold a pair of dumbbells at arm's length next to your sides, your palms facing each other. Stand in a staggered stance, your left foot in front of your right.

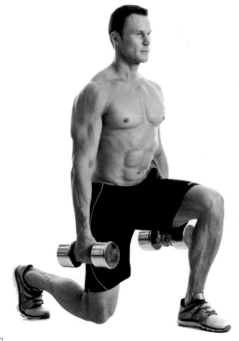

B

- Slowly lower your body as far as you can. Your rear knee should nearly touch the floor.
- Pause, then push yourself back up to the starting position.
- Complete the prescribed number of reps, then do the same number of reps with your right foot in front of your left.

Lower Body Exercises

Single-Arm Dumbbell Squat

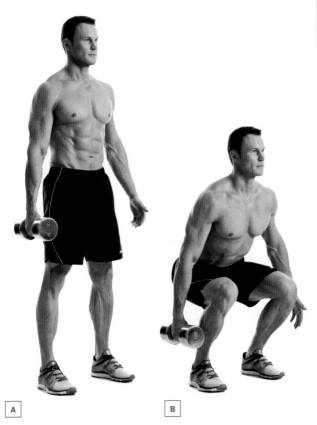

A

B

- Hold one dumbbell at arm's length next to your side, your palm facing your torso, and let your other arm rest at your side.

- Brace your abs, and lower your body as far as you can by pushing your hips back and bending your knees.
- Pause, then push back up to the starting position.
- Do all reps, switch the dumbbell to your other hand, and repeat.

Single-Arm Dumbbell Front Squat

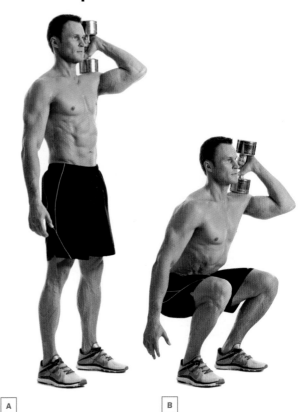

A

B

- Hold a dumbbell in your left hand and let your other arm rest at your side. Rest one of the dumbbell heads on the meatiest part of your left shoulder.
- Keep your body as upright as you can at all times as your left upper arm remains parallel to the floor.

- Brace your abs and lower your body as far as you can by pushing your hips back and bending your knees.
- Pause, then push yourself back to the starting position.
- Do all reps, switch the dumbbell to the other hand, and repeat.

Goblet Squat

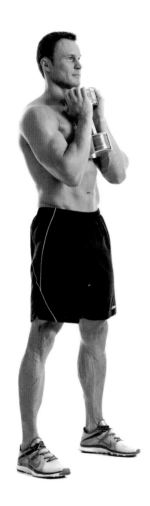

- Hold a dumbbell vertically next to your chest, with both hands cupping the dumbbell head.

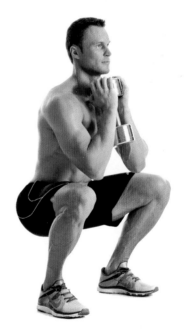

B

- Push your hips back and lower your body into a squat until your upper thighs are at least parallel to the floor. Your elbows should brush the insides of your knees in the bottom position.
- Pause, then press your body back up to the starting position.

Lower Body Exercises

Seal Jack

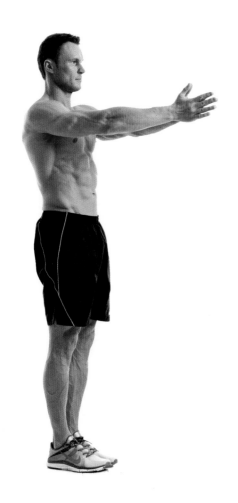
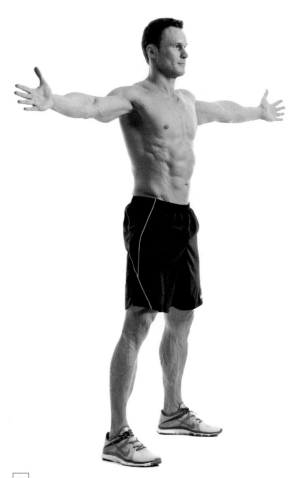

A

- Stand tall with your feet closer than shoulder-width apart, a slight bend in your knees, and your arms at your sides.

B

- Dip your knees and immediately hop up into the air and drop down into a squat so that your feet are wider than shoulder-width apart and your toes are pointing slightly outward. In the bottom position, your hands should be on the inner portion of your thighs and pressing your knees outward.

- Pause, and then jump back up to the starting position.

Box Jump

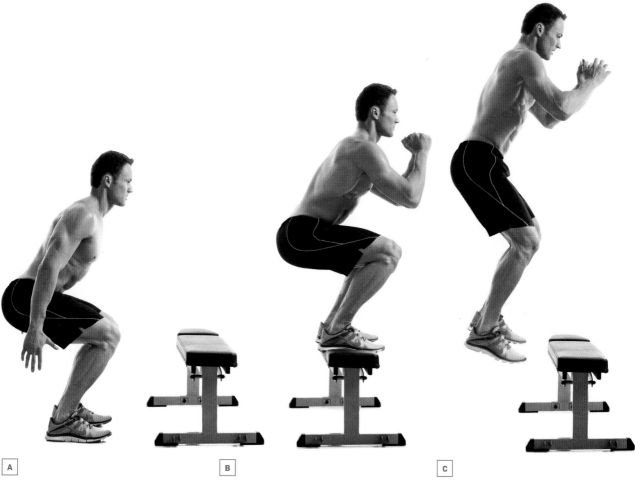

A
- Stand in front of a sturdy, secure box that's high enough so that you have to jump with great effort in order to land on top of it. Your feet should be shoulder-width apart.

B
- Dip your knees, and then explosively jump into the air and land on the top of the box with a "soft" landing.

C
- Step down and return to the starting position.

Lower Body Exercises

Dumbbell Squat Jump

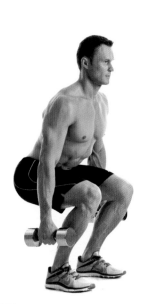
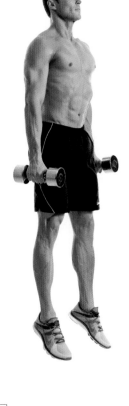

 A

 B

- Grab a pair of dumb-bells and hold them at your sides. Stand in front of a sturdy, secure box that's high enough so that you have to jump with great effort in order to land on top of it. Your feet should be shoulder-width apart.

- Dip your knees, and then explosively jump into the air and land on the top of the box with a "soft" landing.

- Step down and return to the starting position.

One-Arm Dumbbell Sumo Front Squat

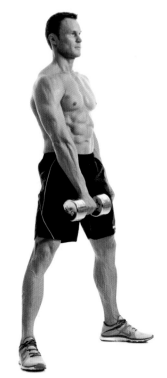
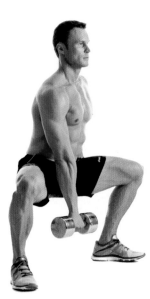

A

B

- Grab a dumbbell in one hand and hold it at arm's length in front of your waist.

- Set your feet about twice shoulder-width with your toes turned slightly outward.

- Push your hips back and lower your body into a squat until your upper thighs are at least parallel to the floor.

- Pause, then press your body back up to the starting position.

Calf Raise

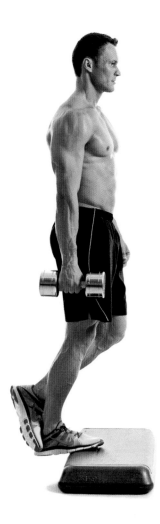

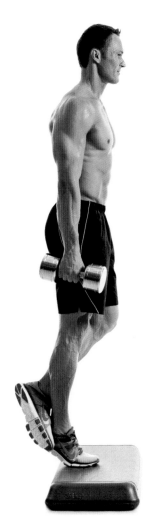

 A

- Grab a dumbbell in your right hand and stand on a step or weight plate.
- Cross your left foot behind your right ankle, and balance your body on the ball of your right foot, with your right heel on the floor or hanging off the step.

 B

- Lift your right heel as high as you can.
- Pause, then lower and repeat.
- Complete the prescribed number of reps with your right leg, then do the same number with your left leg while holding the dumbbell in your left hand.

Lower Body Exercises

Overhead Split Squat

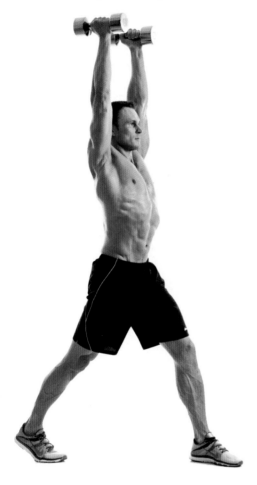

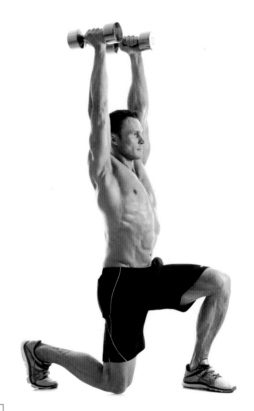

A

- Hold a pair of dumbbells directly over your shoulders, with your arms completely straight. Squeeze your abs tight for the entire exercise. Stand in a staggered stance, your left foot in front of your right foot.

B

- Push your hips back and bend your knees so you lower your body into a squat.
- Pause, then push yourself back up to the starting position.
- Perform the prescribed number of reps, and then do the same number of reps with your right foot in front of your left.

Split Jump

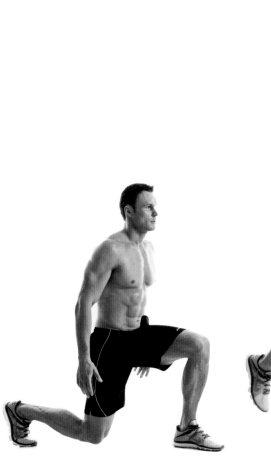

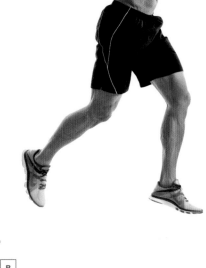

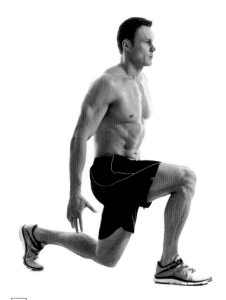

A

- Stand in a staggered stance, your left foot in front of your right foot.
- Lower your body as far as you can.

B

- Quickly jump into the air with enough force that you can switch the direction of your feet in the air.

C

- Land with your right foot in front of your left.
- Lower your body and repeat.
- Continue alternating back and forth with each repetition.

Lower Body Exercises

Dumbbell Split Jump

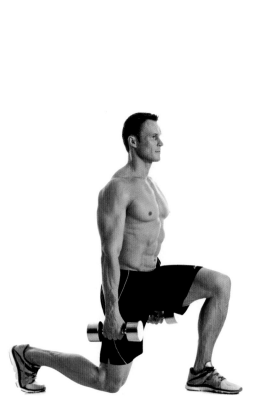
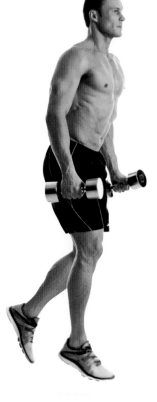
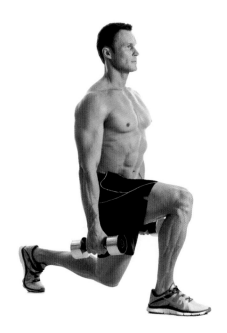

A

- Hold a pair of dumbbells at arm's length next to your sides, your palms facing each other. Stand in a staggered stance, your left foot in front of your right foot.
- Lower your body as far as you can.

B

- Quickly jump into the air with enough force that you can switch the direction of your feet in the air.

C

- Land with your right foot in front of your left.
- Lower your body and repeat.
- Continue alternating back and forth with each repetition.

Dumbbell Walking Lunge

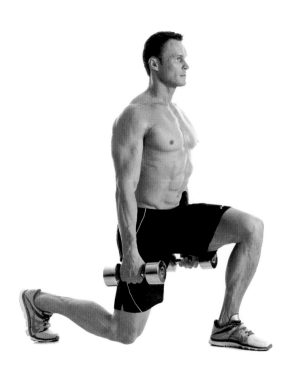

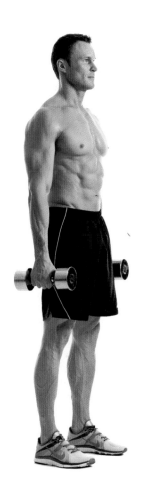

 A

- Grab a pair of dumbbells and hold them at arm's length next to your sides, your palms facing each other.
- Step forward with your left leg and slowly lower your body until your front knee is bent at least 90 degrees.

 B

- Pause, then push yourself to the starting position as quickly as you can.
- Complete the prescribed number of reps with your left leg, then do the same number with your right leg.

Lower Body Exercises

Bodyweight Lunge

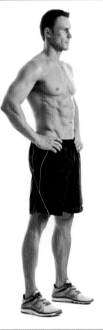

A

- Place your hands on your hips, pull your shoulders back, and stand as tall as you can.

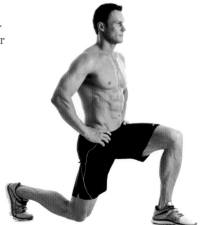

B

- Step forward with your left leg and slowly lower your body until your front knee is bent at least 90 degrees.
- Pause, then push yourself back to the starting position as quickly as you can.
- Complete the prescribed number of reps with your left leg, then do the same number with your right leg.

Dumbbell Lateral Lunge

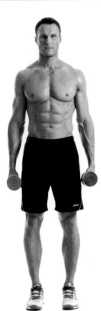

A

- Hold a pair of dumbbells at arm's length next to your sides, your palms facing each other.

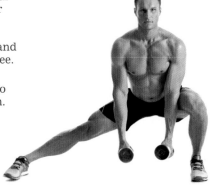

B

- Lift your left foot and take a big step to your left as you push your hips backward and lower your body by dropping your hips and bending your left knee.
- Pause, then quickly push yourself back to the starting position.

▮Bodyweight Lateral Lunge

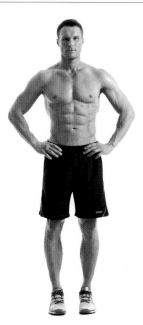

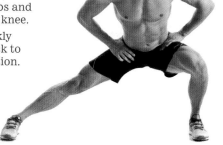

A

- Place your hands on your hips, pull your shoulders back, and stand as tall as you can.

B

- Lift your left foot and take a big step to your left as you push your hips backward and lower your body by dropping your hips and bending your left knee.
- Pause, then quickly push yourself back to the starting position.

▮One-Dumbbell Lunge

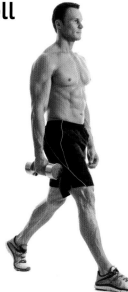

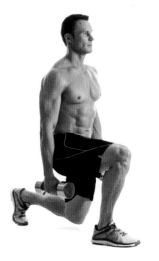

A

- Grab a dumbbell in one hand and hold it at arm's length next to your side, your palm facing your body.
- Step forward with your right leg.

B

- Slowly lower your body until your front knee is bent at least 90 degrees.
- Pause, then push yourself back to the starting position as quickly as you can.
- Repeat with your other leg.
- Complete the prescribed number of reps, alternating legs, then switch the dumbbell to the other hand and repeat.

Lower Body Exercises

█ Cross-Behind Lunge

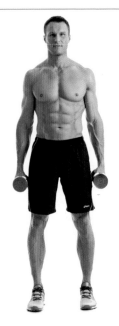

A

- Grab a pair of dumbbells and hold them at arm's length next to your sides, your palms facing each other.

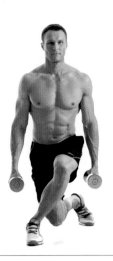

B

- Step forward and to the side so that your lead foot ends up in front of your back foot (like a curtsy).
- Lower your body until your front knee is bent at least 90 degrees.
- Pause, then return to the starting position and repeat with your other leg.

█ Goblet Reverse Lunge

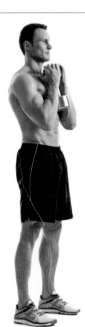

A

- Hold a dumbbell vertically next to your chest, with both hands cupping the dumbbell head.

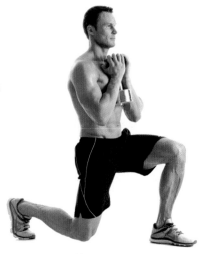

B

- Step backward with your right leg.
- Lower your body into a lunge until your front leg is bent 90 degrees. Pause, then return to the starting position.
- Do all your reps and then repeat with your other leg.

▮One-Dumbbell Reverse Lunge

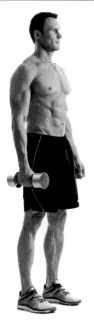

A

- Grab a dumbbell in your right hand.

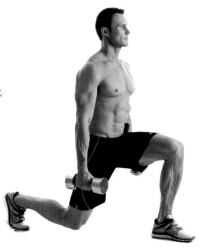

B

- Step backward with your right leg.

- Lower your body into a lunge until your front leg is bent 90 degrees. Pause, then return to the starting position.

- Do all your reps, and then move the weight to your other hand and repeat with your other leg.

▮Reverse Lunge and Rotate

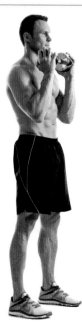

A

- Grab a dumbbell and hold it by the ends, just below your chin. Stand tall with your feet less than shoulder-width apart.

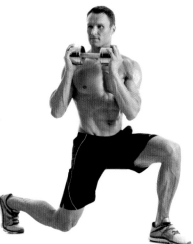

B

- Step backward with your right leg and lower your body into a lunge until your front leg is bent 90 degrees. As you lunge, rotate your upper body toward the same side as the leg you're using to step backward.

- Pause, then return to the starting position.

- Repeat on your other leg, and continue alternating back and forth.

Lower Body Exercises

▍Bulgarian Split Squat

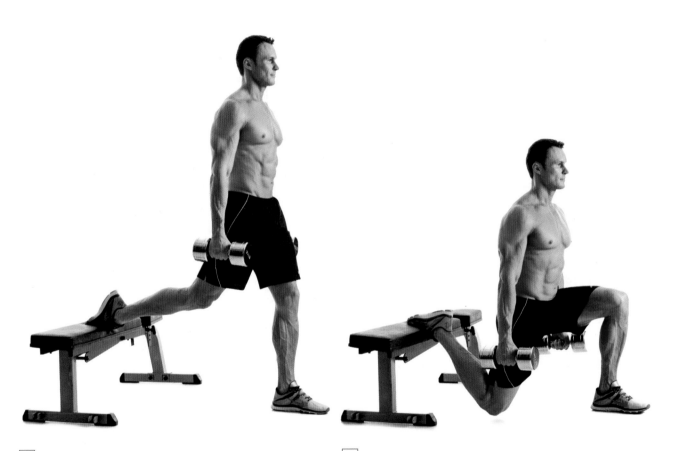

A

- Hold a pair of dumbbells at arm's length next to your sides, your palms facing each other.
- Stand in a staggered stance with your left foot in front of your right, and place the instep of your back foot on a bench.

B

- Lower your body as far as you can, pause, then push your body back up to the starting position.
- Do all reps with your left foot forward, then do the same number with your right foot in front of your left.

Dumbbell Deadlift

A

- Set a pair of dumbbells on the floor in front of you.
- Bend at your hips and knees, and grab the dumbbells with an overhand grip.

B

- Without allowing your lower back to round, stand up with the dumbbells and thrust your hips forward.
- Lower your body back to the starting position.

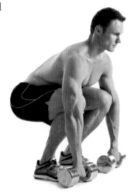

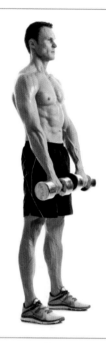

Snatch Grip Deadlift

A

- Load a barbell and roll it up against your shins.
- Bend at your hips and knees, and grab the bar with an overhand grip that's about twice shoulder width.

B

- Without allowing your lower back to round, stand up, thrust your hips forward, and squeeze your glutes.
- Pause, then lower the bar back to the floor while keeping it as close to your body as possible.

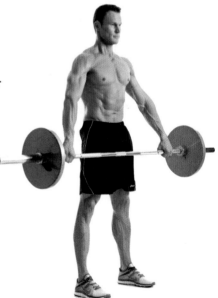

Lower Body Exercises

Barbell Romanian Deadlift

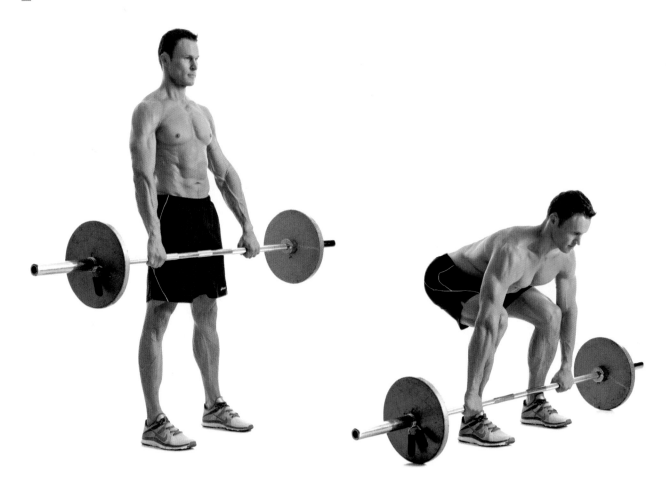

A

- Grab a barbell with an overhand grip that's just beyond shoulder width and hold it at arm's length in front of your hips. Your knees should be slightly bent and chest pushed out. This is the starting position.

B

- Without changing the bend in your knees, bend at your hips and lower your torso until it's almost parallel to the floor.
- Pause, then raise your torso back to the starting position.

One-Dumbbell Single-Leg Romanian Deadlift

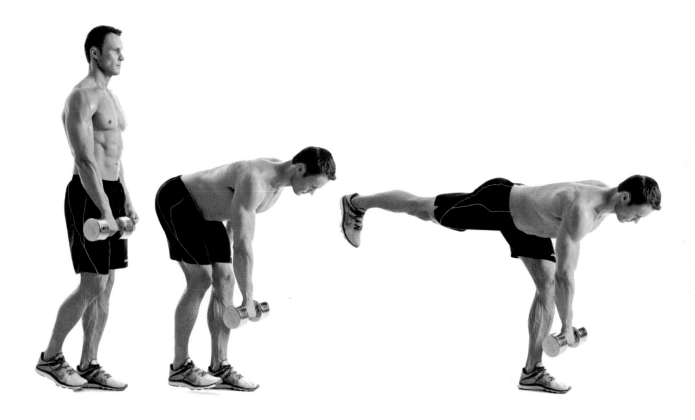

A
- Grab a dumbbell in your right hand, and hold it at arm's length in front of your thighs. Stand with your feet hip-width apart and your knees slightly bent. Balance on your left leg.

B
- Without changing the bend in your knee, bend at your hips and lower your torso until it's almost parallel to the floor.

C
- Pause, then raise your torso back to the starting position.
- Perform all reps, then hold the dumbbell in your left hand and balance on your right leg and repeat.

Lower Body Exercises

Single-Leg Barbell Romanian Deadlift

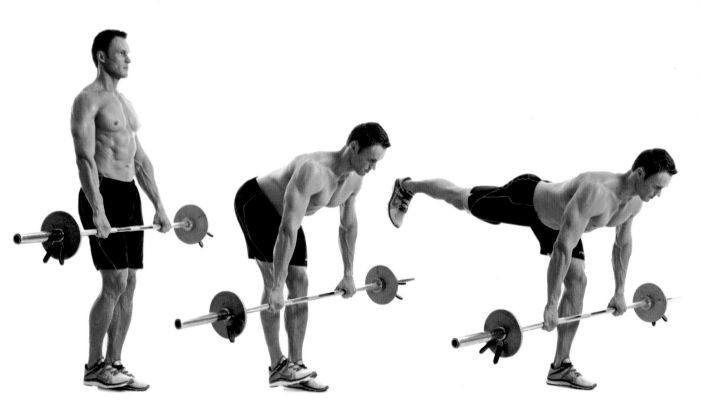

A
- Grab a barbell with an overhand grip that's just beyond shoulder-width and hold it at arm's length in front of your hips. Your knees should be slightly bent and chest pushed out. This is the starting position. Balance on one leg.

B
- Without changing the bend in your knees, bend at your hips and lower your torso until it's almost parallel to the floor.

C
- Pause, then raise your torso back to the starting position.
- Perform all reps, then balance on your other leg and repeat.

■Dumbbell Romanian Deadlift

A

- Grab a pair of dumbbells with an overhand grip and hold them at arm's length in front of your thighs. Stand with your feet hip-width apart and your knees slightly bent.

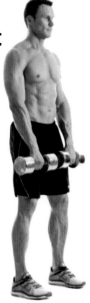

B

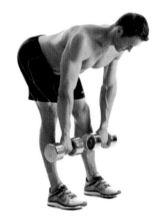

- Without changing the bend in your knees, bend at your hips and lower your torso until it's almost parallel to the floor.
- Pause, then raise your torso back to the starting position.

■Sumo Deadlift

A

- Load a barbell and roll it up against your shins. Set your feet about twice shoulder-width apart with your toes pointed out an angle.
- Bend at your hips and knees, and grab the center of the bar with an overhand grip and your hands about 12 inches apart.

B

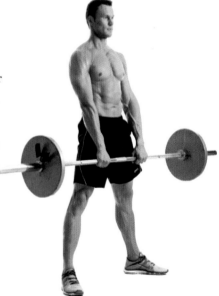

- Without allowing your lower back to round, stand up, thrust your hips forward, and squeeze your glutes.
- Pause, then lower the bar back to the floor while keeping it as close to your body as possible.

Lower Body Exercises

▌Barbell Hip Raise

A

- Sit on the floor with your upper back against a stable bench, your knees bent and feet flat on the floor.
- Put a padded barbell across your hips and grab the barbell with an overhand grip, about shoulder-width apart.

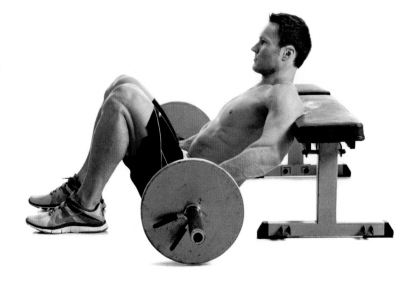

B

- Keeping your back against the bench and the barbell just below your pelvis, raise your hips—while squeezing your glutes—until your hips are in line with your body.
- Return to the starting position and repeat.

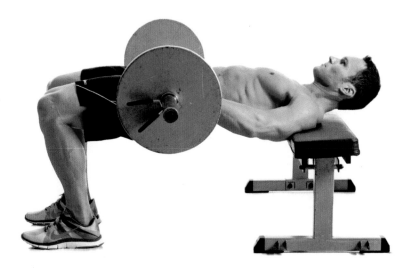

■ Single-Leg Hip Raise

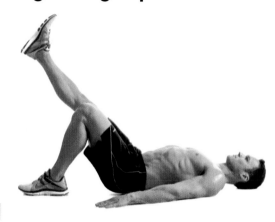

A

- Lie faceup on the floor with your left knee bent and your right leg straight.
- Raise your right leg until it's in line with your left thigh and place your arms out to the sides.

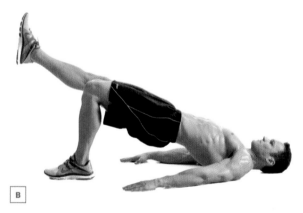

B

- Pushing with your left foot through your heel, push your hips upward, keeping your right leg elevated.
- Pause, then slowly lower your body and leg back to the starting position.
- Complete the prescribed number of reps with your right leg, then switch legs and do the same number with your left leg.

■ Hip Raise

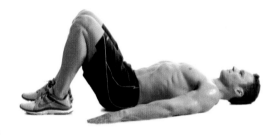

A

- Lie faceup on the floor with your knees bent and your feet flat on the floor.

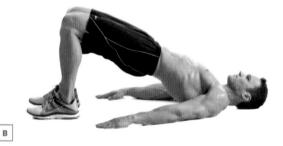

B

- Raise your hips so your body forms a straight line from your shoulders to your knees.
- Pause in the up position, then lower your body back to the starting position.

Lower Body Exercises

▍Resistance Band Hip Raise

- Place a mini resistance band just above your knees, and lie faceup on the floor with your knees bent and your feet flat on the floor.

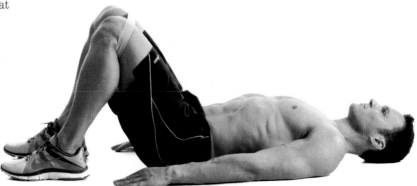

- Press your knees outward against the band and raise your hips so your body forms a straight line from your shoulders to your knees.
- Pause in the up position, then lower your body back to the starting position.

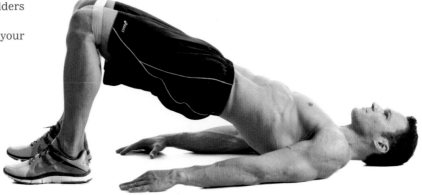

▮ Swiss Ball Hip Raise and Leg Curl

A

- Lie faceup on the floor, and place your lower legs and heels on a Swiss ball.

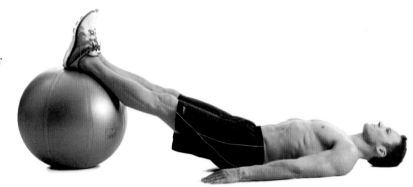

B

- Push your hips up so that your body forms a straight line from your shoulders to your knees.

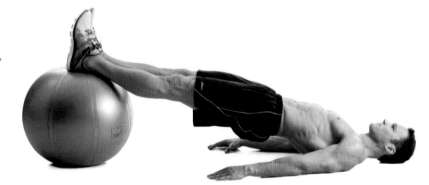

C

- Pull your heels toward your body and roll the ball as close as possible to your butt.
- Pause, then reverse the motion and roll the ball back until your body is in a straight line.
- Lower your hips to the floor and repeat.

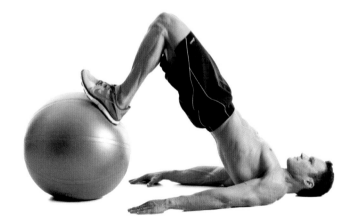

Lower Body Exercises

█ Stepup

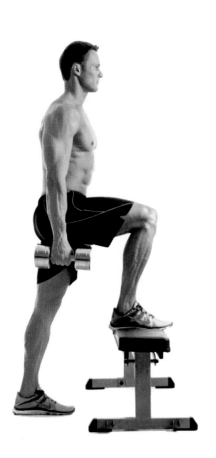

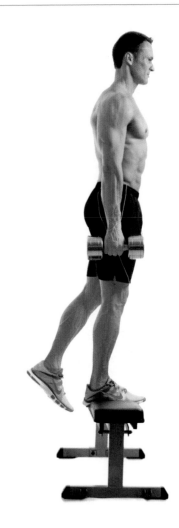

A

- Grab a pair of dumbbells and hold them at arm's length at your sides.
- Stand in front of a step or bench and place your right foot firmly on the step. The step should be high enough that your knee is bent 90 degrees.

B

- Press your right heel into the step, and push your body up until your right leg is straight and you're standing on one leg on the step, keeping your left foot elevated.
- Lower your body back down until your left foot touches the floor. That's 1 rep.
- Complete the prescribed number of reps with your right leg, then do the same number with your left.

Crossover Stepup

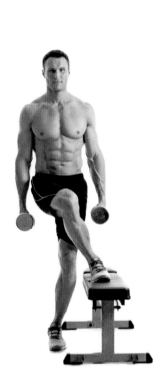
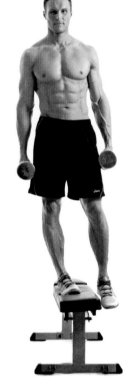

A

- Grab a pair of dumb-bells and stand with your left side next to a step that's at knee height.
- Cross your right foot over your left and place it on the step.

B

- Press through your right heel and push your body up onto the step until both legs are straight.
- Lower your body back to the starting position.
- Perform the prescribed number of reps with your right leg, then switch to your left leg and repeat.

Lateral Band Walk

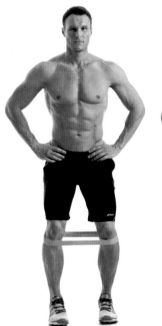
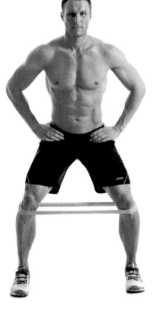

A

- Place both legs between a mini resistance band and position the band just below your knees.

B

- Take small steps to your right for the prescribed number of reps.
- Sidestep back to your left for the same number of reps. That's 1 set.

Lower Body Exercises

█ Side-Lying Clam

A

- Lie on the floor on your left side, with your hips and knees bent 45 degrees. Your right leg should be on top of your left leg, your heels together.

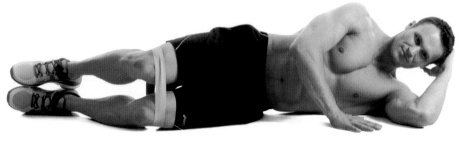

B

- Keeping your feet in contact with each other and your left leg on the floor, raise your right knee as high as you can without moving your pelvis.
- Pause, then return to the starting position.
- Do all reps, then roll to your other side and repeat.

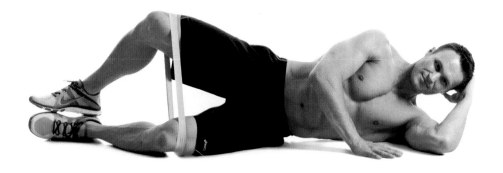

Back Extension

- Position yourself in the back-extension station and hook your feet under the leg anchors.

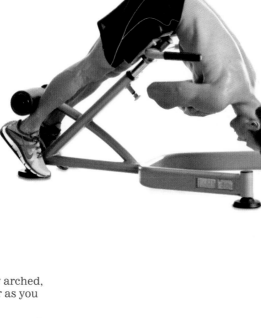

B

- Keeping your back naturally arched, lower your upper body as far as you comfortably can.
- Squeeze your glutes and raise your torso until it's in line with your lower body.
- Pause, then slowly lower your torso back to the starting position.

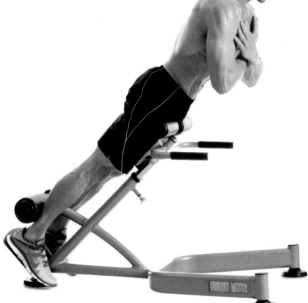

Lower Body Exercises

Three-Way Ankle Mobilization

A

- Set up in a split stance with your front foot about 4 inches away from a wall. You can place your hands on the wall for support.

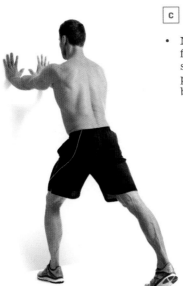

C

- Now drive your knee forward and inward slightly so that it passes over your big toe.

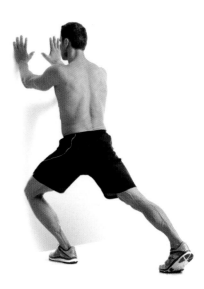

B

- Keeping the heel of your front foot down, slowly drive your knee forward as far as you can. Pause for a second and return to the starting position.

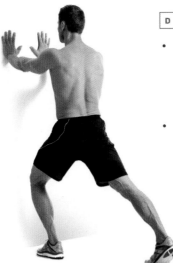

D

- Finally, drive your knee forward and outward slightly so that it passes over your pinky toe. Then switch sides.
- You may feel a stretch in your calves as you drive your knee forward.

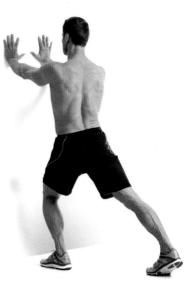

■ Mini-Band Resisted Single-Leg Stance

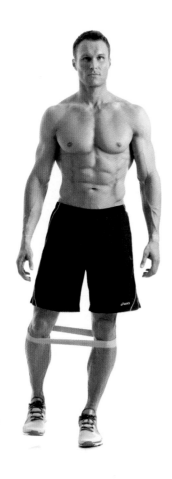

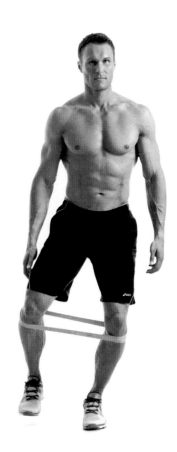

- Stand with your feet shoulder-width apart with a mini-band around your legs just below your knees.
- Lift one foot off the ground and sit down into a quarter squat position with the other leg.

B

- Actively pull the knee of the squatting leg outward so that it points toward your pinky toe. You should feel the outside of that hip engage.
- Hold this position for 10 seconds, then return to the starting position.
- Repeat for each side. Progress to lower depths until you reach a half squat position.

Lower Body Exercises

Rear Foot Elevated Hip Flexor Stretch

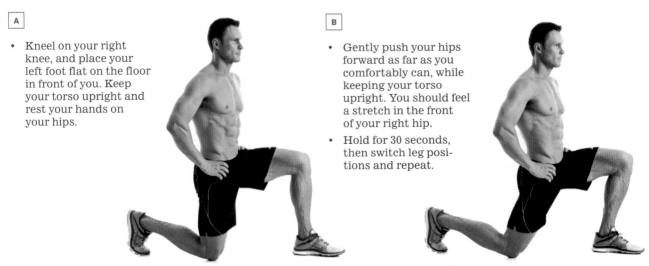

A
- Kneel on your right knee, and place your left foot flat on the floor in front of you. Keep your torso upright and rest your hands on your hips.

B
- Gently push your hips forward as far as you comfortably can, while keeping your torso upright. You should feel a stretch in the front of your right hip.
- Hold for 30 seconds, then switch leg positions and repeat.

Hip Thrust with Bench

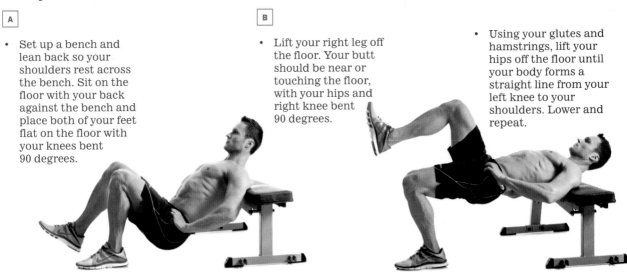

A
- Set up a bench and lean back so your shoulders rest across the bench. Sit on the floor with your back against the bench and place both of your feet flat on the floor with your knees bent 90 degrees.

B
- Lift your right leg off the floor. Your butt should be near or touching the floor, with your hips and right knee bent 90 degrees.
- Using your glutes and hamstrings, lift your hips off the floor until your body forms a straight line from your left knee to your shoulders. Lower and repeat.

Single-Leg Squat

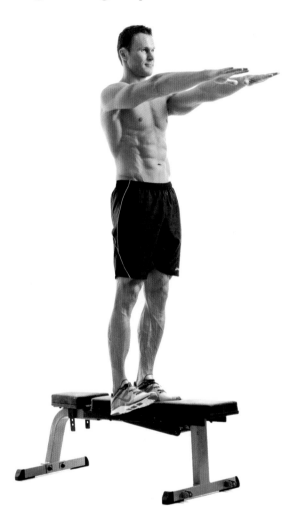

A

- Stand on a bench or box that's about knee height. Hold your arms straight out in front of you.

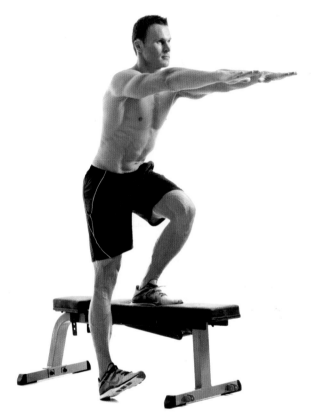

B

- Balancing on your left foot, bend your left knee and slowly lower your body until your right heel lightly touches the floor.
- Pause, then push yourself up.

Lower Body Exercises

▎Spiderman Lunge

A

- Assume the classic pushup position with your hands directly beneath your shoulders, your legs straight, and your abs braced.

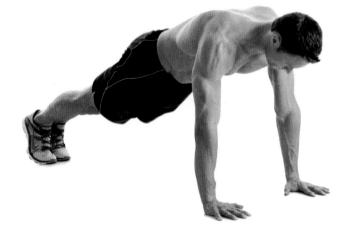

B

- Lift your right foot off the floor, bending your knee, and place the foot outside your right hand.
- Return to the starting position and lunge out with your left leg.

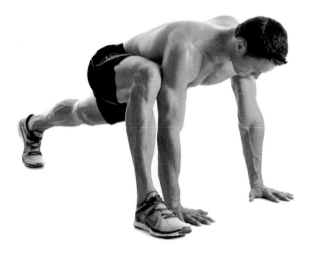

▌Diagonal Hip Rock to Step

- Begin on all fours with your hands beneath your shoulders and your knees beneath your hips.

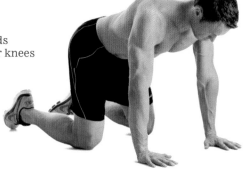

B

- Keep your back flat as you reach back diagonally away from your body with one leg. Pause in this position for a second to feel a stretch in the outside of your front hip.

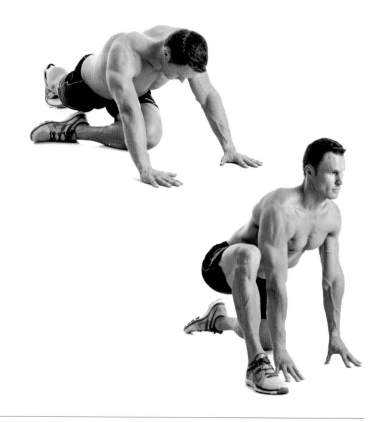

C

- Then pull your leg forward and place your foot on the ground outside your hands.
- Pull your chest forward, and pause for a second to feel a stretch in the front of your back hip and the bottom of your front leg.

Lower Body Exercises

Backward Monster Walk

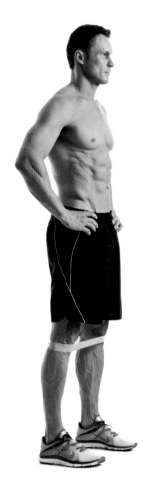

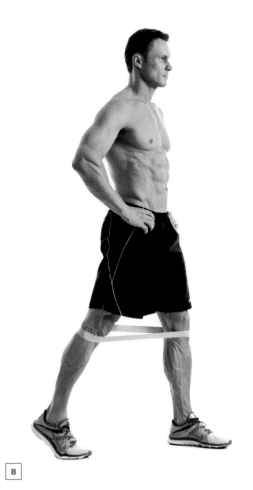

A

- Start with your feet shoulder-width apart, hands on your hips, and a mini-band wrapped around your legs just beneath your knees.

B

- Keeping your hips level with the floor, your knees pulled out, and your feet outside of your shoulders, take a step back with one leg so that the toes of that foot are level with the heel of the front foot.

- Repeat with the other leg. Continue for 15 to 20 yards. You should feel the muscles on the outside and back of your hips engage.

Trap Bar Deadlift

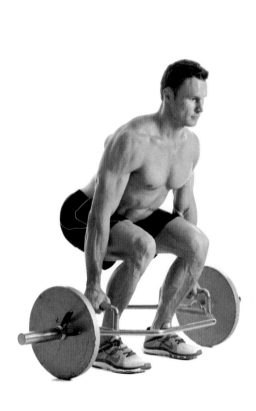

A

- Load a trap bar with weight and stand between the trap bar handles with your feet about hip-width apart.
- Bend down and grab the bar outside your knees. Your shoulders should be over the bar.

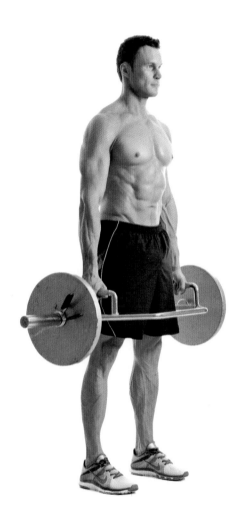

B

- Keeping your lower back in its natural arch, drive your heels into the floor and push your hips forward, lifting the bar until it's in front of your thighs.
- Return to the starting position.

Lower Body Exercises

Kettlebell Squat

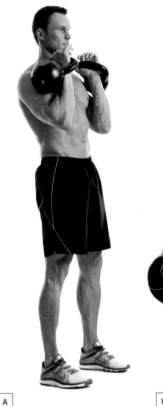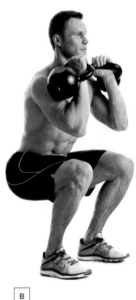

A

- Hold a kettlebell in each hand and raise your arms, with your elbows bent 90 degrees so that the kettlebells rest just above and in front of your shoulders.
- Keep your body as upright as you can at all times as your upper arms remain parallel to the floor.

B

- Brace your abs and lower your body as far as you can by pushing your hips back and bending your knees.
- Pause, then push yourself back to the starting position.

Dumbbell Reverse Lunge

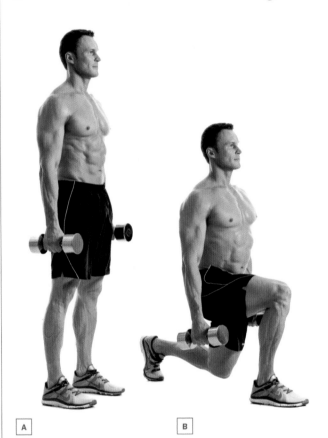

A

- Grab a pair of dumbbells and hold them at arm's length at the sides of your body.
- Step backward with your left leg.

B

- Lower your body into a lunge until your front leg is bent 90 degrees. Pause, then return to the starting position.

■ Barbell Bulgarian Split Squat

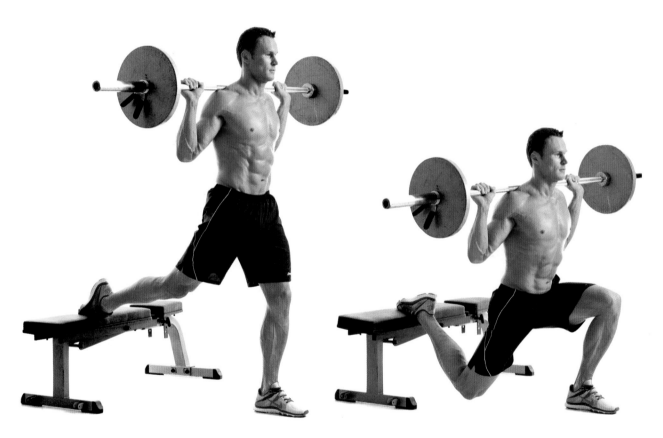

A

- Hold a pair of dumbbells at arm's length next to your sides, your palms facing each other.
- Stand in a staggered stance with your left foot in front of your right. Place the instep of your back foot on a bench.

B

- Lower your body as far as you can, pause, then push your body back up to the starting position.
- Do all reps with your left foot forward, then do the same number with your right foot in front of your left.

Lower Body Exercises

▌Kettlebell Romanian Deadlift

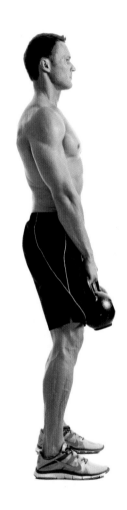

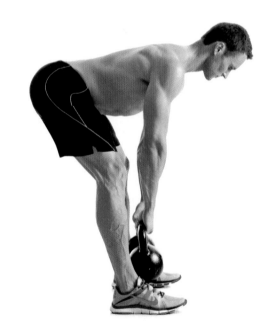

A

- Grab a pair of kettlebells and hold them at arm's length in front of your thighs. Stand with your feet hip-width apart and your knees slightly bent.

B

- Without changing the bend in your knees, bend at your hips and lower your torso until it's almost parallel to the floor.
- Pause, then raise your torso back to the starting position.

Plate Push

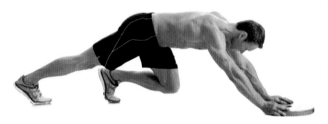

A

- Put a weight plate flat on the floor. Assume a "sprinter's position," making your upper body as close to parallel with the floor as possible. Place your hands on the plate.

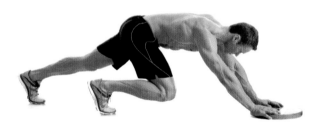

B

- Keeping your back flat and your butt low, drive with your legs to push the plate for the desired distance.

Valslide Hip Raise and Hamstring Curl

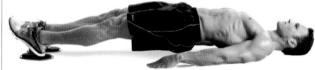

A

- Lie faceup on the floor and place your feet on Valslides.
- Push your hips up so that your body forms a straight line from your shoulders to your knees.

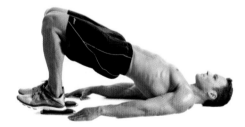

B

- Pull your heels toward your body and as close as possible to your butt.
- Pause, then reverse the motion and push your feet back until your body is in a straight line.
- Lower your hips to the floor and repeat.

Lower Body Exercises

▌Valslide Reverse Lunge

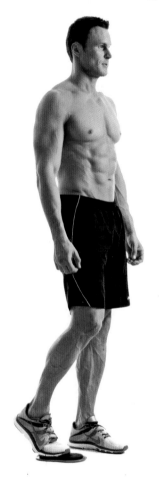

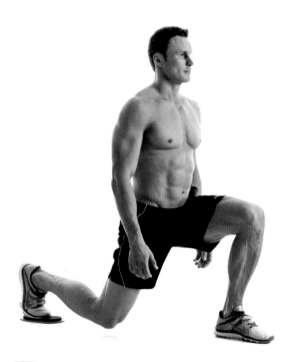

A

- Stand upright and place the ball of your right foot on the middle of the Valslide.

B

- Slide your right foot back until your left knee is bent 90 degrees, then return to the starting position.
- As you stand, press through your left heel, making sure your left leg does all the work bringing your body back to the standing position.
- Do all reps, stand on the Valslide with your left foot, and repeat.

■ Valslide Side Lunge

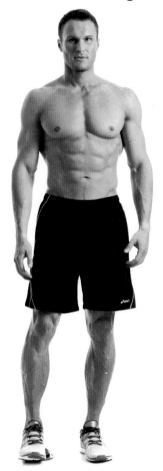

A

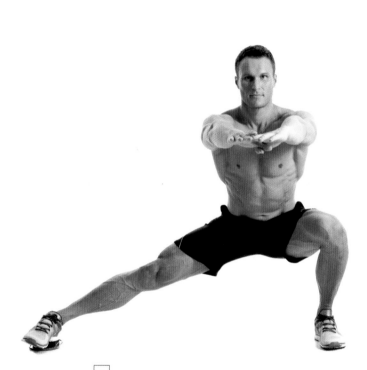

B

- Stand upright and place your right foot on the Valslide.

- Slide your right foot to the side as you push your hips back, bend your left leg, and lower into a squat. Make sure that your toes remain pointing forward and your right leg remains straight.

- Slide your right leg back and return to the starting position.

- Perform all reps and repeat on your other leg.

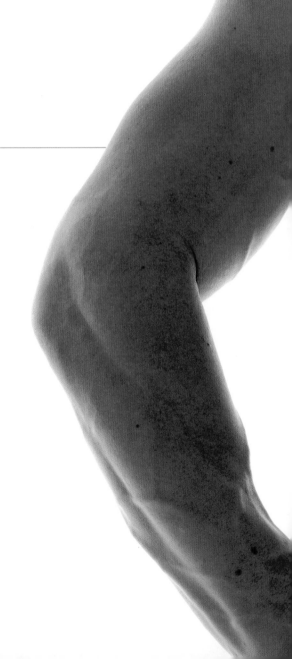

CORE
Exercises

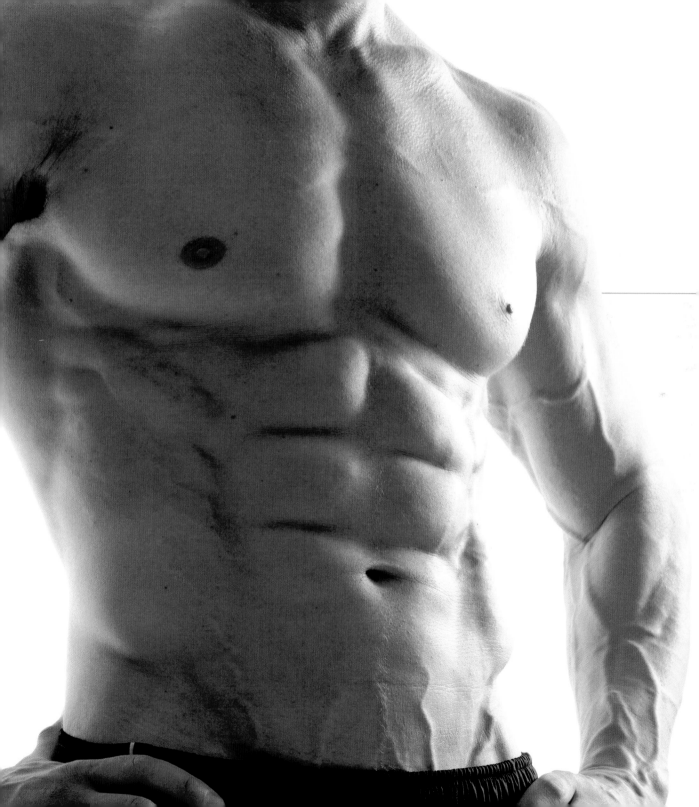

Core Exercises

█ Plank

A

- Start to get in a pushup position, but bend your elbows and rest your weight on your forearms instead of on your hands. Your body should form a straight line from your shoulders to your ankles.

- Brace your core by contracting your abs as if you were about to be punched in the gut.

- Hold this position as directed.

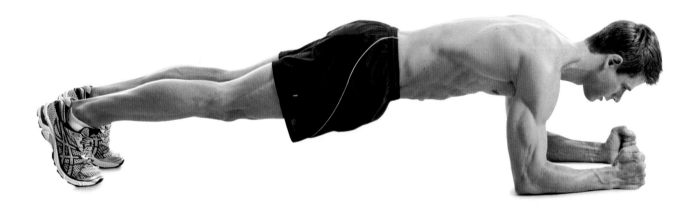

Plank to Pushup

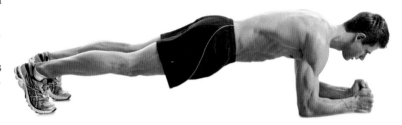

- Start to get in a pushup position, but bend your elbows and rest your weight on your forearms instead of on your hands. Your body should form a straight line from your shoulders to your ankles.
- Brace your core by contracting your abs as if you were about to be punched in the gut.

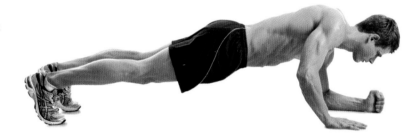

- Press your body up into the top position of a pushup by extending your arms one at a time.

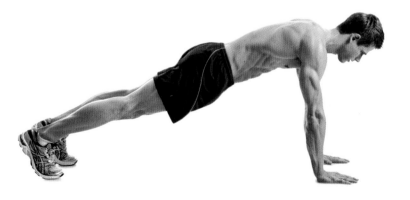

- Pause, then reverse the movement and return to your elbows. That's 1 rep.

Core Exercises

Front Plank with Weight Transfer

A

- Assume the plank position with a light weight to the outside of your right elbow.

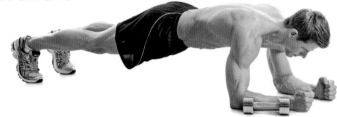

B

- Pick up the weight with your right hand and pass it to your left hand.

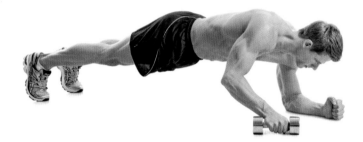

C

- Place the weight to the outside of your left elbow.

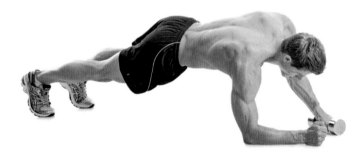

D

- With your left hand, move the weight back to the other side. That's 1 rep.
- Make sure you brace your abs to keep your torso from rotating as you lift the weight.

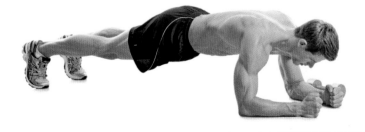

Hands-Free Side Plank

- Lie on your left side with your knees straight.
- Place both of your feet on a bench and cross both of your arms across your chest, so your left shoulder is on the floor.
- Squeeze your glutes and prop your upper body up on your left shoulder. Brace your core by contracting your abs forcefully as if you were about to be punched in the gut.
- Raise your hips until your body forms a straight line from your ankles to your shoulders. Hold for the required duration, then switch sides and repeat.

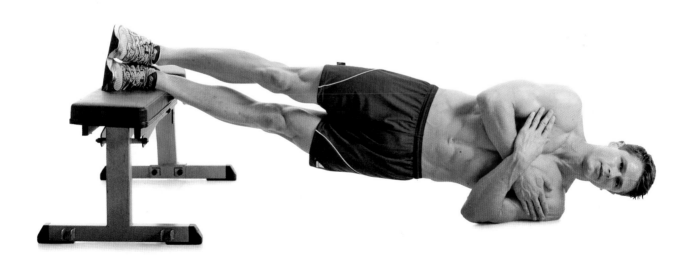

Core Exercises

█ Mountain Climber

A

- Assume a pushup position with your arms completely straight. Your body should form a straight line from your shoulders to your ankles.

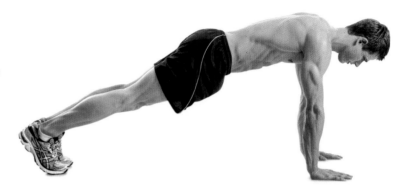

B

- Lift your right foot off the floor and slowly raise your knee as close to your chest as you can.

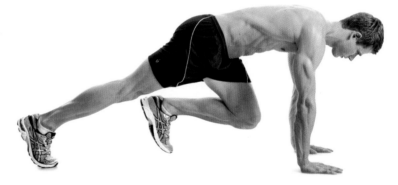

C

- Return to the starting position and repeat with your left leg.
- Continue alternating for the prescribed number of reps or time.

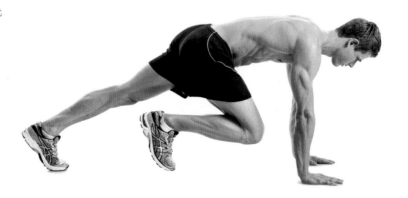

▮Side Plank

A

- Lie on your left side with your knees straight.
- Prop your upper body up on your left elbow and forearm.
- Brace your core by contracting your abs forcefully as if you were about to be punched in the gut.
- Raise your hips until your body forms a straight line from your ankles to your shoulders.
- Hold as directed, then switch sides and repeat.

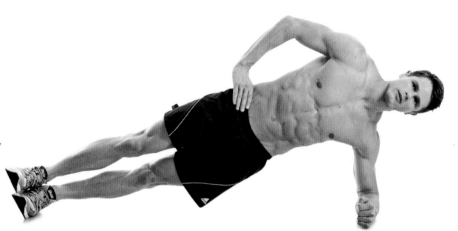

▮Side Plank and Rotate

A

- Lift your body into a side plank, and start with your right arm raised straight above you so that it's perpendicular to the floor.

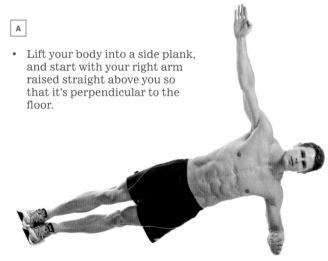

B

- Reach under and behind your torso with your right hand, keeping your abs braced.
- Lift your arm back up to the starting position. That's 1 rep.
- Do all reps, roll onto your other side, and repeat.

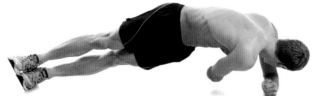

Core Exercises

█Plank Jumping Jack

A

- Start to get in a pushup position, but bend your elbows and rest your weight on your forearms instead of on your hands. Your body should form a straight line from your shoulders to your ankles.
- Brace your core by contracting your abs as if you were about to be punched in the gut.

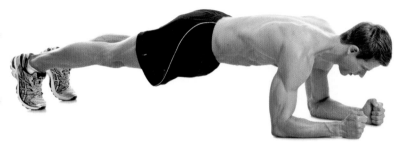

B

- Jump your feet out to the sides as if you were performing a jumping jack, making sure that your upper body doesn't rotate.

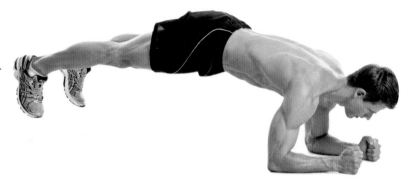

C

- Quickly return your feet to the starting position. That's 1 rep.

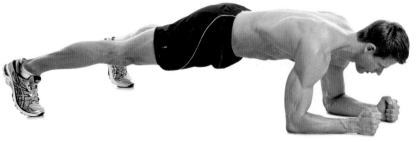

Plank with Arm Extension

A

- Start to get in a pushup position, but bend your elbows and rest your weight on your forearms instead of on your hands. Your body should form a straight line from your shoulders to your ankles.
- Brace your core by contracting your abs as if you were about to be punched in the gut.

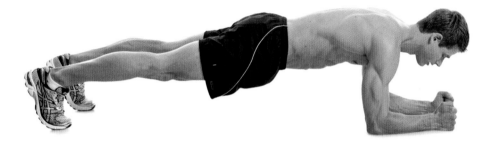

B

- Raise and straighten your left arm, and hold it so that it's parallel to the rest of your body.
- Hold as directed, lower to the starting position, then raise your other arm and repeat.

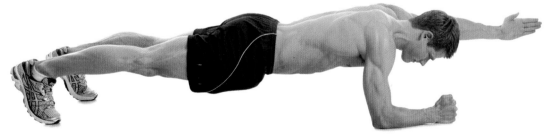

Core Exercises

Lateral Plank Walk

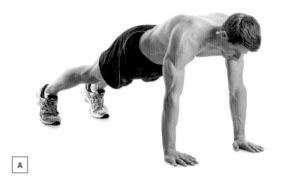

A

- Lower onto all fours and place your weight on your hands so you're in the start position of a pushup.

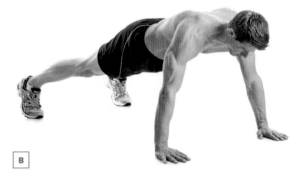

B

- "Walk" your right hand and right foot to the right, followed by your left hand and foot.
- Continue this process for 10 steps. Make sure you keep your abs tight and don't allow your body to rotate.
- Reverse the direction and walk your way back to the starting position.

Alternating Superman Plank and Reach

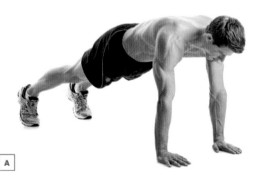

A

- Lower onto all fours and place your weight on your hands so you're in the start position of a pushup. Move your feet so that they're about shoulder-width apart. Your body should form a straight line from your shoulders to your ankles.

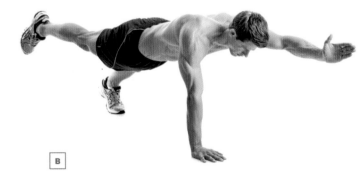

B

- Raise your right foot and left arm off the floor and hold.
- Return to the floor and repeat with your left foot and right arm. That's 1 rep.
- Make sure that when you raise your arm and leg, your body doesn't rotate and your hips don't rise.

■ Planking Frog Tuck

A

- Start in a pushup position with your body straight from your shoulders to your ankles.

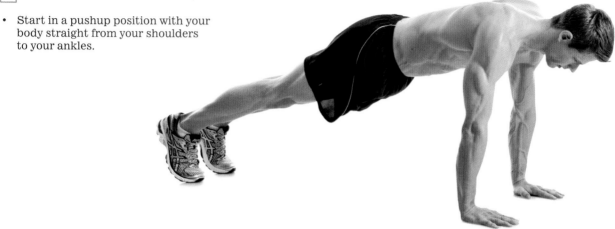

B

- Bring your right foot forward and place it next to your right hand (or as close as you can). Try to prevent your hips from sagging or rising.
- Return your leg to the starting position and repeat with your left leg. That's 1 rep.

Core Exercises

Cross-Body Mountain Climber

A

- Assume a pushup position with your arms completely straight. Your body should form a straight line from your shoulders to your ankles.

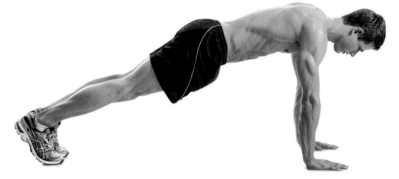

B

- Lift your left knee toward your right elbow before returning back to starting position.

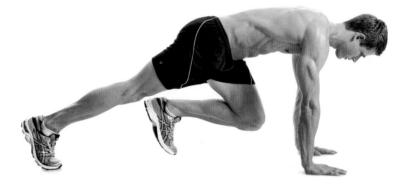

C

- Raise your right knee toward your left elbow. Return back to the starting position. That's 1 rep.

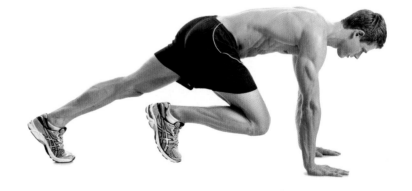

■ One-Leg Plank

- Start to get in a pushup position, but bend your elbows and rest your weight on your forearms instead of on your hands. Your body should form a straight line from your shoulders to your ankles.

B

- Brace your core by contracting your abs as if you were about to be punched in the gut.
- Raise one foot a few inches off the floor and hold.
- Lower your foot and repeat with your other foot. That's 1 set.

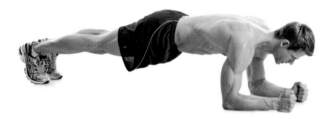
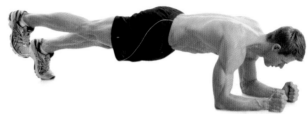

■ Extended Plank

A

- Lower onto all fours and place your weight on your hands so you're in the start position of a pushup. Your body should form a straight line from your shoulders to your ankles.
- Squeeze your abs as if you're about to be punched in the stomach, and hold for the prescribed time.

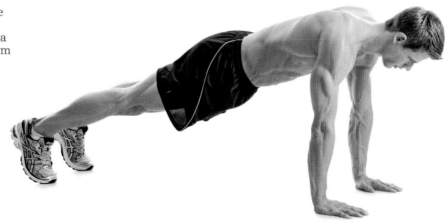

Core Exercises

Side Plank with Row

A

- Attach a handle to the low pulley of a cable machine and grab it with your right hand.
- Brace your core and raise your body into a side plank on your left side.

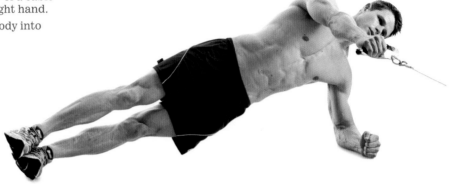

B

- Bend your right elbow and pull the handle to your rib cage, keeping your hips pushed up and forward.
- Slowly straighten your arm back in front of you.
- Complete all reps on your left side, then switch to your right side, grab the handle with your left hand, and repeat.

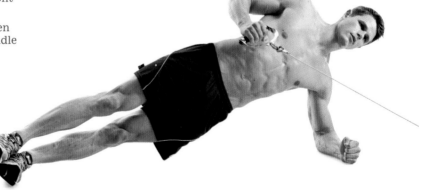

Bird Dog

- Get down on your hands and knees with your palms flat on the floor and shoulder-width apart. Your thighs should be perpendicular to the floor.

B

- Without allowing your lower back to rise or round, squeeze your abs, and raise your left arm and right leg until they're in line with your body.
- Hold for 5 seconds, then return to the starting position.
- Repeat with your right arm and left leg. Continue alternating back and forth.

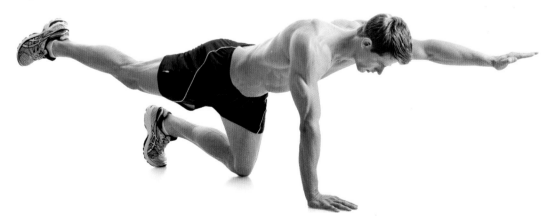

Core Exercises

Rolling Plank

- Begin in a plank position with your body forming a straight line from your shoulders to your ankles.

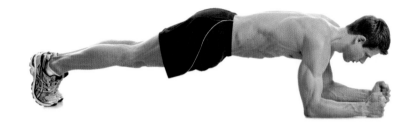

- Rotate to your left side and into a side plank.
- Hold for 10 seconds.

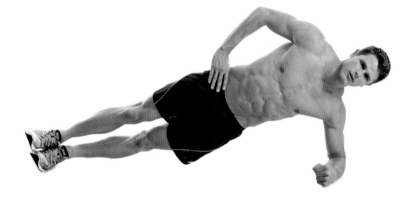

- Rotate into a right side plank and hold for another 10 seconds. That's 1 rep.
- Return to a plank position and repeat.

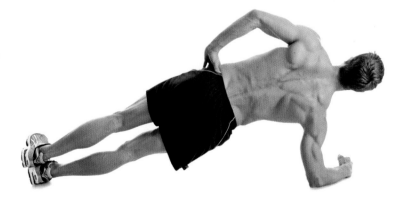

■ Ab Wheel Rollout

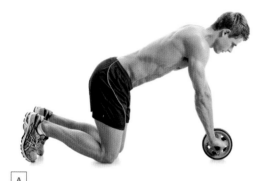

A

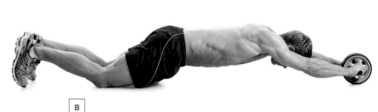

B

- Sit on your knees in front of an ab wheel, and grab the handles of the ab wheel with your arms straight and your body upright.

- Keeping your core braced, slowly roll the wheel forward, straightening your arms and extending your body as far as you can without allowing your lower back to collapse.
- Use your abs to pull the wheel back to your knees.

■ Kneeling Barbell Rollout

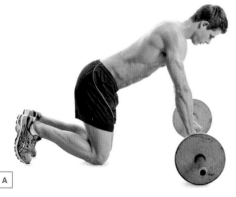

A

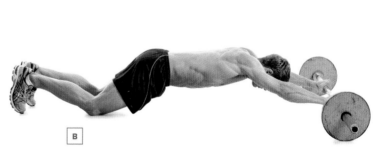

B

- Sit on your knees in front of a loaded barbell, and grab the bar with your hands shoulder-width apart, arms straight, and your body upright.

- Keeping your core braced, slowly roll the barbell forward. Keep your arms straight and extend your body as far as you can without allowing your lower back to collapse.
- Use your abs to pull the barbell back to your knees.

Core Exercises

Lying Scap and Chin Retraction

A

- Lie on your back with your knees bent and feet flat on the ground. Interlock your fingers behind your head.
- Keeping your hands behind your head, actively push your elbows down into the ground. You should feel your shoulder blades squeeze together in the back.
- From here, think of getting tall through the back of your neck as you pull your chin in. Your head should still be on your hands, which are on the ground, and you should feel your neck engage in the front and possibly stretch in the back.
- Hold this position, with your elbows pushed into the ground and chin pulled in, for 5 seconds.

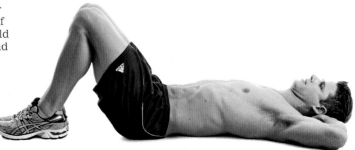

Extension Rotation

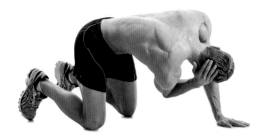

A

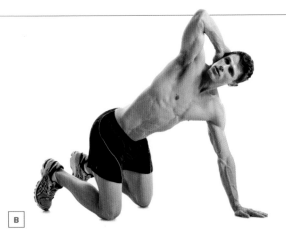

B

- Set up on all fours with your hands beneath your shoulders and your knees beneath your hips.
- Place one hand behind your head. Rotate your eyes and head away from the side of the raised arm and follow through with the arm so that your elbow pulls across your body and under the opposite arm.

- Rotate your eyes and head back toward the side of your raised arm, and follow through with your elbow so that your elbow is pointed up toward the ceiling.
- Your hips and lower back should remain stable throughout the motion. You should feel the rotation of your thoracic spine as you move through the exercise.
- Repeat for 6 to 8 reps, then switch sides.

Knee-Grab Situp

- Lie on your back with your legs straight and arms at your sides, keeping your elbows bent at 90 degrees.

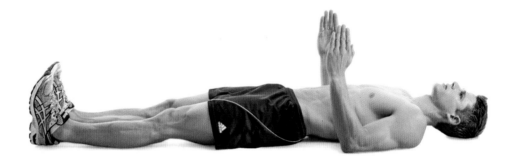

- Perform a situp. As you sit up, bring your knees toward your chest and try to grab just below your kneecaps.
- Lower your body to the starting position, and repeat.

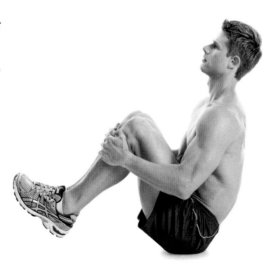

Core Exercises

Tall Kneeling Kettlebell Halo

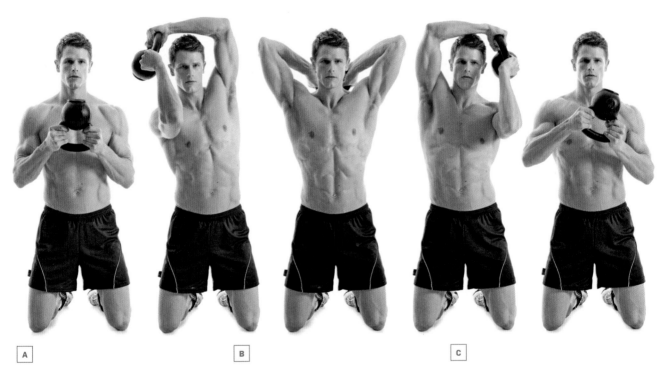

A

- Sit on your knees with your body upright and your core tight. Hold a kettlebell in both hands with the bottom of the bell facing the ceiling.

B

- Your elbows should be bent about 90 degrees and your hands in front of you. In one movement, move the kettlebell in a circular fashion around your head while keeping your elbows bent. Keep your core tight and try to avoid any movement in your upper body.

C

- Make sure you stay as tall as possible, squeeze your glutes, and make the rotation as tight as possible by keeping the bell close to your body. Continue until you complete all reps.

▮Dumbbell Saxon Side Bend

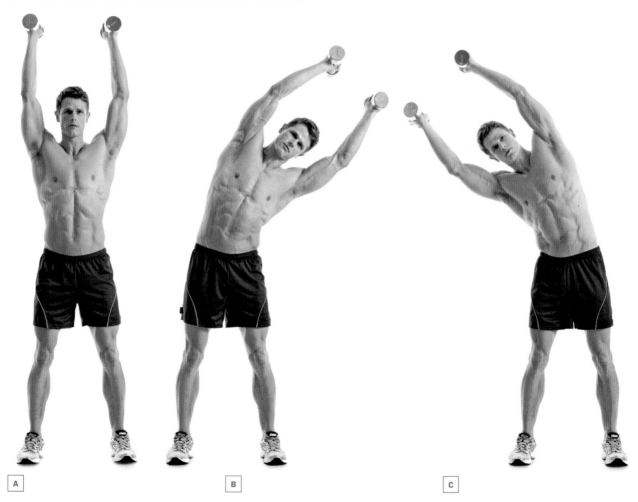

A

- Hold a pair of lightweight dumbbells over your head, in line with your shoulders, with your elbows slightly bent.

B

- Keep your back straight and slowly bend directly to your left side as far as possible without twisting your upper body.

C

- Pause, return to an upright position, then bend to your right side as far as possible.

Core Exercises

Stability Ball Plank with Mini Rollout

A

- Set up in a plank position with your feet shoulder-width apart and your forearms on a stability ball. Your spine should be neutral and your eyes should be looking straight through your hands.
- Think of getting tall through your chest to pull your shoulder blades back and together slightly.

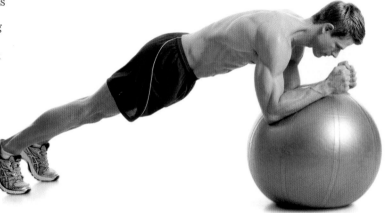

B

- Without losing this position, slowly push the ball a few inches away from you until you feel your core engage.
- Pause here for a second and then return to the starting position.

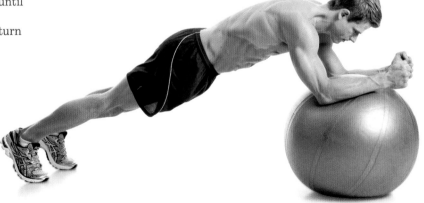

■ Swiss Ball Mountain Climber

- Place your hands on a Swiss ball and assume a pushup position with your arms completely straight. Your body should form a straight line from your shoulders to your ankles.

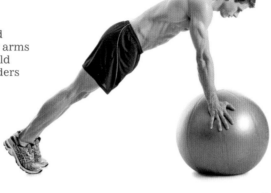

B

- Lift your right foot off the floor and slowly raise your knee as close to your chest as you can.

C

- Return to the starting position and repeat with your left leg.
- Continue alternating for the prescribed number of reps or time.

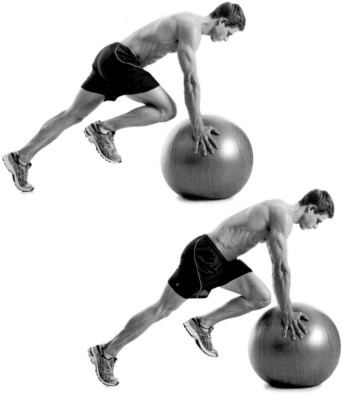

Core Exercises

▌Stability Ball Jackknife

A

- Assume a pushup position with your arms completely straight.
- Rest your shins on a Swiss ball so that your body forms a straight line from your shoulders to your ankles.

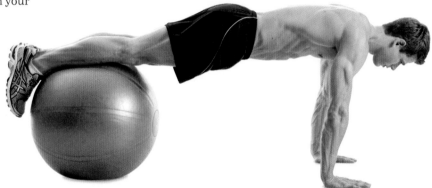

B

- Without changing your lower back posture, roll the Swiss ball toward your chest by pulling it forward with your feet.
- Pause, then return the ball to the starting position by rolling the ball backward.

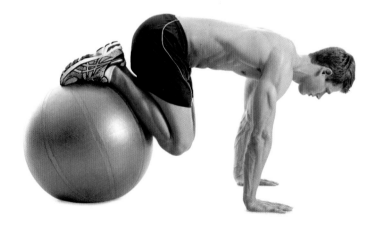

Stability Ball Reverse Leg Lift

A

- Lie on a Swiss ball with your legs bent. Hold on to a sturdy object for support. Your lower back should be in the middle of the ball and your knees slightly bent.

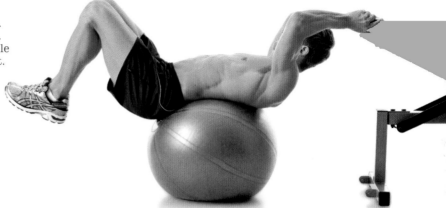

B

- Lift your hips up and bring your knees toward your chest until your legs are perpendicular to the floor.
- Pause, then lower your legs back to the starting position.

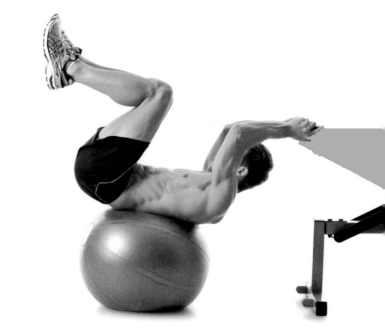

Core Exercises

▌Stability Ball Reaching Crunch

A

- Lie with your hips, lower back, and shoulders in contact with a Swiss ball and hold a weight plate across your chest.

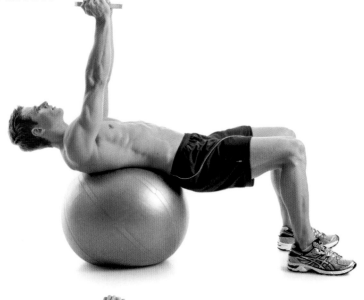

B

- Raise your head and shoulders, and crunch your rib cage toward your pelvis.
- Pause, then return to the starting position.

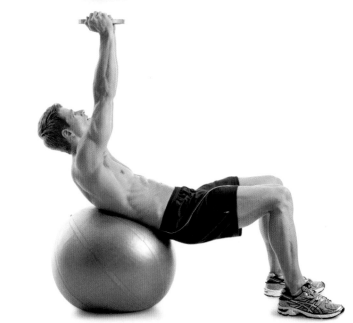

Stability Ball Side Crunch

A

- Lie sideways on your right side on a Swiss ball and brace your right foot against a wall or a heavy object. Place your fingers behind your ears.

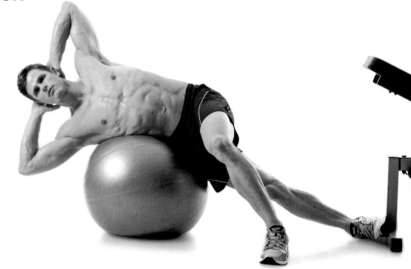

B

- Lift your shoulders and crunch sideways toward your hip.
- Pause, then return to the starting position.
- Complete the prescribed number of reps on that side, then do the same number on your other side.

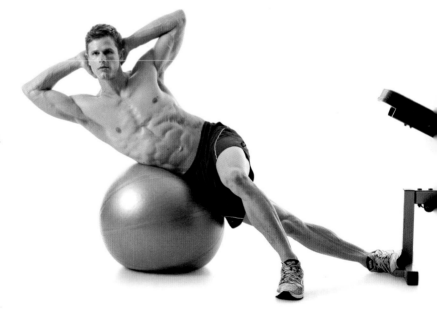

Core Exercises

High Cable Chop

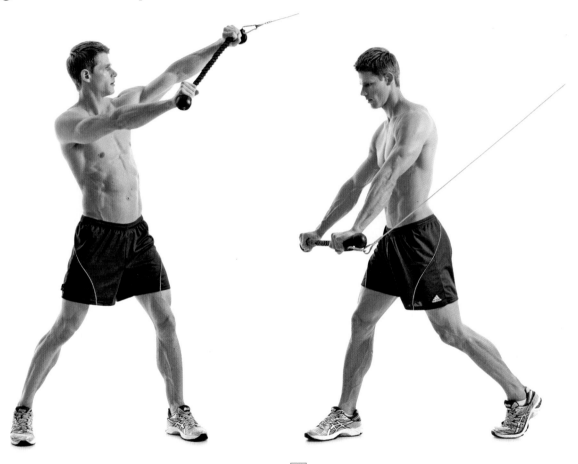

A

- Attach a rope handle to the high pulley of a cable station.
- Stand in a staggered stance with the left side of your body facing the stack and your inside foot in front of your outside foot. Rotate your body to grip the rope with both hands. Your torso should be turned toward the cable machine.

B

- In one movement, pull the rope down and past your left hip as you simultaneously rotate your torso.
- Reverse the movement to return to the starting position.
- Complete the prescribed number of repetitions to your right side, then do the same number with your right side facing the stack, pulling toward your right.

▍Low Cable Lift

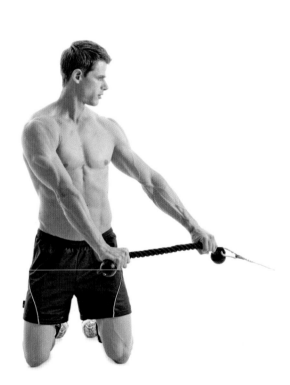

- Attach a rope handle to the low pulley of a cable station.
- Kneel down next to the handle so that your left side faces the weight stack.

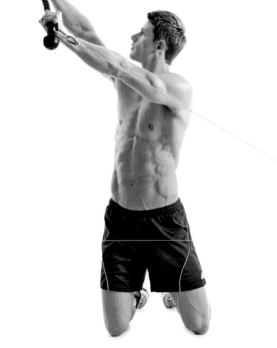

- Brace your core and rotate your body to grip the rope with both hands. Your shoulders should be turned toward the cable machine. Keep your torso upright for the entire movement.
- In one movement, pull the rope past your right shoulder as you simultaneously rotate your torso to the right.
- Reverse the movement to return to the starting position.

Core Exercises

▊Dumbbell Chop

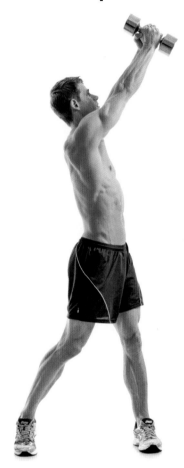

- Grab a dumbbell and hold it with both hands above your left shoulder. Rotate your torso to your left.

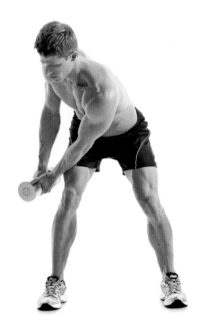

- Swing the dumbbell down and to the outside of your right knee by rotating to the right and bending at your hips.
- Reverse the movement to return to the start.
- Complete the prescribed number of reps toward your right side, then do the same number on your left side, holding the dumbbell over your right shoulder.

◼ Dumbbell Reverse Chop (Low to High)

◼ Resistance Band Chop

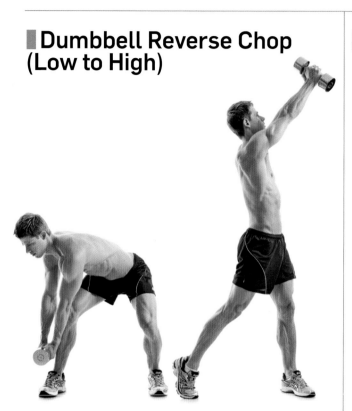

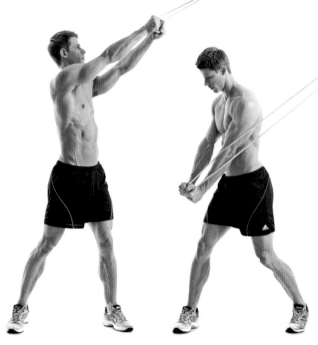

A

B

A

B

- Stand with your feet shoulder-width apart. Grab a dumbbell and hold it with both hands just outside and below your knee.

- Brace your core, and in one movement pull the dumbbell up past your left shoulder as you simultaneously rotate your torso to the left.

- Reverse the movement to return to the starting position.

- Complete the prescribed number of reps to your left side, then do the same number starting with the dumbbell just outside your left ankle, rotating to your right.

- Loop one end of a large resistance band around a chinup bar and then pull it through the other end of the band.

- Clasp both hands around the band and step away so that your left side faces the anchor point. Your shoulders should be turned toward the band.

- In one movement, while keeping your arms straight, rotate your torso and pull the band across your body so your hands end up outside your right hip.

- Pause, then return to the starting position.

- Do all reps to your right side, then repeat with your right side facing the anchor point.

Core Exercises

Split Stance Cable Chop

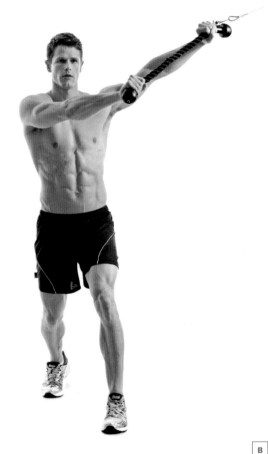

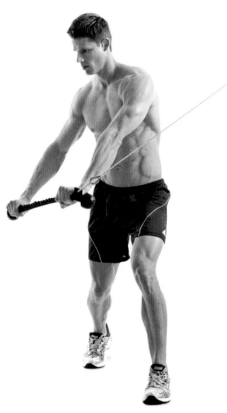

A

- Attach a rope handle to the high pulley of a cable station.
- Stand in a staggered stance with your left foot in front of your left foot, your left side facing the cable station. Rotate your body to grip the rope with both hands.

B

- In one movement, pull the rope down and past your right hip as you simultaneously rotate your torso right.
- Reverse the movement to return to the starting position.
- Complete the prescribed number of repetitions to your right side, then do the same number with your right side facing the stack, pulling toward your left.

▊Band Tight Rotation

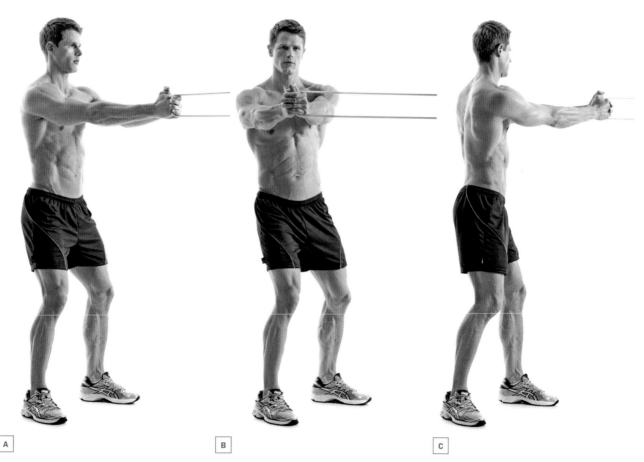

A

B

C

- Attach a resistance band to a stable object at waist height.
- Clasp the band with both hands and stand so that you face the anchor, holding the band in front of your chest with your arms extended. Step away until you feel light tension.

- Keeping your hips square and your core engaged, rotate your upper body to the right so your arms are in line with your right shoulder. That's 1 rep.

- Quickly reverse, twisting all the way to the left so your arms are in line with your left shoulder.
- Continue alternating as fast as you can for the prescribed number of reps.
- On the next set, stand with your right side facing the anchor.

Core Exercises

Tight Rotation

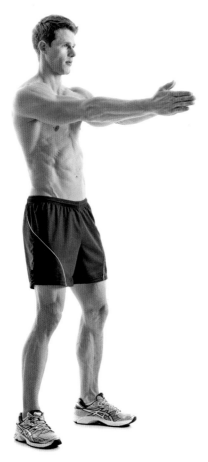

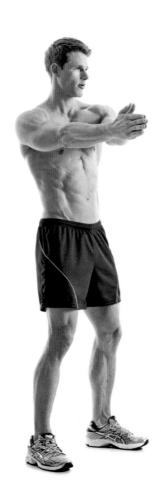

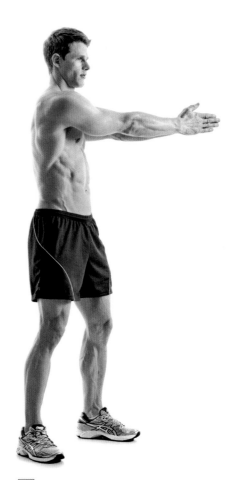

 A

- Stand with your feet more than hip-width apart and your arms extended in front of you, palms together.

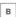 **B**

- Keeping your hips square and your core engaged, rotate your upper body to the right so your arms are in line with your right shoulder. That's 1 rep.

C

- Quickly reverse, twisting all the way to the left so your arms are in line with your left shoulder.
- Continue alternating as fast as you can for the prescribed number of reps.

▮Dumbbell Seated Core Stabilization

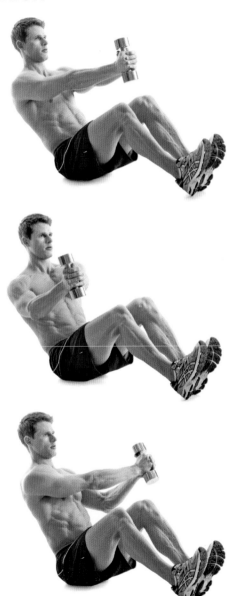

A

- Sit on the floor with your knees bent.
- Hold a dumbbell with both hands straight out in front of your chest.
- Lean back so your torso is at a 45-degree angle to the floor, and brace your core.

B

- Without moving your torso, slowly (take 2 seconds) rotate your arms to the right as far as you can.
- Pause for 3 seconds.

C

- Slowly rotate your arms to the left as far as you can.
- Pause again, then continue to alternate back and forth for the allotted time.

Core Exercises

Side Pillar Jack

A

- Lie on your left side with your knees straight.
- Prop your upper body up on your left elbow and forearm.
- Raise your hips until your body forms a straight line from your shoulders to your ankles.

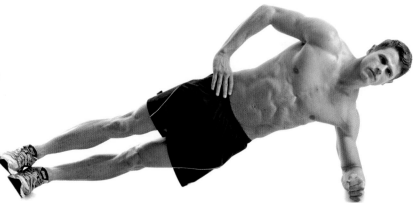

B

- Raise your top leg as high as you can and hold it that way for 2 seconds.
- Lower it back to the starting position. That's 1 rep.
- Perform the prescribed number of reps, then turn around so that you're lying on your right side and repeat.

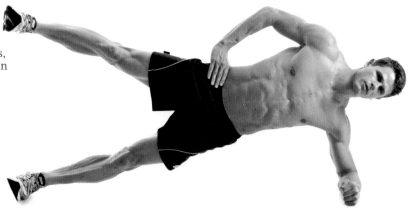

Seated Twist

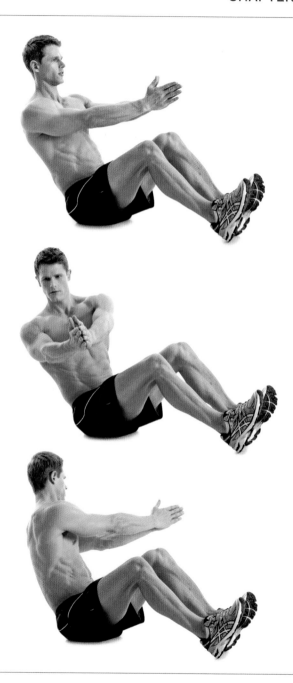

A

- Sit on the floor with your knees bent and your feet flat.
- Hold your arms straight out in front of your chest with your palms together.
- Lean back so your torso is at a 45-degree angle to the floor.

B

- Brace your core and rotate your arms to the right as far as you can.

C

- Pause, then reverse your movement and twist all the way back to the left as far as you can.

Core Exercises

Swiss Ball Rollout

A

- Sit on your knees in front of a Swiss ball, and place your forearms and fist on the ball. Your elbows should be bent about 90 degrees.

B

- Keeping your core braced, slowly roll the ball forward, straightening your arms and extending your body as far as you can without allowing your lower back to collapse.
- Use your abs to pull the ball back to your knees.

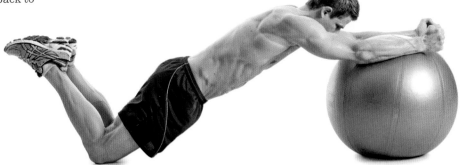

Swiss Ball Stir the Pot

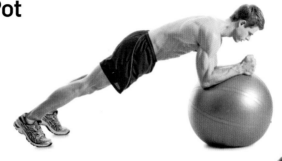

A

- Assume a plank position with your forearms on a Swiss ball. Your body should form a straight line from your shoulders to your ankles.
- Squeeze your abs and glutes as hard as you can.

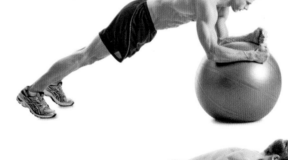

B

- Use your forearms to move the ball in small circles while keeping the rest of your body in the original position.

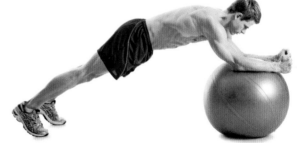

C **D**

- Make one circle moving to the right and then one to the left. That's 1 rep.

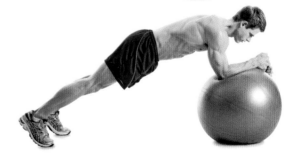

Core Exercises

Swiss Ball Pike

A

- Assume a pushup position with your arms completely straight. Position your hands slightly wider than and in line with your shoulders.

- Rest your shins on a Swiss ball. Your body should form a straight line from your shoulders to your ankles.

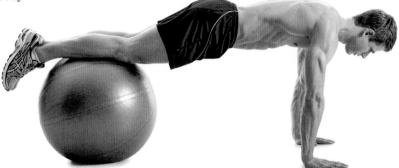

B

- Without bending your knees, roll the Swiss ball toward your body by raising your hips as high as you can.

- Pause, then return the ball to the starting position by lowering your hips and rolling the ball backward.

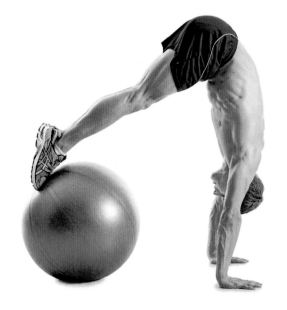

▌Cable Core Press

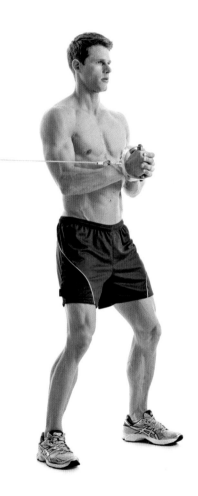

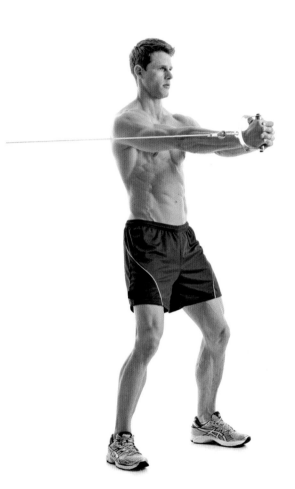

 A

- Attach a handle to a cable machine at chest height.
- Grab the handle with your hands clasped and stand with your right side facing the weight stack. Spread your feet about shoulder-width apart.
- Holding the handle against your chest, step away from the stack until you feel tension in the cable.

 B

- Slowly press your arms in front of you until they're completely straight.
- Hold for 2 seconds, then return your hands to the starting position.
- Do all your reps, then turn around and repeat with your left side facing the weight stack.

Core Exercises

Resistance Band Core Press

A

- Attach a resistance band to a cable machine at chest height.
- Grab the band with your hands clasped and stand with your right side facing the weight stack. Spread your feet about shoulder-width apart.
- Step away from the stack until you feel tension in the cable.

B

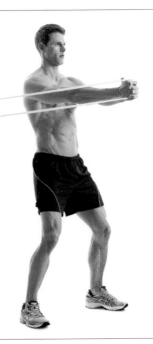

- Hold the band against your chest and slowly press your arms in front of you until they're completely straight.
- Hold for 2 seconds, then return your hands to the starting position.
- Do all your reps, then turn around and repeat with your left side facing the cable machine.

Slide Out

A

- Kneel on the floor and place both hands on a Valslide. Your hands should be under your shoulder.

B

- Slowly push the Valslide forward, extending your body as far as you can without allowing your hips to sag.
- Use your abs to pull your hands back to below your shoulders.

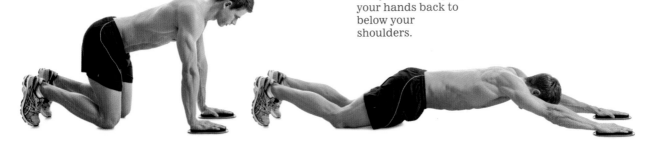

▮ Garhammer Raise

A

- Lie on your back with your hips bent 90 degrees and your legs straight, with your feet pointing toward the ceiling.

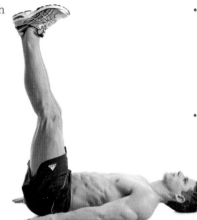

B

- With your hands flat on the floor and your arms at your sides, roll your hips up off the floor and toward your chest, while keeping your legs in the same position.
- Pause when your feet are just above your chest, then slowly lower back to the starting position.

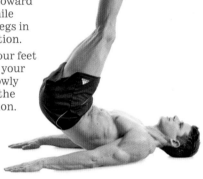

▮ Reverse Crunch

A

- Lie faceup on the floor with your palms facing down.
- Bend your knees 90 degrees.
- Raise your hips off the floor and crunch them toward your chest.

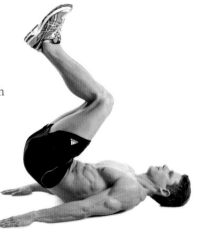

B

- Pause, then slowly lower your legs until your heels nearly touch the floor.

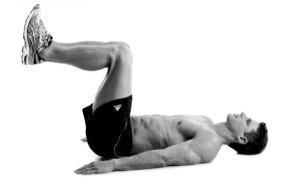

323

Core Exercises

█ Med Ball Side Rotation

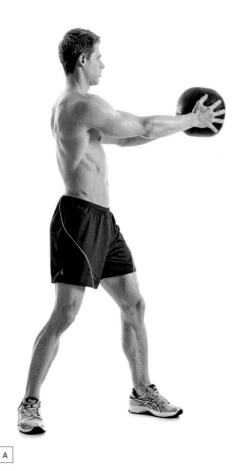

A

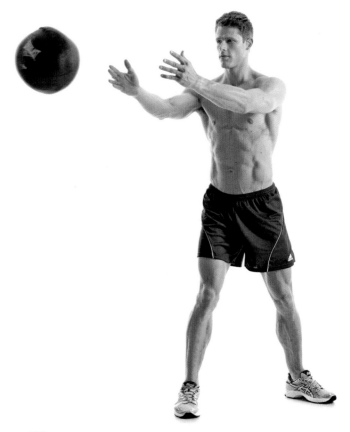

B

- Grab a medicine ball and stand sideways about 3 feet from a brick or concrete wall, with your right side facing the wall.
- Hold the ball at chest level with your arms straight and rotate your torso to your left.

- Quickly switch directions and throw as hard as you can against the wall to your right.
- As the ball rebounds off the wall, catch it and repeat the movement.
- Complete the prescribed number of repetitions, then repeat with your left side facing the wall.

▮Med Ball Slam

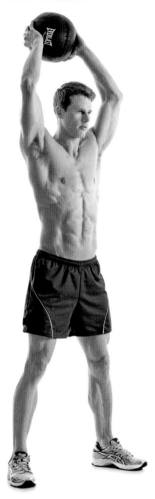

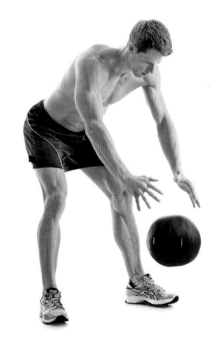

- Grab a medicine ball and hold it above your head. Your arms should be slightly bent and your feet shoulder-width apart.

B

- Forcefully slam the ball to the floor in front of you as hard as you can.
- Pick the ball up and repeat.

Core Exercises

Med Ball Russian Twist

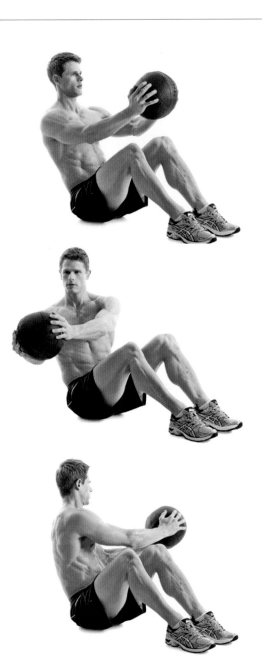

A

- Sit on the floor with your knees bent and your feet flat.
- Hold a medicine ball, with your arms straight out in front of your chest.
- Lean back so your torso is at a 45-degree angle to the floor.

B

- Brace your core and rotate to the right as far as you can.

C

- Pause, then reverse your movement and twist all the way back to the left as far as you can.

Swiss Ball Body Saw

- Assume a plank position, but place your elbows and forearms on a Swiss ball. Your body should form a straight line from your shoulders to your ankles.

B

- Squeeze your abs and glutes as tight as you can, then move your forearms forward and backward just a few inches in a sawing motion. That's 1 rep.

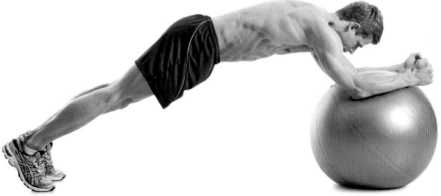

Core Exercises

▌ Med Ball Extension with Breath

A

- Lie on the floor with your knees bent, feet flat on the ground, and a small medicine ball in your midback, right between the base of your shoulder blades.
- Interlock your hands behind your head and pull your elbows in by your ears.

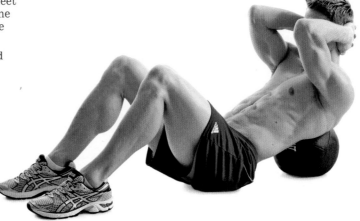

B

- Exhale and point your elbows backward over your head as you slowly extend back over the ball. Only go as far as you can without your lower back arching or your ribs flaring up in the front.
- From this position, take a deep breath in through your nose, and feel your thoracic spine and chest open up.
- Exhale through your mouth as you return to the starting position.

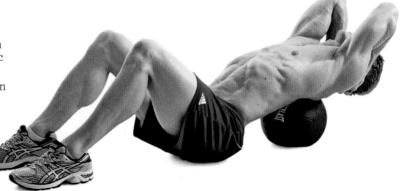

▊ Med Ball Single-Leg Kick

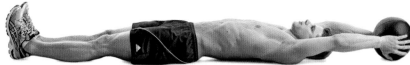

A

- Hold a medicine ball in both hands, and lie faceup on the floor with your legs and arms straight. Your arms should be straight above the top of your head.

B

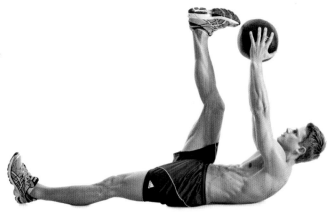

- In one movement, lift your torso and one of your legs, and try to touch your toes.

C

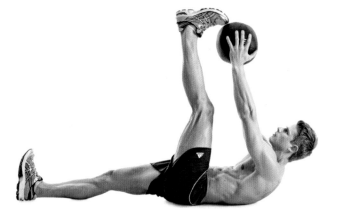

- Lower your body back to the starting position, and repeat with your other leg.

Core Exercises

Med Ball Side Slam

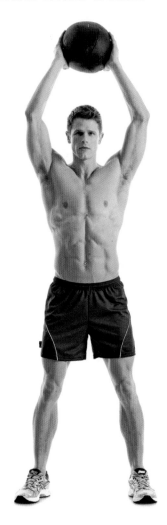

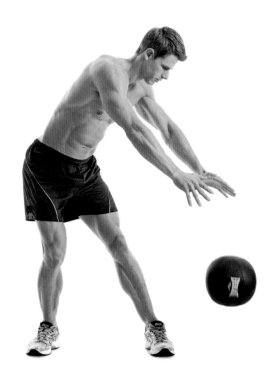

- Grab a medicine ball and hold it above your head. Your arms should be slightly bent and your feet shoulder-width apart.

B

- Forcefully slam the ball toward the outside of your left foot as hard as you can.
- Pick the ball up and repeat, this time slamming toward the outside of your right foot. That's 1 rep.

■ Around the World

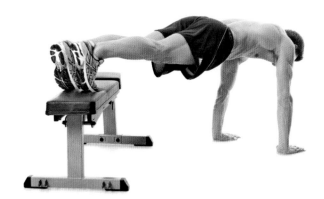

A

- Place both feet on a bench and assume a pushup position. Your body should form a straight line from your shoulders to your ankles.

B **C**

- Brace your core and, without dropping your hips or moving your feet, make a full revolution around the bench by "walking" your hands all the way around it. That's 1 rep.

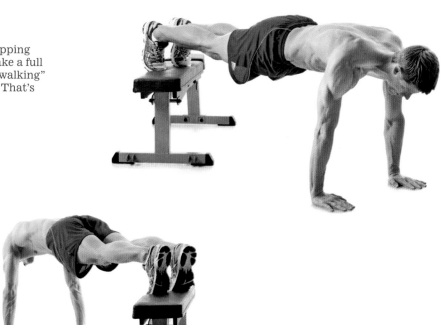

Core Exercises

Valslide Body Saw

A

- Stand with each foot in the middle of the Valslide.
- Lower your body into pushup position, but place your weight on your elbows and keep your feet on the Valslide. Your body should be in a straight line from your shoulders to your ankles.

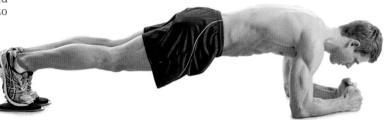

B

- Squeeze your abs as if you're about to be punched in the stomach, and then slightly slide both of your feet backward.

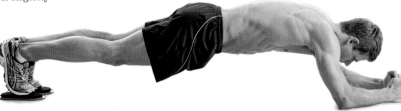

C

- Return to the starting position. Your entire body should create a slightly "sawing" motion.

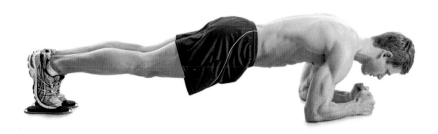

■ Valslide Mountain Climber

A

- Stand with each foot in the middle of the Valslide.
- Lower your body into pushup position, keeping your feet on the Valslide.

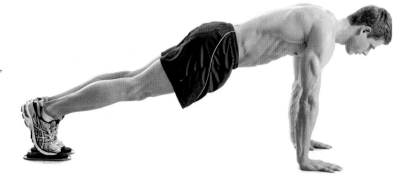

B

- With your body in a straight line from your shoulders to your ankles, slide your right knee toward your chest.
- Slide back to the start and repeat with your left knee.

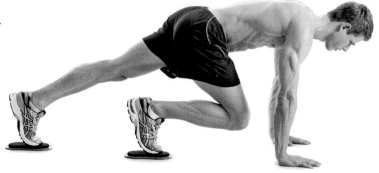

C

- Alternate between both legs until you finish all reps.

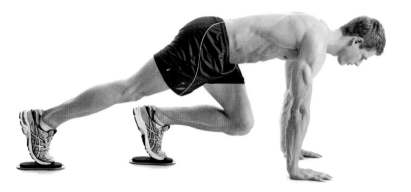

Core Exercises: Back

▎Chinup

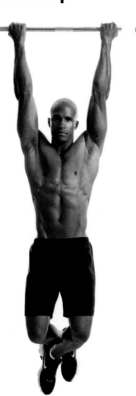 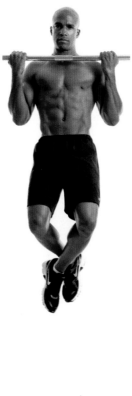

A

- Grab a chinup bar with a shoulder-width underhand grip.
- Hang at arm's length and pull your shoulder blades down and back so that your shoulders are as far from your ears as possible.

B

- Pull your chest to the bar as you squeeze your shoulder blades together.
- Pause, then lower your body back to a dead hang.

▎Chinup L-Sit Hold

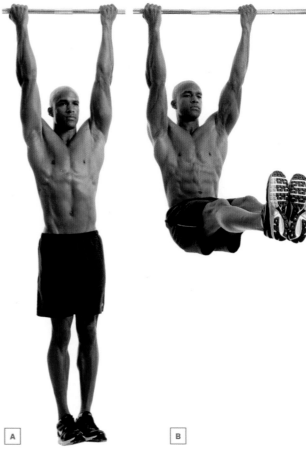

A

- Grab a chinup bar with a shoulder-width underhand grip.
- Hang at arm's length and pull your shoulder blades down and back so that your shoulders are as far from your ears as possible.

B

- Keeping your legs straight, raise your hips and rotate your pelvis so that your legs are perpendicular to your torso. Hold for the prescribed time.
- Pause, then lower your body back to a dead hang.

Hanging Leg Raise

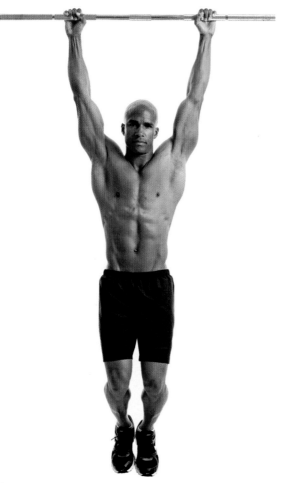

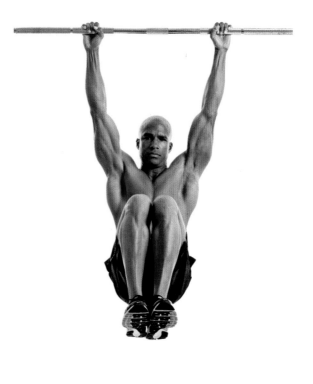

- Grab a chinup bar with an overhand, shoulder-width grip and hang from the bar with your knees slightly bent and feet together.

- Simultaneously bend your knees, raise your hips, and curl your lower back underneath you as you lift your thighs toward your chest.
- Pause when the fronts of your thighs reach your chest, then slowly lower your legs back to the starting position.

Chapter 10
Revolutionize Your Training

All exercise routines are not created equal.

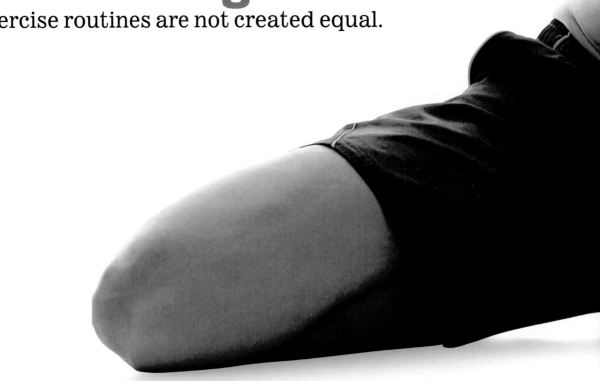

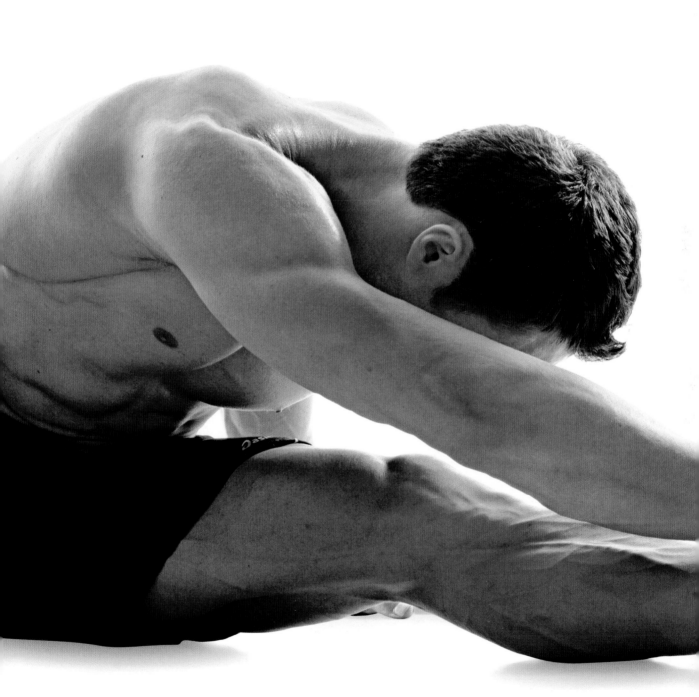

Revolutionize Your Training

Just as you have good and bad diets, the same could be said about your gym routine. Anyone can put together a bunch of exercises and call it a workout. It's done every day in gyms around the world. But those same programs have caused years of fitness frustration. You don't need trainers yelling and screaming for you to drop weight fast (although some barking can help motivate you). There's an art and science to designing a program. Each exercise needs to serve a purpose and help you reach your goals. A plan also needs to be structured in a way that keeps you working hard and improving.

That's why we took the guesswork out of exercise so that you could confidently take on any goal and succeed. We found the world's top fitness experts and had them put together a list of their best workouts, which you'll find in Chapter 11. Whether you want to get ready for the beach, channel your inner athlete, or never perform a crunch again (and still lose weight), anything is possible. All you need to do is follow the step-by-step plans and work hard. The results will follow.

But here's the key: Don't change the exercises unless noted by the experts. These workouts were specifically designed to help you melt away fat, reveal those abs, and get in the best shape of your life. They'll be fun, fast, and effective. But when you reach an exercise that's difficult, don't default back to what you know or avoid the learning curve.

Be patient and follow this guide with complete trust. Your faith will be rewarded with complete body transformation—and the confidence of knowing that you finally cracked the weight loss code. Your fittest body starts here.

Your Guide to Every Workout

Follow these rules to help simplify your workouts and see results fast

Workout 101

• Always perform the exercises in the order shown.

• Exercises will be ordered by number. Do all of the sets of a particular number before moving on to the next one.

• When you see a number and a letter combined, it indicates that the exercises are part of a group (such as 1A, 1B, 1C). That is, do 1 set of the first exercise (1A), 1 set of the second exercise (1B), and so on. Follow this pattern until you've finished all sets of each exercise with the same number. Do this regardless of how many exercises share the same number (it will be anywhere from two to five exercises). Perform all of these exercises before moving on to the next number (2, 3, and 4).

• Each exercise contains specific guidelines for reps, sets, and rest periods.

• The reps are the number of times you will perform an exercise before taking a break. Sometimes the number of reps will not be a number (like 8), but instead be a period of time (30 seconds). In these instances, perform as many reps as you can in the time specified. Or for certain moves, like the plank, hold the exercise until time is up.

• The sets are how many times you will repeat a series of reps.

• The rest periods indicate your breaks after each exercise. Sometimes a rest period will say "0." When this occurs, there is no rest, and you should move immediately to the next exercise.

• Very important: Before each workout, perform The Total Body Jump Start (page 340). It's a warmup designed to prepare your body for each plan and prevent injury. Don't skimp on this.

BENEFITS OF WARMUP

• Prime your central nervous system and increase mental alertness

• Increase core temperature

• Improve pliability of the soft tissues of your body

• Improve overall mobility and movement

• Activate inhibited muscle groups

• Amp you up!

The Total Body Jump Start (7 to 10 minutes)

A great workout doesn't start with your first rep—it begins with your warmup. After all, a "cold" muscle can end up an injured muscle or can limit your potential results. Your muscles are like a rubber band. When they are cold, they easily snap. But a warm muscle is more pliable and can generate more force. And a more forceful muscle is one that can shred fat and tone every inch of your body.

This warmup, designed by Jim Smith, CSCS, should take about 7 to 10 minutes. Perform each of the exercises once, and when you're done, move on to your workout.

This plan involves four steps—all designed to help you make the most of every workout and prevent injury.

STEP 1

Self-myofascial release: Everyone likes massages. And that's exactly what this is for your muscles. Some areas will hurt during the process, while others will feel good. But this entire sequence will make your body feel great. The goal here is to improve the quality, extensibility, and elasticity of your soft tissues (think cold taffy versus warm taffy); relax the tension in your muscles; improve movement; and remove aches and pains.

STEP 2

Dynamic mobility: Now you're targeting movement, introducing lost range of motion and creating stability. You'll also improve posture by mobilizing your hip and upper back restrictions.

STEP 3

Activation: It's time to restore muscular balance to your joints by taking you through exercises that challenge your range of motion and target those hard-to-reach muscles that you probably miss during your workouts. You'll also reactivate muscle groups that you've ignored and reestablish proper muscle contraction so that your primary muscles can do their job during the workout and you can see better results.

STEP 1

Preworkout light work sets: The final step allows you to focus on your grooving pattern for your first exercises and have you ready to make every workout your best workout.

Revolutionize Your Training

SEQ	TARGET	EXERCISE	SETS	REPS	WEIGHT
1A	Full Body	Self-Myofascial Release (page 343)	1	30–60 seconds each area	Bodyweight
1B	Hip Mobility	Hip Thrust with Bench (page 266)	1	8–10 each leg	Bodyweight
1C	Hip Mobility	Rear Foot Elevated Hip Flexor Stretch (page 266)	1	30 seconds each leg	Bodyweight
1D	Upper Back Mobility	Side-Lying Windmill (page 157)	1	8 each side	Bodyweight
1E	Upper Back Mobility/ Glute Activation	Lunge and Reach (page 218)	1	10	Bodyweight
1F	Glute Activation	Hip Thrust with Bench (page 266)	1	10	Bodyweight
1G	Upper Back Activation	Wall Slide (page 192)	1	10	Bodyweight
1H	Upper Back Activation	Face Pulls (page 166)	1	20	Bodyweight
1I	CNS Activation	Box Jump (page 239)	1	20	Bodyweight
1J	Preworkout Priming	Light work sets of first exercise*	1–2	1–2	bar, 30–50%

* Light work sets = doing 3 to 4 sets with 50–65% of the weight you'd use for your actual "working" sets.

ABOUT THE EXPERT

Jim Smith, CSCS, is a highly respected, world-renowned strength and conditioning specialist who has been called one of the most innovative strength coaches in the fitness industry by *Elite FTS*—one of the leading voices in the strength training industry. Training athletes, fitness enthusiasts, and weekend warriors, Smith has dedicated himself to helping them reach "beyond their potential." He holds multiple national fitness certifications and is a consultant and lecturer, giving seminars all over the country. He is also the creator of the Amped Warm-Up (www.ampedwarmup.com). You can find his work at http://dieselsc.com.

Self-Myofascial Release

UPPER BACK

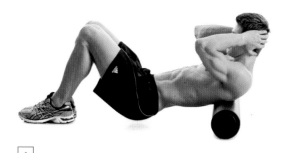

A

- Lie faceup with a foam roller under your midback, at the bottoms of your shoulder blades.
- Clasp your hands behind your head and pull your elbows toward each other.

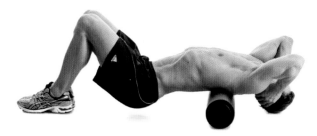

B

- Raise your hips off the floor slightly.
- Slowly lower your head and upper back to your upper back bends over the foam roller. Raise back to the start, roll forward a couple of inches, and repeat.

LOWER BACK

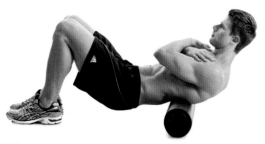

A

- Lie faceup with a foam roller under your midback.
- Cross your arms over your chest, with your knees bent and feet flat on the floor.

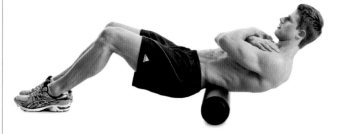

B

- Raise your hips off the floor slightly, and roll back and forth over your lower back.

Revolutionize Your Training

IT BAND

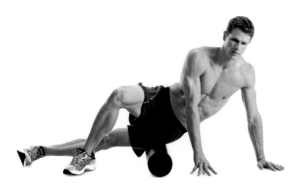

A

- Lie on your left side and place a foam roller under your left hip.
- Put your hands on the floor for support, cross your right leg over your left, and place your right foot flat on the floor.

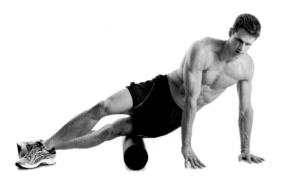

B

- Roll your body forward until the roller reaches your knee. Then roll back and forth.
- Lie on your right side and repeat with the roller under your right hip.

QUADS AND HIP FLEXORS

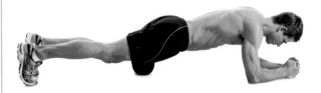

A

- Lie facedown on the floor with a foam roller positioned above your right knee.
- Cross your left leg over your right ankle and place your elbows on the floor for support.

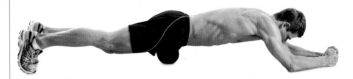

B

- Roll your body backward until the roller reaches the top of your right thigh. Then roll back and forth. Repeat with the roller above your left knee.

HAMSTRINGS

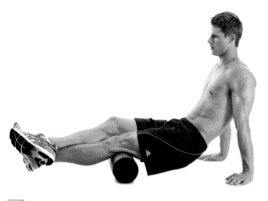

A

- Lie faceup and place a foam roller under your left knee with your leg straight. Cross your right leg over your left ankle and put your hands flat on the floor for support.

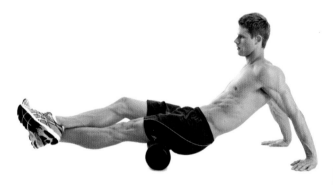

B

- Roll your body forward until the roller reaches your glutes, then roll back and forth. Repeat with the roller under your right knee.

GLUTES

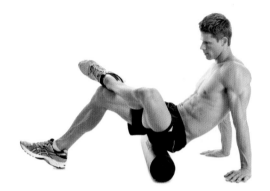

A

- Sit on a foam roller with it positioned on the back of your left thigh, just below your glutes. Cross your left leg over the front of your right thigh and put your hands flat on the floor for support.

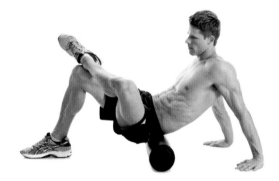

B

- Roll your body forward until the roller reaches your lower back, then roll back and forth.
- Repeat with the roller under your right thigh.

The Best Abs Workouts

Ever Created

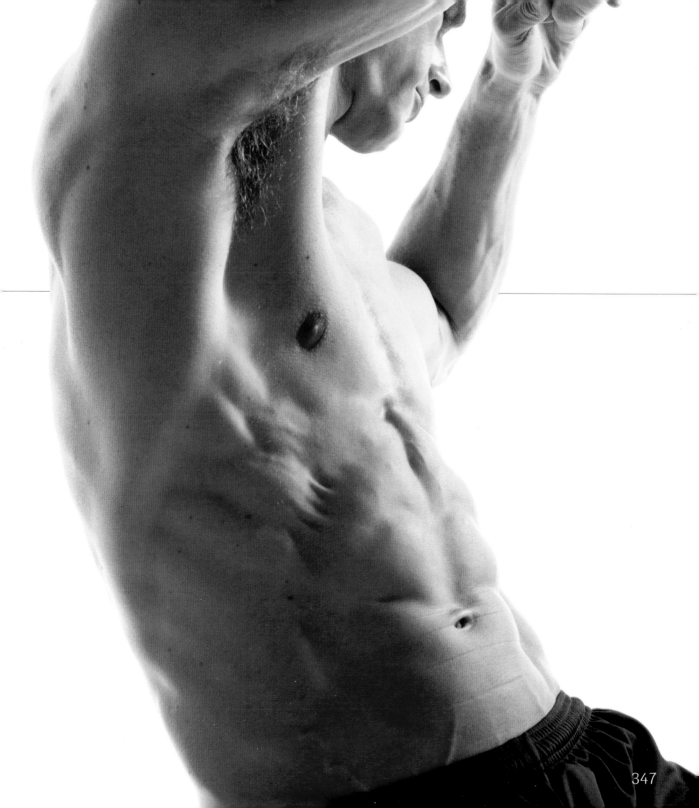

The Warrior's Workout

Martin Rooney, the creator of the Training for Warriors system, spent the last 15 years perfecting his conditioning techniques to create a workout that simulates the cardiovascular demands of a fight while still building muscle and burning fat. His approach is known as "hurricane training." Think you can survive it?

HOW TO DO IT

■ Perform a hurricane 3 days a week, resting at least a day between each session. So you might complete this routine on Monday, Wednesday, and Friday.

■ Treadmill running is incorporated into each round. If the recommended speed is too fast or the incline grade is too intense, start at a comfortable level until you build up to the recommended pace.

■ Prior to the workout, complete the "The Total Body Jump Start" warmup on page 340.

■ Each hurricane consists of three rounds: A round is 3 sets of three exercises, performed back-to-back with only a short period of rest between movements. Once you do all three sets, that's one round. Rest for 2 minutes between rounds. Complete all of the pre-scribed sets in a round before moving on to the next series of exercises.

■ Rooney created three categories of hurricanes for *The Men's Health Big Book: Getting Abs*. Each category increases in difficulty from category 1 to 3.

Category 1 This hurricane uses two simple bodyweight activities in place of recovery after each sprint. Classic choices of activities to perform for this category are pushups, situps, or medicine ball slams.

Category 2 This hurricane uses two light resistance exercises after each sprint. Classic choices of activities to perform for this category are barbell curls and rows, dumbbell presses, and triceps work.

Category 3 This hurricane increases in intensity and uses two heavy resistance exercises after each sprint. Classic choices of activities to perform for this category are barbell presses, chinups, and dips.

Category 1 Workout

Perform the following three exercises as a circuit. That is, after you complete 1 set of the first exercise, immediately move to the next. After you've completed 1 set of each exercise, rest as little as possible (no rest, if you can) and then start the process over. You'll complete the circuit a total of three times. After you finish the third set, rest for 2 minutes and then move on to the next round. Follow the same pattern for all three rounds.

Round 1

EXERCISE	SETS	REPS	Rest
1A Treadmill: 9 mph at 10% grade	3	20 seconds	0
1B Knee-Grab Situp (page 299)	3	10	0
1C Knee to Elbow Pushup (page 141)	3	10	0

Round 2

EXERCISE	SETS	REPS	REST
2A Treadmill: 10 mph at 10% grade	3	20 seconds	0
2B Med Ball Single-Leg Kick (page 329)	3	8	0
2C Knee to Elbow Pushup (page 141)	3	10	0

Round 3

EXERCISE	SETS	REPS	REST
3A Treadmill: 10.5 mph at 10% grade	3	20 seconds	0
3B Med Ball Russian Twist (page 326)	3	50	0
3C Pushup (page 132)	3	10	0

Category 2 Workout

Perform the following three exercises as a circuit. That is, after you complete 1 set of the first exercise, immediately move to the next. After you've completed 1 set of each exercise, rest as little as possible (no rest, if you can) and then start the process over. You'll complete the circuit a total of three times. After you finish the third set, rest for 2 minutes and then move on to the next round. Follow the same pattern for all three rounds.

Round 1

EXERCISE	SETS	REPS	REST
1A Treadmill: 9.5 mph at 10% grade	3	25 seconds	0
1B Push Jerks (page 207)	3	10	0
1C Dumbbell Snatch (page 209)	3	10	0

Round 2

EXERCISE	SETS	REPS	REST
2A Treadmill: 10.5 mph at 10% grade	3	25 seconds	0
2B Dumbbell Bent-Over Row (page 161)	3	10	0
2C Dumbbell High Pull (page 214)	3	10	0

Round 3

EXERCISE	SETS	REPS	REST
3A Treadmill: 11.5 mph at 10% grade	3	25 seconds	0
3B Dumbbell Biceps Curl (page 175)	3	10	0
3C Standing Overhead Dumbbell Triceps Press (page 177)	3	10	0

Category 3 Workout

Perform the following three exercises as a circuit. That is, after you complete 1 set of the first exercise, immediately move to the next. After you've completed 1 set of each exercise, rest as little as possible (no rest, if you can) and then start the process over. You'll complete the circuit a total of three times. After you finish the third set, rest for 2 minutes and then move on to the next round. Follow the same pattern for all three rounds.

Round 1

EXERCISE	SETS	REPS	REST
1A Treadmill: 10.5 mph at 10% grade	3	30 seconds	0
1B Close-Grip Bench Press (page 150)	3	8	0
1C Chinup (page 334)	3	8	0

Round 2

EXERCISE	SETS	REPS	REST
2A Treadmill: 12 mph at 10% grade	3	30 seconds	0
2B Dips (page 156)	3	8	0
2C Dumbbell Overhead Press (page 189)	3	8	0

Round 3

EXERCISE	SETS	REPS	REST
3A Treadmill: 13 mph at 10% grade	3	30 seconds	0
3B Dumbbell Bent-Over Row (page 161)	3	10	0
3C Dumbbell Biceps Curl (page 175)	3	10	0

ABOUT THE EXPERT

Martin Rooney is an internationally recognized fitness expert and author, known for training some of the greatest athletes in the world. He has a master's degree in health science and a bachelor's degree in physical therapy from the Medical University of South Carolina, and he also holds a bachelor's degree in exercise science from Furman University. He is the creator of the Training for Warriors system (www.trainingforwarriors.com); the author of *Training for Warriors, Ultimate Warrior Workouts,* and *Warrior Cardio;* and is the COO of the Parisi Speed School, a national franchise.

The Summer Abs Workout

Most guys are stuck talking too much at the gym and not focusing on the work needed to look great at the beach, in the boardroom, and in the bedroom. All of that ends now.

This is a no-nonsense plan that uses a total reps approach to making sure that every workout is a successful one. Rather than setting predetermined sets and reps, you have a goal number of reps to perform for each exercise. This emphasizes quality and will ensure that you build strength, pack on muscle, and have a body designed to impress.

HOW TO DO IT

▌ Perform this full body workout 3 days a week, resting at least a day between each session. So you might do it on Monday, Wednesday, and Friday.

▌ Prior to the workout, complete "The Total Body Jump Start" warmup on page 340.

▌ This plan uses the total reps method. It focuses on the total number of reps performed for a given exercise, rather than specifying the number of sets. You pick a targeted volume goal and perform as few sets as possible (AFAP, see chart) to reach the goal—maintaining focus on good form.

▌ Be sure to focus on the quality of your reps. As fatigue sets in, intensity and good form will be crucial. Keep 1 rep in the tank (reserve) for each set and don't perform to complete failure.

▮ You're going to start this workout on the treadmill—and it won't be easy. After your warmup, you'll perform 6 to 8 sets of treadmill sprints. This will wake up your entire nervous system, fry some fat, and have you ready to perform. If you need to build up to those 6 to 8 sets, be smart and either start at a slower pace or do fewer total sets. Try to maintain the work-to-rest ratio.

▮ 2A, 2B, 2C, and 2D should be performed as a circuit with as many good reps as possible for each exercise before moving to the next. Once you reach 2D, go back to 2A and continue until you reach the goal number of reps.

▮ For the pushups, you can use a variety of hand positions (close, wide, staggered) and foot positions (elevated, one foot), or overload the movement with a band, weight plate, or a partner providing resistance.

SEQ	TARGET	EXERCISE	SETS	REPS	REST
1	Speed, power	Sprints Treadmill on incline, speed greater than 8 mph Rest to work ratio 2:1 (15-second sprint/30-second rest)	6–8	One 15-second sprint	30 seconds per sprint
2A	Full body	Barbell Clean and Press (page 213)	AFAP	50	30–60 seconds
2B	Upper back mass	Pullup (page 171)	AFAP	50	30–60 seconds
2C	Full body	Barbell Deadlift (page 272)	AFAP	50	30–60 seconds
2D	Upper body mass	Pushup (page 132)	AFAP	100	30–60 seconds
3	Core stability and strength	Ab Wheel Rollout (page 297)	4	12	30 seconds

The Best Abs Workouts Ever Created

The Cardio-Strength Workout

Running, jogging, cycling—they're all great cardio activities. But none of them are designed to shed body fat and get you fit fast. Why settle for one goal when you can have both? By using traditional resistance training exercises and performing them at a high tempo, you turn your metabolism into a gut-melting furnace, while also improving your cardiovascular performance. Complete a session and you'll realize this is the fastest way to change your body.

HOW TO DO IT

▮ Perform this workout 3 days a week, resting at least a day between each session. So you might go Monday, Wednesday, and Friday.

▮ Prior to the workout, complete "The Total Body Jump Start" warmup on page 340.

▮ The workout consists of three complexes, each consisting of three exercises. For each complex, perform the exercises in succession. That is, you will do one exercise after another without rest. Once you complete all three exercises, that's one complex.

▮ Your goal is to complete the number of sets and reps within each complex using the chart below. For instance, if your goal is to perform 3 sets of 6 reps, you will complete 3 circuits of complex 1, rest, and then move on to complex 2 for another 3 sets. Do not move on to the next complex until you have finished the prescribed number of sets.

▮ You will time each set and rest exactly as long as it takes to complete that set before starting your next set.

▮ Use the table to determine how many reps you should perform each workout and every week.

Exercises

COMPLEX 1	COMPLEX 2	COMPLEX 3
1A Kettlebell Squat (page 274)	2A Pullup (page 171)	3A Spiderman Pushup (page 153) using Valslide
1B Kettlebell Romanian Deadlift (page 276)	2B Divebomber Pushup (page 142), explosive	3B Valslide Hip Raise and Hamstring Curl (page 277)
1C Kettlebell Swing (page 210)	2C Squat Thrust (page 201)	3C Valslide Body Saw (page 332)

	WEEK 1	WEEK 2	WEEK 3	WEEK 4
SETS X REPS	3 x 6	3 x 7	3 x 8	3 x 10
REST TIME	1:1	1:1	1:1	1:1

ABOUT THE EXPERT

Robert dos Remedios, MA, CSCS, SCCC, is an international speaker on many topics in strength and conditioning, ranging from Olympic lifts to cardio strength training. He has written two best-selling books, *Men's Health Power Training* and *Cardio Strength Training*, and is the 2006 NSCA Collegiate Strength and Conditioning Coach of the Year. He can be found at www.coachdos.com.

The Best Abs Workouts Ever Created

The No-Crunch Abs Workout

Your plan to shred your abs is almost *too* predictable. Finish your cardio? Work your abs? Done with your lifting session? Hit them again. Just brushed your teeth? One more set of crunches won't hurt. But that's just a mind game. The real secret is combining heavy, multimuscle exercises and high-intensity intervals that will scorch the fat off your body. Add in a few challenging core exercises and you have a plan that will actually work—rather than crunching your way to soreness that doesn't show.

HOW TO DO IT

▌Perform this workout 3 days a week, resting at least a day between each session. So you might go on Monday, Wednesday, and Friday.

▌Prior to the workout, complete "The Total Body Jump Start" warmup on page 340.

▌This workout will require some space. If you're limited, use the distance you have available and perform more reps to meet the equivalent that is prescribed.

▌The training plan calls for 3 circuits consisting of three exercises each. You will complete all of the sets within a given circuit before moving on to the next group of exercises.

▌When you see a number with a letter next to it (such as 1A, 1B), that indicates the order that the exercises should be performed for each circuit. For every circuit, do 1 set of each exercise listed in succession. For example, complete 1 set of exercise 1A, rest as directed, and then perform 1 set of exercise 1B and rest again before completing a set of 1C. Follow this pattern until you've completed all sets of each exercise in the group, and then progress to the next circuit.

▌Be sure to select a weight that is challenging for the lower rep range, but does not bring you to complete failure at the higher rep range. That means you should still be able to squeeze out one more rep with perfect form at the end of each exercise. Completely exhausting your muscles on each set is not the goal of this workout.

EXERCISES	SETS	REPS	REST
1A Barbell Front Squat (page 232)	4	6–8	30 seconds
1B Dumbbell Renegade Crawl (page 219)	4	20 yards	30 seconds
1C Plate Push (page 277)	4	40 yards	60 seconds
2A Barbell Romanian Deadlift (page 252)	4	6–8	30 seconds
2B Spiderman Pushup (page 153), weighted	4	20 yards	30 seconds
2C Force treadmill sprints	4	80 yards	60 seconds
3A Hanging Leg Raise (page 335)	3	6–8	30 seconds
3B Ab Wheel Rollout (page 297)	3	10–12	30 seconds
3C Cable Core Press (page 321)	3	60	90–120 seconds

ABOUT THE EXPERT

Rob Sulaver, CSCS, owns and operates Bandana Training. His advice on training, nutrition, and lifestyle is full of intelligence and humor—a welcome marriage in an industry divided between "all-too-serious scientists and models-turned-trainers-turned-bloggers." Sulaver's approach to being a "dumb jock" underscores what Bandana Training is all about: "Taking care of yourself is vitally important and virally amusing." Read more about him at BandanaTraining.com or http://Facebook.com/BandanaTraining.

The Athlete's Core Workout

There's a saying that goes, "Athletes aren't born. They're made." Nothing could be more accurate once you realize how much a strong core influences your sports performance. Whether you want to help your company softball team, improve the distance on your golf drive, or compete at a high level, your core is the key to unlocking your potential on the playing field. This workout is designed for the athlete in us all. It focuses on core stability and on making sure that you generate more power in your upper and lower body so that you can succeed in any game at any level.

HOW TO DO IT

▌ This plan is split into 2 days. Do each workout twice per week and never train on 3 consecutive days. For instance, you might do Workout A on Monday, Workout B on Wednesday, and then repeat the sequence on Friday and Sunday. Or, you could do Workout A on Monday and Workout B on Tuesday. Rest on Wednesday, and repeat the workouts on Thursday and Friday.

▌ Prior to the workout, complete "The Total Body Jump Start" warmup on page 340.

▌ Both workouts should be performed as circuits. For each circuit, perform 1 set of each exercise in the order listed. Rest the amount of time suggested, and then repeat the circuit.

▌ For Workout A, rest 90 seconds after you complete the circuit. Perform a total of 3 to 4 circuits.

▌ For Workout B, rest 60 seconds after you complete the circuit. Perform a total of 3 to 4 circuits.

Workout A

EXERCISE	SETS	REPS	REST
1A Kettlebell Suitcase Carry (page 226) with Squat Thrust (page 201)	3–4	10	0
1B Dumbbell Renegade Crawl (page 219)	3–4	5/side	0
1C Tall Kneeling Kettlebell Halo (page 300)	3–4	5/side	0

Workout B

EXERCISE	SETS	REPS	REST
2A Front Plank with Weight Transfer (page 284)	3–4	10/side	0
2B Dumbbell T-Pushup (page 135)	3–4	5/side	0
2C Swiss Ball Body Saw (page 327)	3 to 4	20–30 seconds	0

ABOUT THE EXPERT

Tony Gentilcore, CSCS, is one of the co-founders of Cressey Performance, one of the premiere strength and conditioning facilities in the country, located just outside of Boston. He holds a degree in health education from the State University of New York at Cortland, and his collegiate baseball experience helps him relate to student and professional athletes. For more information, check out his Web site at http://tonygentilcore.com.

The Stubborn Fat Loss Workout

Let's be honest: Sometimes even the best workout seems to leave you wanting more—especially when it comes to your abs. If you ever feel like you need a little more focus on your core and a few more calories burned, then this plan is for you. This is what you call an "abs finisher," and it's specifically designed to push you to your goal without accepting failure. By plugging in these challenging and unique abs finishers after your main workout and into your success plan, you'll find yourself leaner in less time.

HOW TO DO IT

▌Perform the following workout at the end of your normal training day. You should not do this workout more than three to four times per week.

▌Prior to the workout, complete "The Total Body Jump Start" warmup on page 340.

▌Do all six exercises as a circuit. That is, perform one after the other, trying to rest as little as possible between each set.

▌Once you have finished all of the exercises, rest for 20 seconds and then repeat the circuit one to two more times.

FASTER FAT LOSS

If you grow tired of body-weight fat loss finishers, these options are for you. Specifically designed by Jason Ferruggia, strength coach and owner of Renegade Training Center, these exercises are ideal for after your workout. Add them to crank up your metabolism and melt away unwanted pounds in the most efficient of ways. Known for creating some of the most effective workout programs, these options from Ferruggia can turn any workout into a fat loss plan.

Add any of these workouts at the end of your training:
Sprints
Find a patch of grass that's about 60 yards long (or 30 yards, and go back and forth) and perform the following workouts:
The plan: 10 sets of 6-yard sprints, resting for 60 to 90 seconds between sets.

Kettlebell swings
Grab a heavy kettlebell that you can use for 20 to 30 reps.
The plan: Do 30 seconds of swings, followed by 60 seconds of rest. Repeat this pattern for 10 to 15 minutes.

Jump rope

Perform the following circuit:
1A) Jump with both legs for 30 seconds, followed by 30 seconds of rest.

1B) Jump only on your right leg for 15 to 20 seconds, followed by 30 seconds of rest.

1C) Jump only on your left leg for 15 to 20 seconds, followed by 30 seconds of rest.

Repeat this cycle as many times as possible for 10 to 20 minutes.

EXERCISE	SETS	REPS	REST
Squat Thrust (page 201) to Chinup (page 334)	2–3	5	0
Spiderman Pushup (page 153)	2–3	6/side	0
Split Jump (page 243)	2–3	7/side	0
Plyo Pushup (page 144)	2–3	8	0
Swiss Ball Rollout (page 318)	2–3	9	0
Kettlebell Swing (page 210)	2–3	10	0

ABOUT THE EXPERT

Mike Whitfield, certified Turbulence Trainer, is the author of *Workout Finishers* and *Ab Finishers*. He lost 105 pounds, propelling him into the fitness industry, which is now his passion. His unique approach of using metabolic workout finishers has helped thousands of people lose fat through his online and offline programs. He is known across the fitness industry for his "finishers" and runs http://workoutfinishers.com and http://abfinishers.com.

The Perfect Posture Workout

Sit up straight and listen up: While you might assume that slouching only leads to back pain, bad body alignment can alter your joints, weaken your ligaments, and even decrease your muscle tone. That adds up to a slumped-over body and sagging skin around your chest, lower abs, and arms. That's why the Perfect Posture Workout is just what your overworked body needs. When you realign your body to its proper position, you restore the tension in your muscles, which gives your body the muscular and masculine look you've been searching for.

HOW TO DO IT

▌Perform this workout three times a week. Alternate between Workout A and Workout B 3 days a week, resting at least a day between each session. That means, you'd perform Workout A on Monday, Workout B on Wednesday, and Workout A again on Friday. The next week you'd perform Workout B on Monday, Workout A on Wednesday, and Workout B on Friday.

▌Prior to the workout, complete "The Total Body Jump Start" warmup on page 340.

▌When you see a number with a letter next to it (such as 1A, 1B), that means the exercises are performed as a circuit. For each circuit, do 1 set of each exercise in succession. For example, complete 1 set of exercise 1A, rest as directed, and then perform 1 set of exercise 1B and rest again. Follow this pattern until you've completed all sets of each exercise in the group, and then progress to the next circuit.

▌This workout also includes Energy System Training, a bonus workout that you can complete at the end of your workout if one of your primary goals is fat loss. This portion consists of one exercise (Squat Thrust, for example) that will be performed for timed intervals. You'll do exercise for the amount of time prescribed, rest as indicated, and then repeat for the number of sets listed.

▌Each exercise includes a prescription for tempo—that is, the speed at which you move the weight. Each tempo includes three numbers that each refer to a lifting speed (in seconds).

The first number represents how much time you should take to lower the weight. So if the first number is 3, then you should take 3 seconds to lower the weight.

The second number represents how long you should pause at the bottom of a rep. If that number is 0, then there is no pause.

The last number is how quickly you should lift or press the weight. For instance, a 1 would mean an explosive lift that takes just 1 second.

The Best Abs Workouts Ever Created

Workout A

Strength Training

EXERCISE	TEMPO	WEEK 1	WEEK 2	WEEK 3	WEEK 4	REST
1A Goblet Squat (page 237)	3, 0, 1	2 sets of 8–12 reps	3 sets of 8–12 reps	3 sets of 8–12 reps	3 sets of 8–12 reps	60–90 seconds
1B Pushup (page 132)	2, 0, 2	2 sets of 8–12 reps	3 sets of 8–12 reps	3 sets of 8–12 reps	3 sets of 8–12 reps	60–90 seconds
2A Dumbbell Romanian Deadlift (page 255)	3, 0, 1	2 sets of 10 reps	3 sets of 10 reps	3 sets of 8 reps	3 sets of 8 reps	60 seconds
2B Cable Core Press (page 321)	3, 0, 1	2 sets of 12 reps	3 sets of 12 reps	3 sets of 10 reps	3 sets of 10 reps	60 seconds
3A Wall Slide (page 192)	2, 0, 2	2 sets of 8 reps	2 sets of 8 reps	2 sets of 10 reps	2 sets of 10 reps	45–60 seconds
3B I Raise (page 188), T Raise (page 186), Y Raise (page 187); perform these as a sequence	1, 2, 1	2 sets of 6–12 reps	2 sets of 6–12 reps	2 sets of 6–12 reps	2 sets of 6–12 reps	45–60 seconds

Energy System Training (optional to increase fat loss)

SQUAT THRUST (page 201)	INTENSITY	RECOVERY	SETS	COMMENTS
WEEK 1	30 seconds	90 seconds	4	
WEEK 2	30 seconds	90 seconds	5	
WEEK 3	30 seconds	90 seconds	6	
WEEK 4	30 seconds	60 seconds	6	

Workout B

Strength Training

EXERCISE	TEMPO	WEEK 1	WEEK 2	WEEK 3	WEEK 4	REST
1A Dumbbell Deadlift (page 251)	3, 0, 1	2 sets of 12 reps	3 sets of 12 reps	3 sets of 10 reps	3 sets of 10 reps	60–90 seconds
1B Dumbbell Bent-Over Row (page 161)	3, 0, 1	2 sets of 12 reps	3 sets of 12 reps	3 sets of 10 reps	3 sets of 10 reps	60–90 seconds
2A Barbell Hip Raise (page 256)	2, 1, 2	2 sets of 12 reps	3 sets of 12 reps	3 sets of 10 reps	3 sets of 10 reps	60 seconds
2B Split Stance Cable Chop (page 312)	3, 1, 1	2 sets of 12 reps	3 sets of 12 reps	3 sets of 10 reps	3 sets of 10 reps	60 seconds
3A Side Plank (page 287)	1, 5, 1	2 sets of 8 reps	2 sets of 8 reps	2 sets of 10 reps	2 sets of 10 reps	45–60 seconds
3B Three-Point Dumbbell Row (page 167)	1, 4, 1	2 sets of 12 reps	2 sets of 12 reps	2 sets of 12 reps	2 sets of 12 reps	45–60 seconds

Energy System Training (optional to increase fat loss)

DUMBBELL CLEAN (page 211)	INTENSITY	REST	SETS
WEEK 1	10 swings/minute	0	8
WEEK 2	10 swings/minute	0	8
WEEK 3	10 swings/minute	0	10
WEEK 4	10 swings/minute	0	10

ABOUT THE EXPERT

Bill Hartman is co-owner of Indianapolis Fitness and Sports Training (http://indianapolis-fitnessandsport-straining.com/). He has been a physical therapist and sports performance coach for more than 17 years. Hartman has received advanced training in treatment of spinal disorders including spinal mobilization, treatment of lumbo-pelvic disorders, shoulder rehabilitation, knee rehabilitation, core conditioning, and treatment of soft tissue disorders. He is also an Active Release Techniques Practitioner with credentials to treat upper extremity, lower extremity, and spinal disorders.

The Two-Exercise Abs Builder

Guys hate gimmicks, especially when it comes to empty promises regarding their body. Electrical belts. Rotating chairs. Creams that magically make your stomach ripple. That's all BS. But you might be surprised to find out that a workout consisting of just two exercises might be the fastest way to jump-start a fat loss plan. This isn't a hard sell: It's an eye-opening look at a new, more efficient way to build your body in no time. Do this plan for 4 weeks to burn off some serious fat, and then shift your goals to continue on your better body mission.

HOW TO DO IT

▌ Perform this workout 3 days a week, resting at least a day between each session. So you might perform on Monday, Wednesday, and Friday.

▌ Prior to the workout, complete "The Total Body Jump Start" warmup on page 340.

▌ The routine consists of just two exercises: stepups and getups. Alternate between 60 seconds of work and 30 seconds of rest. That is, do the first exercise for 60 seconds and rest 30 seconds. Then move to the second exercise and do that for another 60 seconds, followed by another 30 seconds of rest. That's one round.

▌ Perform a total of eight rounds, rest 1 minute, and then complete the entire sequence a second time. If you really want to scorch more calories, you can try for a third cycle.

EXERCISE	SETS	REPS	REST
Stepup (page 260), using a dumbbell or kettlebell	8 rounds	60 seconds	30 seconds
Dumbbell Getup (page 227), or use a kettlebell	8 rounds	60 seconds	30 seconds

ABOUT THE EXPERT

BJ Gaddour, CSCS, is a fitness boot camp and metabolic training expert. He is the CEO of StreamFIT (http://StreamFIT.com), which provides unlimited streaming follow-along workouts from the top trainers in the game. He is also a regular contributor to *Men's Health* and a consultant to New Balance.

The 4-Day Core Transformation Plan

Guys like simplicity and speed. It's why things like microwaves, iPhones, and SportsCenter Top 10 were made for men. No question about it: They get the job done in a way that you approve. The same can be said about this workout plan. It's to the point. Four exercises. Four days per week completed over a 4-week span. And it targets the four areas of focus you need to build abs: a total body approach, cardio conditioning, more intensity, and a varied plan that will keep it fun and challenging. The simplicity? Well, you don't even have to count reps. Combine it all together, and you have a routine designed to build muscle, condition your body, and take your metabolism to the next level. Consider this the new generation of a guy-friendly training plan that won't disappoint.

HOW TO DO IT

▌ This routine consists of three workouts: A, B, and C. Perform Workouts A and B on back-to-back days, rest a day, and then do Workouts A and C on back-to-back days. For example, you'll do Workout A on Monday and Workout B on Tuesday. You'll take a day off on Wednesday. On Thursday you'll repeat Workout A and then do Workout C on Friday.

▌ Prior to the workout, complete "The Total Body Jump Start" warmup on page 340.

▌ Workout A consists of 3 circuits. Start with the first circuit and perform 1 set of each exercise in the order listed. That's one round. Rest for 60 seconds, and then repeat the circuit another two times. Once you have completed 3 sets of the circuit, then move on to the next circuit and repeat.

▌ Workouts B and C consists of supersets. When you see a number with a letter next to it—such as 1A and 1B—it means the exercises should be performed as a group. Do 1 set of the first exercise, rest for the prescribed amount of time, and then do 1 set of the next exercise in the group. Repeat until you've completed all of your sets for each exercise, and then move on to the next group.

The Best Abs Workouts Ever Created

Workout A: Metabolic Circuit 9 rounds = 45 minutes total

Circuit 1

EXERCISE	SETS	REPS	REST
Dumbbell Uppercut (page 193)	3	30 seconds	15 seconds
Dumbbell Walking Lunge (page 245)	3	30 seconds	15 seconds
Dumbbell Pushup Row (page 155)	3	30 seconds	15 seconds
Jump rope/run/shadow box	3	90 seconds	60 seconds

Circuit 2

EXERCISE	SETS	REPS	REST
Dumbbell or Kettlebell Swing (page 210)	3	30 seconds	15 seconds
Squat Jump (page 234)	3	30 seconds	15 seconds
Inchworm (page 224)	3	30 seconds	15 seconds
Jump rope/run/shadow box	3	90 seconds	60 seconds

Circuit 3

EXERCISE	SETS	REPS	REST
Spiderman Pushup (page 153)	3	30 seconds	15 seconds
Dumbbell Deadlift (page 251) + Calf Raise (page 241) + Dumbbell Shrug (page 190)	3	30 seconds	15 seconds
T Raise (page 186)	3	30 seconds	15 seconds
Jump rope/run/shadow box	3	30 seconds	15 seconds

Workout B: Push/Pull Strength Workouts

EXERCISE	SETS	REPS	REST
1A Dumbbell Chest Press (page 145)	4–5	6–8	60 seconds
1B Dumbbell Bent-Over Row (page 161)	4–5	6–8	60 seconds
2A Barbell Shoulder Press (page 184)	4–5	6–8	60 seconds
2B Pullup (page 171)	4–5	6–8	60 seconds
3A Dumbbell Skull Crusher (page 181)	3	10–12	60 seconds
3B Dumbbell Biceps Curl (page 175)	3	10–12	60 seconds
4 Dumbbell Farmer's Walk (page 226)	4–5	1 minute	60 seconds

Workout C: Legs/Hips/Abs Strength Workouts

EXERCISE	SETS	REPS	REST
1A Barbell Deadlift (page 272)	4–5	6–8	60 seconds
1B Stability Ball Reaching Crunch (page 306)	4	6–8	60 seconds
2A Dumbbell Walking Lunge (page 245)	3–4	6–8	60 seconds
2B Band Tight Rotation (page 313)	3–4	15–20	60 seconds
3A Barbell Front Squat (page 232)	3	10–12	60 seconds
3B Swiss Ball Hip Raise and Leg Curl (page 259)	3	10–15	60 seconds
4 Dumbbell Farmer's Walk (page 226)	4–5	1 minute	60 seconds

ABOUT THE EXPERT

Nick Tumminello is the owner of Performance University International, which provides hybrid strength training and conditioning in Ft. Lauderdale, Florida. He trains the trainers and athletes all over the world. Nick writes a very popular fitness blog at http://NickTumminello.com.

The Better Sex Workout

The money line. The love line. Penis line. No matter what you call it, everyone knows what's you're talking about: the inguinal crease. It's the one bit of erotic body definition that everyone recognizes. Every guy wants them. Every woman wants to explore them. Now it's time to have them.

It's speculated that you'll need to drop to about 8 percent body fat to make the magical lines appear.

While you might have trouble believing that a workout in the gym could improve your workout in bed, it's true. This plan will arm you with stronger abs, hips, and glutes—all of the muscles you need to thrust, grind, and please. Plus, the added strength will help you hold positions longer *and* hold your partner in ways that will open up a whole new world of sexual possibilities. And your improved conditioning in the gym will lead to more stamina in the sack, meaning you can finally last longer with your lady.

ABOUT THE EXPERT

Roger Lawson, CSCS, is a personal trainer at All-Access Fitness Academy in Shrewsbury, Massachusetts. He is a highly sought-after coach for advanced athletes to beginners because of his relaxed approach to fitness, and he specializes in fat loss and muscle gain. Lawson is also the author of RogLawFitness (www.roglawfitness.com) where he writes weekly fitness advice, blending hilarity, nerd references and an unyielding sense of positivity with the goal of "sexifying" the world one person at a time.

HOW TO DO IT

▮ Perform this workout 3 days a week, resting at least a day between each session. So you might go on Monday, Wednesday, and Friday.

▮ Prior to the workout, complete "The Total Body Jump Start" warmup on page 340.

▮ When you see a number with a letter next to it—such as 1A and 1B—it means the exercises should be performed as a group. Do 1 set of the first exercise, rest for the prescribed amount of time, and then do 1 set of the next exercise in the group. Repeat until you've completed all of your sets for each exercise, and then move on to the next group.

▮ Use the following guide to your rest:

Exercises 1 and 2: 2 minutes rest between sets

Exercises 3, 4, and 5: 45 seconds between sets

Exercise 6: 60 seconds between sets

EXERCISE	SETS	REPS	REST
1 Barbell Front Squat (page 232)	2–3	6–8	2 minutes
2 Chinup L-Sit Hold (page 334)	2–3	6–8	2 minutes
3A One-Dumbbell Reverse Lunge (page 249)	2–3	8–10/side	45 seconds
3B Kneeling Barbell Rollout (page 297)	2–3	8–10	45 seconds
4A Single-Arm Dumbbell Chest Press (page 149), neutral grip	2–3	6–8	45 seconds
5A Dumbbell Saxon Side Bend (page 301)	2–3	8–10	45 seconds
5B Stability Ball Jackknife (page 304)	2–3	10–12	45 seconds
6 Bird Dog (page 295)	2–3	15–30 seconds	60 seconds

The Strong and Lean Workout

It doesn't matter if you've never visited the gym before or have been pumping iron for 20 years. The formula for a better body depends on a few simple concepts: Pick the right exercises, improve each workout, and bring the intensity. This workout was designed for all three of those purposes: The exercises not only are some of the most effective you'll find, but also are designed to make you stronger with each visit to the gym and force you to bring your A-game with each rep. If your workouts ever go astray, this plan will get you back on track and build a killer row of abs—and pack on definition to your back, shoulders, arms, and legs.

HOW TO DO IT

▌ Perform this workout 3 days a week, resting at least a day between each session. So you might go on Monday, Wednesday, and Friday.

▌ Prior to the workout, complete "The Total Body Jump Start" warmup on page 340.

▌ On the first exercise (Trap Bar Deadlift), you'll be working up to a top-level set. That is, you'll warm up until you do 1 set of 3 to 5 reps using 85 to 90 percent of your 1-rep max. Then, you'll reduce the load by 5 percent for each subsequent set, making sure you rest 2 minutes between sets.

▌ For the second exercise, you'll be using the "rest-pause" technique. Pick a weight you can manage for 10 to 12 reps on your first set. Do the first set, but stop about 1 to 2 reps short of failure. Then, rest for 20 seconds and again perform as many reps as you can, stopping about 1 rep short of failure. Continue this pattern until you complete 30 total reps. Add more weight when you can do more than 12 reps on the first set.

EXERCISE	SETS	REPS	REST
1 Trap Bar Deadlift (page 273)	5	3–5	2 minutes
2 Barbell Bent-Over Row (page 160)	Rest-pause	30 total reps	20 seconds between pauses
3 Cable Core Press (page 321)	3	6–8	60 seconds
4 Med Ball Slam (page 325)	3	45 seconds	30 seconds

ABOUT THE EXPERT

JC Deen, founder of JCDFitness.com, is a Nashville-based strength coach, consultant, and writer. Deen has been featured in Forbes.com and has written for the *Alan Aragon Research Review* as well as Bodybuilding.com. He's known for his no-BS, science-based approach to training, with an emphasis on looking great naked.

The Rapid Fat Loss Workout

Spartacus. 300. The Immortals. All of these movies highlight the lean, chiseled bodies of warriors—and the look that most modern men want. The problem? Most guys don't put themselves through the gauntlet of challenges needed to build *that* type of hard body. That's why we approached Craig Ballantyne, the founder of Turbulence Training, to create a gauntlet-style workout routine that constantly challenges and rechallenges your muscles to provide the fastest results possible. We'll warn you: Performing this workout might feel like you're going to battle. And while your life doesn't require that you prepare for actual war, the end result will have you looking the part of a real warrior.

HOW TO DO IT

▐ Perform this workout 3 days a week, resting at least a day between each session. So you might go on Monday, Wednesday, and Friday.

▐ Prior to the workout, complete "The Total Body Jump Start" warmup on page 340.

▐ This routine consists of 3 circuits of three exercises each. Perform 1 set of each exercise in the order listed, trying to rest as little as possible between exercises. Once you finish 1 set of each move, rest for 1 minute and then repeat two more times. After you have finished all sets, move on to the next circuit.

▐ The final circuit is a metabolic finisher. Perform each exercise for 30 seconds with no rest between exercises (but rest if needed). Do this entire circuit three times, resting 1 minute between rounds.

EXERCISE	SETS	REPS	REST
1A Barbell Deadlift (page 272)	3	8	0
1B Single-Arm Dumbbell Chest Press (page 149)	3	8	0
1C Three-Point Dumbbell Row (page 167)	3	15	0

EXERCISE	SETS	REPS	REST
2A Swiss Ball Rollout (page 318)	3	12	0
2B High Cable Chop (page 308)	3	12	0
2C Swiss Ball Rollout (page 318)	3	8	0

EXERCISE	SETS	REPS	REST
3A Inchworm (page 224)	3	30 seconds	0
3B Cross-Body Mountain Climber (page 292)	3	30 seconds	0
3C Inchworm (page 224)	3	30 seconds	0

ABOUT THE EXPERT

Craig Ballantyne is a strength and conditioning coach in Toronto, author of *Turbulence Training*, and a *Men's Health* magazine training expert. Ballantyne is also the editor of www.EarlytoRise.com. Each day, he sends a wisdom essay, showing you how to live a better life and how to achieve the American Dream. He has an advanced research background with a master's in exercise physiology from McMaster University in Hamilton, Ontario. Ballantyne's fat loss, muscle-building Web site, www.TurbulenceTraining.com, features his best-selling Turbulence Training for Fat Loss program; www.TTmembers.com offers access to all of his Turbulence Training workouts and videos.

The Best Abs Workouts Ever Created

Burn Your Spare Tire

Hey, gut! Yeah, you hear me. I'm talking to you—the belly. Listen up, because this program was specifically designed for YOU.

Imagine if you could burn fat 24 hours a day, 7 days a week. How much easier would it be to eat your favorite foods and still look like you bust your ass in the gym? While we can't guarantee nonstop fat burning, this workout is the closest thing you'll find to the gut-eliminator. At first glance, it doesn't look like much. But each one of these "traditional" exercises has been modified to work your abs more than they've ever been challenged before. And they've been adjusted to recruit your larger muscles even more than usual, so you're stripping away layers of fat and replacing it with real muscle. It's a scientific approach: Two days a week you'll be packing on new size, and the other two you'll be targeting unwanted pounds. Take this workout for a test drive, and you'll be in the fast lane to your new body.

▌This routine consists of four workouts: A, B, C, and D. Perform Workouts A and B on back-to-back days, rest a day, and then do Workouts C and D on back-to-back-days. Make sure that you never train on three consecutive days. For instance, you'll do Workout A on Monday, Workout B on Tuesday, and then rest on Wednesday. On Thursday you'll do Workout C, Friday Workout D, and then follow with more rest before repeating the sequence.

▌Prior to the workout, complete "The Total Body Jump Start" warmup on page 340.

▌When you see a number with a letter next to it—such as 1A and 1B—it means the exercises should be performed as a group. Do 1 set of the first exercise, rest for the prescribed amount of time, and then do 1 set of the next exercise in the group. Repeat until you've completed all of your sets for each exercise, and then move on to the next group.

▌On your off days, it's recommended that you perform the foam-rolling routine shown in the warmup or do light cardio to burn some extra calories.

The Best Abs Workouts Ever Created

Workout A

EXERCISE	SETS	REPS	REST
1A Single-Arm Dumbbell Push Press (page 206)	3	8–10/side	60–90 seconds
1B Barbell Front Squat (page 232)	3	6–10	60–90 seconds
2A Single-Arm Dumbbell Chest Press (page 149)	3	8–10/side	60–90 seconds
2B Single-Leg Squat (page 267)	3	6–8/side	60–90 seconds
3A Cable Punch (page 152)	3	15–20/side	60–90 seconds
3B Dumbbell Chop (page 310)	3	15–20/side	60–90 seconds
4A Side-to-Side Pushup (page 143)	3	15–20/side	60–90 seconds
4B Plyo Pushup (page 144)	3	6–10	60–90 seconds
4C Pushup (page 132)	3	6–10	60–90 seconds

Workout B

EXERCISE	SETS	REPS	REST
1A Med Ball Slam (page 325)	4	40 seconds	90–120 seconds
1B Kettlebell or Dumbbell Suitcase Carry (page 226), right arm	4	30 meters	90–120 seconds
1C Med Ball Side Rotation (page 324)	4	40 seconds	90–120 seconds
1D Dumbbell Suitcase Carry (page 226), left arm	4	30 meters	2 minutes
2 Dumbbell Thruster (page 380)	8	20 seconds	10 seconds

Workout C

EXERCISE	SETS	REPS	REST
1A Chinup (page 334)	3	6–8	60–90 seconds
1B Single-Leg Barbell Romanian Deadlift (page 254)	3	6–8	60–90 seconds
2A Hanging Leg Raise (page 335)	3	8–10	60–90 seconds
2B Split Stance Single-Arm Cable Row (page 165)	3	10–12	60–90 seconds
3A Rope High Pull (page 215)	3	12–15	60–90 seconds
3B Resistance Band Core Press (page 322)	3	20–30/side	60–90 seconds
4A Seated Dumbbell Biceps Curl (page 175)	3	6–8	60–90 seconds
4B EZ Bar Curl (page 179)	3	6–8	60–90 seconds
4C Reverse Grip EZ Bar Curl (page 180)	3	6–8	60–90 seconds

Workout D

EXERCISE	SETS	REPS	REST
1A Dumbbell Farmer's Walk (page 226)	4	40 meters	90–120 seconds
1B Dumbbell Clean (page 211)	4	8–10	90–120 seconds
1C Dumbbell Pushup Row (page 155)	4	10–20	90–120 seconds
1D Dumbbell Farmer's Walk (page 226)	4	40 meters	90–120 seconds
2 Dumbbell or Kettlebell Swing (page 210)	8	20 seconds	10 seconds

ABOUT THE EXPERT

Jon Goodman, CSCS, is the founder and head coach of the Personal Trainer Development Center (www.theptdc.com) and the senior trainer at Body + Soul Fitness in Toronto, Canada. His book, *Ignite the Fire: The Secrets to Building a Successful Personal Training Career*, is a must-have resource for any new or existing personal trainer striving to improve. You can find Goodman on Facebook (www.facebook.com/CoachJonGoodman), and he maintains a personal blog at www.jongoodman.ca.

The Best Abs Workouts Ever Created

The Hollywood Abs Workout

You know that the abs on the silver screen can be deceiving. It's not that actors don't work themselves into top shape—it's just that they have a few unfair advantages. They have all day to dedicate to training, the best trainers, and a rock-solid diet plan. While we can't pay you to hit the gym, we can provide the same type of expert diet and training advice typically reserved for the stars. This plan, from celeb supertrainer Joe Dowdell, delivers what you want: a kick-ass workout that will make your body look like an A-List talent.

HOW TO DO IT

▌Perform this workout 3 days a week, resting at least a day between each session. So you might lift weights on Monday, Wednesday, and Friday.

▌Prior to the workout, complete "The Total Body Jump Start" warmup on page 340.

▌This workout is split into 3 separate circuits. Each circuit contains three exercises. Perform 1 set of each exercise in succession, resting just 30 seconds between moves. Once you finish the third exercise in the circuit, rest and restart the process. After you have completed the circuit three times, move on to the next group of exercises and repeat the same process.

EXERCISE	SETS	REPS	REST
1A Goblet Squat (page 237)	3	10–12	30 seconds
1B Three-Point Dumbbell Row (page 167)	3	10–12	30 seconds
1C Plank (page 282)	3	60 seconds	30 seconds
2A Swiss Ball Hip Raise and Leg Curl (page 259)	3	10–12	30 seconds
2B Pushup (page 132)	3	AMAP	30 seconds
2C Jumping Jack (page 198)	3	10–12	30 seconds
3A Dumbbell Push Press (page 205)	3	10–12	30 seconds
3B Dumbbell Zottoman Curl (page 178)	3	10–12	30 seconds
3C Mountain Climber (page 286)	3	60 seconds	30 seconds

ABOUT THE EXPERT

Joe Dowdell, CSCS, is the co-owner of Peak Performance in New York City. Dowdell makes his living training celebrities, professional athletes, and cover models, and is widely recognized as one of the best strength coaches in the world. He is also the co-author of *Ultimate You.* You can find more from Joe at http://JoeDowdell.com.

Index

Boldface page references indicate photographs. <u>Underscored</u> references indicate boxed text.

A

Abdominal muscles
  activation of, 104
  assessing weaknesses, 122–25
  frequency of training, 28
Abs Workout, 100–119
  Bodyweight Training (Workout 3),
    112–13, **112–13**
  Bodyweight Training (Workout 6),
    118–19, **118–19**
  Cardio Workout
    high-intensity interval training
      (HIIT), 120
    20-minute moderate-intensity, 121
  Descending Pyramids (Workout 2),
    110–11, **110–11**
  Descending Pyramids (Workout 5),
    116–17, **116–17**
  Heavy Training (Workout 1), 108–9,
    108–9
  Heavy Training (Workout 4), 114–15,
    114–15
  program explained, 104, 106
  schedule, 107
Ab wheel rollout, 297, **297**
Alcohol, 19
Alignment. *See also* Exercise movement
    patterns
  anterior pelvic tilt, 34, **34**
  importance of, 35
  normal spinal, **34**
Almonds
  Beef, Vegetable, and Almond Stir-Fry, 88

Alternating superman plank and reach,
  290, **290**
Ankle mobility, 41
Anterior pelvic tilt, 34, **34**
Aragon, Alan, <u>28</u>
Arms, exercises for, 172–81
Around the world, 331, **331**
Arthritis, <u>15</u>
Artificial sweeteners, 26
Assisted chinup, 165, **165**
Athlete's Core Workout, 358–59
Avocado
  Egg and Avocado Breakfast Sandwich,
    84

B

Back
  exercises for, 158–71
  pain, 30, 36
Back extension, 263, **263**
Backward monster walk, 37, **37**, 270,
  270
Ballantyne, Craig, 376, 377
Bananas
  Strawberry-Banana Protein Smoothie,
    91
Band pull-apart, 164, **164**
Band tight rotation, 313, **313**
Barbell bench press, 151, **151**
Barbell bent-over row, 160, **160**
Barbell clean and press, 213, **213**

Barbell deadlift, 272, **272**
Barbell front squat, 232, **232**
Barbell hack squat, 271, **271**
Barbell high pull, 212, **212**
Barbell hip raise, 256, **256**
Barbell Romanian deadlift, 252, **252**
Barbell shoulder press, 184, **184**
Barbell squat, 230, **230**
Basal metabolic rate (BMR), 11
Beans
  Chipotle Glazed Steak with Black
    Bean Salad, 86
  Roast Salmon with White Bean
    Compote, 90
Beef
  Beef, Vegetable, and Almond Stir-Fry,
    88
  Chipotle Glazed Steak with Black
    Bean Salad, 86
Beer, 13, 19, <u>73</u>
Bench press, form for, 46, **46**
Better Sex Workout, 372–73
Beverages, calorie-rich, 13
Bird dog, 295, **295**
Black tea, <u>59</u>, 70
Blood sugar, 57
Blueberries, <u>82</u>
  Berry Goat Cheese Salad, 85
  High-Protein Blueberry Yogurt Shake,
    90
BMR, 11
Body fat percentage, 28

Bodyweight exercises. *See also specific exercises*
  Bodyweight Training workouts, 112–13, **112–13**, 118–19, **118–19**
  efficacy of, 106
  lateral lunge, 247, **247**
  lunge, 246, **246**
  squat, 231, **231**
Bok choy
  Rice Bowls with Shrimp and Bok Choy, 86
Box jump, 239, **239**
Breakfast
  eating plan, 59, 60–63
  recipes, 83–84
  skipping, 78
Breathing assessment, 122–23
Bulgarian split squat, 250, **250**
Burn Your Spare Tire workout, 378–81

C

Cable core press, 321, **321**
Cable punch, 152, **152**
Caffeine, 25, 71
Calcium, 94, 96
Calf raise, 241, **241**
Calories
  burned by
    cardio, 54, 55
    digestion, 57
    exercise, 44
    fat in diet, 14
    intervals, 55
    non-exercise activity thermogenesis (NEAT), 25
    protein, 73
    thermic effect of food (TEF), 73
    vegetables in diet, 72
    weight training, 14, 55
  counting, 23, 53, 54, 77
  empty, 54
  sources of
    beverages, 13
    dairy products, 25
    eating out, 99
    low-protein diets, 59

  protein shakes, 23
  snacks, 12–13
  vegetables, 56
Cancer, 13
Carbohydrates
  overeating, 23, 97
  thermic effect of food (TEF), 73
  in vegetarian diet, 96
Cardio
  interval training, 26
  weight training compared, 24, 26, 54–55, 56
  workouts
    Cardio-Strength Workout, 354–55
    high-intensity interval training (HIIT), 120
    20-minute moderate-intensity, 121
Casein, 18
Celiac disease, 98
Chest, exercises for, 131–57
Chewing your food, 16, 59
Chicken
  Chicken Lettuce Cups, 87
  Chicken with Walnuts and Spinach, 88
  Grilled Chicken and Pineapple Sandwich, 85
  Hoisin-Orange Glazed Chicken, 89
Chinup, **44**, 44–45, 334, **334**
Chinup L-sit hold, 334, **334**
Chitosan, 71
Chocolate
  Chocolate-Peanut Butter Smoothie, 91
  dark, 82
  Mint Chocolate Chip Smoothie, 91
Cholesterol, 74–75
Closed kinetic chain exercises (CKCE), 106
Close-grip bench press, 150, **150**
Compound exercises, 26–27, 31
Conjugated linoleic acid (CLA), 71
Cooldown, 120
Core muscles, 103
  Athlete's Core Workout, 358–59
  exercises for, 27–28, 280–335
  strength for back health, 30
Corrective exercise, 35
Cortisol, 14, 18, 73

Cottage cheese, 95
Cravings, 13, 15, 16, 17, 28
Creatine, 97
Cressey, Eric, 28–29
Cross-behind lunge, 248, **248**
Cross-body mountain climber, 292, **292**
Crossover stepup, 261, **261**
Crunches, 26, 103

D

Dairy
  benefits of, 18, 24–25
  lactose intolerance, 94–96
  shopping list, 65
Deadlift, 27, 31, 38, **38**
  barbell, 272, **272**
  barbell Romanian, 252, **252**
  dumbbell, 251, **251**
  dumbbell Romanian, 255, **255**
  kettlebell Romanian, 276, **276**
  one-dumbbell single-leg Romanian, 253, **253**
  single-leg barbell Romanian, 254, **254**
  snatch grip, 251, **251**
  sumo, 255, **255**
  trap bar, 273, **273**
Deen, J.C., 375
Dehydration, 70
Descending Pyramids workouts, 110–11, **110–11**, 116–17, **116–17**
Desk, getting up from, 25
Dessert, 16–17, 73
DHA, 97
Diabetes, risk decrease with lower body fat, 15
Diagonal hip rock to step, 37, **37**, 269, **269**
Diaphragmatic breathing, 122
Diet(s)
  Abs Formula, 77
  eating out, 99
  exercise as complement to, 5, 19
  gluten-free, 97, 98, 99
  guidelines
    protein, 72–74
    snacks, 74, 76, 78

Diet(s) (*cont.*)
  guidelines (*cont.*)
    vegetables, 70, 72
    water, 69–70
  lactose intolerant, 94–96
  vegetarian, 96–97
Diet foods, 15
Dieting, restrictive, 53, 55, 93–94
Dinner
  eating plan, 59, 60–63
  recipes, 87–90
Dips, 156, **156**
Divebomber pushup, 142, **142**
Docosahexaenoic acid (DHA), 97
Dopamine, 16
Dos Remedios, Robert, 355
Dowdell, Joe, 382, 383
Dumbbell bent-over row, 161, **161**
Dumbbell bent-over row (neutral grip),
  162, **162**
Dumbbell biceps curl, 175, **175**
Dumbbell Bulgarian split squat, 275, **275**
Dumbbell chest press, 145, **145**
Dumbbell chop, 310, **310**
Dumbbell clean, 211, **211**
Dumbbell curl to squat to press, 200, **200**
Dumbbell deadlift, 251, **251**
Dumbbell farmer's walk, 39, **39**, 227, **227**
Dumbbell front raise, 191, **191**
Dumbbell front squat, 231, **231**
Dumbbell getup, 27–28, 222, **222**
Dumbbell hang jump shrug, 217, **217**
Dumbbell high pull, 214, **214**
Dumbbell jump, 234, **234**
Dumbbell lateral lunge, 246, **246**
Dumbbell lateral shoulder raise,
  185, **185**
Dumbbell overhead press, 189, **189**
Dumbbell push press, 205, **205**
Dumbbell pushup row, 155, **155**
Dumbbell rear lateral raise, 186, **186**
Dumbbell renegade crawl, 219, **219**
Dumbbell reverse chop (low to high), 311,
  311
Dumbbell reverse lunge, 274, **274**
Dumbbell Romanian deadlift, 255, **255**
Dumbbell row with rotation, 168, **168**

Dumbbell Saxon side bend, 301, **301**
Dumbbell seated core stabilization, 315,
  315
Dumbbell shrug, 190, **190**
Dumbbell skull crusher, 181, **181**
Dumbbell snatch, 209, **209**
Dumbbell split jump, 244, **244**
Dumbbell split squat, 235, **235**
Dumbbell squat jump, 240, **240**
Dumbbell squat thrust, 204, **204**
Dumbbell suitcase carry, 226, **226**
Dumbbell swing, 210, **210**
Dumbbell T-pushup, 135, **135**
Dumbbell uppercut, 193, **193**
Dumbbell walking lunge, 245, **245**
Dumbbell Zottoman curl, 178, **178**

E

Eating
  after workout, 29
  flexible guide, 65
  late-night, 28
  with people having similar goals, 17
  social, 59
  speed of, 16, 59
  stress effect on, 16
  tips for eating less, 59
Eating plan, 59, 60–63
Eggs
  Better-For-You Egg Salad, 86
  Egg and Avocado Breakfast Sandwich,
    84
  fat in, 75
  Flat Green Chile and Goat Cheese
    Omelet, 84
  Huevos Rancheros, 83
  Smoked Salmon and Scrambled Eggs
    on Toast, 83
Eicosapentaenoic acid (EPA), 82
Elliptical, 13
Energy System Training, 363–65
Ephedrine, 25
Epigallocatechin gallate, 71
Erectile dysfunction, 17
Exercise ball, sitting on, 28–29
Exercise machines, 14, 55, 102–3

Exercise movement patterns, 36–49,
  36–49
  lower body pulling, 38–39, **38–39**
  lower body pushing, 36–37, **36–37**
  lower body split stance/lunge, 40–41,
    40–41
  upper body horizontal pulling, 42–43,
    42–43
  upper body horizontal pushing, 46–47,
    46–47
  upper body vertical pulling, 44–45,
    44–45
  upper body vertical pushing, 48–49,
    48–49
Exercises. *See also* Workouts; *specific
    exercises*
  compound, 26–27, 31
  for core, 280–335
  for fat loss, 361
  frequency of, 22–23
  lower body, 228–79
  for movement correction
    backward monster walk, 37, **37**
    diagonal hip rock to step, 37, **37**
    dumbbell farmer's walk, 39, **39**
    lying scap and chin retraction, 39, **39**
    med ball extension with breath, 45, **45**
    mini-band resisted single-leg stance,
      41, **41**
    one-arm waiter's walk, 49, **49**
    quadruped extension-rotation, 43, **43**
    scap pushup, 47, **47**
    stability ball front plank with mini
      rollout, 47, **47**
    standing hips flexed Ts and Ws, 43,
      43
    3-way ankle mobilization, 41, **41**
    wall slide, 45, **45**
    wall snow angel, 49, **49**
  rotational, 31
  total body, 196–227
  upper body
    arms, 172–81
    back, 158–71
    chest, 131–57
    shoulders, 182–95
Extended plank, 293, **293**

Extension rotation, 298, **298**
EZ bar curl, 179, **179**

F

Face pulls, 166, **166**
Fartlek, 26
Fat loss
  by high-protein dieters, 57
  optional exercises for faster, 361
  sources of
    diet, 23
    exercise, 22, 24
    high-fiber vegetables, 72
    late-night meals, 78
    protein in diet, 73
    vitamin D, 18
    weight training, 54–55, 56
    whey protein in diet, 17
    yogurt, 95
  supplements, 25, 71
  thermic effect of food (TEF), 73
  workouts
    Burn Your Spare Tire, 378–81
    Energy System Training for, 364–65
    Rapid Fat Loss Workout, 376–77
    Stubborn Fat Loss Workout, 360–61
Fats
  calories in, 77
  monounsaturated fats (MUFAs), 15, 75
  as percentage of diet, 15, 75
  saturated, 15, 24, 75
  shopping list, 65
  sources of, 15, 24, 75
  trans, 15, 24
Feta cheese
  Spinach and Feta Frittata, 83
Fish
  Asian Salmon Burgers, 87
  Chili-Spiced Fish Tacos, 88
  Peruvian Seafood Stew, 84–85
  Roast Salmon with White Bean
    Compote, 90
  Smoked Salmon and Scrambled Eggs
    on Toast, 83
Fish oil, 14, 71, 97
Food journal, 12

Foods. *See also* Diet; Recipes
  "diet," 15
  fat-free, 4
  favorite in diet, 4
  lean-body, 82
  low-fat, 75
  processed, 58
  recipes, 83–91
  shopping list, 65
  thermic effect of food (TEF), 73
  worst for abs, 25
Form. *See* Exercise movement patterns
45-degree cable row, 170, **170**
4-Day Core Transformation Plan, 368–71
  Legs/Hips/Abs Strength Workouts, 371
  Metabolic Circuit, 370
  Push/Pull Strength Workouts, 371
Front plank with weight transfer, 284, **284**
Fruits, 57, 65

G

Gaddour, B.J., 367
Garhammer raise, 323, **323**
Gentilcore, Tony, 359
Ghrelin, 16
Gluten-free diet, 97, 98, 99
Glutes, self-myofacial release for, 345, **345**
Goals, setting, 18
Goat cheese
  Berry Goat Cheese Salad, 85
  Flat Green Chile and Goat Cheese
    Omelet, 84
Goblet reverse lunge, 248, **248**
Goblet squat, 237, **237**
Goblet squat to press, 203, **203**
Goodman, Jon, 381
Grains, 65
Grasshopper pushup, 140, **140**
Greens, 56–57, 71, 72
Green tea, 70
Gyros, 89

H

Hamstrings, self-myofacial release for,
  345, **345**

Hands-free side plank, 285, **285**
Hanging leg raise, 335, **335**
Hard Body Rules, 54–57
Hartman, Bill, 365
Heart disease, risk decrease with lean
  bellies, 12
Hernia, 27
High cable chop, 308, **308**
High incline dumbbell press, 147, **147**
Hip flexors, self-myofacial release for,
  344, **344**
Hip mobility/stability, 37
Hip raise, 257, **257**
Hip thrust with bench, 266, **266**
Hollywood Abs Workout, 382–83
Hurricane training, 348

I

Inchworm, 224–25, **224–25**
Incline barbell bench press, 151, **151**
Incline dumbbell press, 146, **146**
Injury
  from crunches, 104
  from exercise machines, 103
Insulin, 14, 15, 58
Intensity, workout, 28, 55
Intervals, 26, 55
Inverted row, 161, **161**
I raise, 188, **188**
IT band, self-myofacial release for, 344, **344**

J

Journal, food, 12
Jumping jacks, 198, **198**
Jump rope, 361

K

Kefir, 95
Kettlebell Romanian deadlift, 276, **276**
Kettlebell squat, 274, **274**
Kettlebell suitcase carry, 226, **226**
Kettlebell swing, 210, **210**
Kettlebell swings, 361
Kettlebell windmill, 223, **223**

Knee-grab situp, 299, **299**
Kneeling barbell rollout, 297, **297**
Kneeling mixed-grip pulldown, 169, **169**
Knee movement, 40–41
Knee to elbow pushup, 141, **141**

L

Lactase, 95
Lactose intolerance, 94–96
Lasagna, 87
Lateral band walk, 261, **261**
Lateral plank walk, 290, **290**
Lawson, Roger, 372
Laying posture, 51
Lettuce
    Chicken Lettuce Cups, 87
    Special Shrimp Salad, 86
Low cable lift, 309, **309**
Lower back
    pain, 30
    self-myofacial release, 343, **343**
Lower body
    exercises, 228–79
    pulling (movement pattern), 38–39,
        38–39
    pushing (movement pattern), 36–37,
        36–37
    split stance/lunge (movement pattern),
        40–41, **40–41**
Low incline dumbbell neutral grip chest
    press, 148, **148**
Lunch
    eating plan, 59, 60–63
    recipes, 84–87
Lunge, form for, 40, **40**
Lunge and reach, 218, **218**
Lying scap and chin retraction, 39, **39**
Lying scap and chin rotation, 298, **298**

M

Machines, exercise, 14, 55, 102–3
Meals
    cheat, 25
    eating plan (4 week), 59, 60–63
    flexible eating guide, 65

floating, 76
    late-night, 78–79
    number/frequency of, 12, 24, 59, 64, 76
    recipes, 83–91
    size of, 24
Med ball extension with breath, 45, **45**,
    328, **328**
Med ball Russian twist, 326, **326**
Med ball side rotation, 324, **324**
Med ball side slam, 330, **330**
Med ball single-leg kick, 329, **329**
Med ball slam, 325, **325**
Metabolic syndrome, 15–16, 58
Metabolism
    basal metabolic rate (BMR), 11
    boost with
        water consumption, 70
        weight training, 14, 22, 55
    sleeping, 14
    slowed by processed foods, 58
Microtrauma, 106
Milk, 18
Mini-band resisted single-leg stance, 41,
    41, 265, **265**
Monounsaturated fats (MUFAs), 15, 75
Mountain climber, 286, **286**
Movement correction. *See* Exercise
    movement patterns
MUFAs, 15, 75
Muscle tone
    increase with heavy weight load, 106
    myogenic, 106
    neurogenic, 106
Myofacial release. *See* Self-myofacial
    release

N

No-Crunch Abs Workout, 356–57
Non-exercise activity thermogenesis
    (NEAT), 25
Nuts, 65, 96

O

Obesity, 4, 75, 78
Obliques, rotational exercises for, 31

Omega-3 fatty acids, 14, 24, 82
One-arm dumbbell sumo front squat,
    240, **240**
One-arm overhead press, 189, **189**
One-arm waiter's walk, 49, **49**
One-dumbbell lunge, 247, **247**
One-dumbbell reverse lunge, 249, **249**
One-dumbbell single-leg Romanian
    deadlift, 253, **253**
One-leg plank, 293, **293**
Open kinetic chain exercises (OKCE), 106
Oranges
    Hoisin-Orange Glazed Chicken, 89
Overeating, 16, 23, 56, 64, 72
Overhead press, form for, 48, **48**
Overhead split squat, 242, **242**
Overhead waiter's carry, 208, **208**

P

Pain
    back, 30, 36
    posture problems as cause, 34, 35
Pasta
    Polenta Lasagna, 87
Peanut butter
    Chocolate-Peanut Butter Smoothie,
        91
    Peanut Butter Strawberry Wrap, 84
Perfect Posture Workout, 362–65
Pike pushup, 134, **134**
Pineapple
    Grilled Chicken and Pineapple
        Sandwich, 85
Pizza, 73
Plank, 29, 30, 282, **282**
Planking frog tuck, 291, **291**
Plank jumping jack, 288, **288**
Plank test, 123, **123**
Plank to pushup, 283, **283**
Plank with arm extension, 289, **289**
Plateau, 29, 69
Plate push, 277, **277**
Plyo pushup, 144, **144**
Pork
    Pork Gyros, 89
Portion control, 13, 17

Posture
  desk job effect on, 25
  exercise movement patterns, 36–49,
    36–49
  importance of, 34
  outside the gym
    laying, 51
    sitting, 50–51
    standing, 50
    24-hour rule, 50–51
  Perfect Posture Workout, 362–65
  problems of poor, 34–35
Probiotics, 95
Processed foods, 58
Protein
  before/after workout, 22, 29, 73
  benefits of, 14, 57, 73
  calories in, <u>77</u>
  in every meal, 57
  high-protein foods, 99
  role in diet plan, 72–74
  shopping list, 65
  sources of, 18, 73–74
  thermic effect of food (TEF), 73
  whey, 17, 18, 95
Protein powder, 17, 22, 95, 96
Protein shakes, 17, 23
Pulling (movement pattern)
  lower body, 38–39, **38–39**
  upper body horizontal, 42–43, **42–43**
  upper body vertical, 44–45, **44–45**
Pullup, 44, **44**, 171, **171**
Pulse repetitions, 112
Pumpkin seeds, <u>82</u>
Pushing (movement pattern)
  lower body, 36–37, **36–37**
  upper body horizontal, 46–47, **46–47**
  upper body vertical, 48–49, **48–49**
Push jerks, 207, **207**
Pushup, 46, 132, **132**
  divebomber, 142, **142**
  dumbbell pushup row, 155, **155**
  dumbbell T-pushup, 135, **135**
  grasshopper, 140, **140**
  with hand raise, 138, **138**
  knee to elbow, 141, **141**
  pike, 134, **134**

  plank to pushup, 283, **283**
  plyo, 144, **144**
  scap, 47, **47**
  side-to-side, 143, **143**
  single-leg, 137, **137**
  single-leg with shoulder touch, 139, **139**
  spiderman, 153, **153**
  Valslide spiderman, 154, **154**
Pushup and stepout, 136, **136**
Pushup jack, 137, **137**
Pushup plus, 133, **133**
Pushup test, **124**, 124–25
Pushup with hand raise, 138, **138**
Pyramid training, 105, 110–11, **110–11**,
  116–17, **116–17**

Q

Quadruped extension-rotation, 43, **43**
Quads, self-myofacial release for, 344, **344**

R

Rainbow trout, <u>82</u>
Rapid Fat Loss Workout, 376–77
Raspberry ketones, <u>71</u>
Rate of perceived exertion, 121
Rear foot elevated hip flexor stretch, 266,
  266
Recipes, 83–91
  breakfast, 83–84
    Egg and Avocado Breakfast
      Sandwich, 84
    Flat Green Chile and Goat Cheese
      Omelet, 84
    Huevos Rancheros, 83
    Peanut Butter Strawberry Wrap, 84
    Smoked Salmon and Scrambled
      Eggs on Toast, 83
    Spinach and Feta Frittata, 83
  dinner, 87–90
    Asian Salmon Burgers, 87
    Beef, Vegetable, and Almond Stir-
      Fry, 88
    Chicken Lettuce Cups, 87
    Chicken with Walnuts and Spinach,
      88

    Chili-Spiced Fish Tacos, 88
    Hoisin-Orange Glazed Chicken, 89
    Pork Gyros, 89
    Roast Salmon with White Bean
      Compote, 90
  lunch, 84–87
    Berry Goat Cheese Salad, 85
    Better-For-You Egg Salad, 86
    Chipotle Glazed Steak with Black
      Bean Salad, 86
    Grilled Chicken and Pineapple
      Sandwich, 85
    Peruvian Seafood Stew, 84–85
    Polenta Lasagna, 87
    Rice Bowls with Shrimp and Bok
      Choy, 86
    Special Shrimp Salad, 86
    Tangy Turkey Ciabatta, 85
  smoothies, 90–91
    Chocolate-Peanut Butter Smoothie,
      91
    High-Protein Blueberry Yogurt
      Shake, 90
    Mint Chocolate Chip Smoothie, 91
    Mixed Fruit Breakfast Smoothie, 90
    Strawberry-Banana Protein
      Smoothie, 91
Rectus abdominis, 27, 28
Repetitions
  high-rep workouts, 29–30
  number of, 106
  pulse, 112
  in pyramid training, 105
Resistance band biceps curl, 177, **177**
Resistance band chop, 311, **311**
Resistance band core press, 322, **322**
Resistance band hip raise, 258, **258**
Resistance band overhead triceps press,
  176, **176**
Resistance band pulldown, 170, **170**
Resistance training. *See* Weight training
Rest, 105, 374
Restaurants, eating at, 99
Reverse crunch, 27, 323, **323**
Reverse grip EZ bar curl, 180, **180**
Reverse lunge and rotate, 249, **249**
Reverse lunge and SA cable row, 216, **216**

Rice
    Rice Bowls with Shrimp and Bok Choy, 86
Ricotta cheese, 82
Robertson, Mike, 122
Rolling plank, 296, **296**
Romaniello, John, 104, 115
Rooney, Martin, 348, 351
Rope high pull, 215, **215**
Rotational exercises, 31
Roussell, Mike, 99
Row, form for, 42, **42**
Running, 13, 26, 54, 55

S

Salad
    Berry Goat Cheese Salad, 85
    Better-For-You Egg Salad, 86
    Chipotle Glazed Steak with Black
        Bean Salad, 86
    Special Shrimp Salad, 86
Salmon
    Asian Salmon Burgers, 87
    Roast Salmon with White Bean
        Compote, 90
    Smoked Salmon and Scrambled Eggs
        on Toast, 83
Saturated fats, 15, 24, 75
Scap pushup, 47, **47**
Seafood
    Peruvian Seafood Stew, 84–85
    Rice Bowls with Shrimp and Bok Choy,
        86
    Special Shrimp Salad, 86
Seal jump, 238, **238**
Seated dumbbell biceps curl, 175, **175**
Seated lat pulldown, 168, **168**
Seated twist, 317, **317**
Self-myofacial release, 341, 343–45,
        343–45
    glutes, 345, **345**
    hamstrings, 345, **345**
    IT band, 344, **344**
    lower back, 343, **343**
    quads and hip flexors, 344, **344**
    upper back, 343, **343**

Sex
    Better Sex Workout, 372–73
Shakes
    High-Protein Blueberry Yogurt Shake,
        90
    meal-replacement, 98
    protein, 17, 23
Shopping list, 65
Shoulder press, form for, 48, **48**
Shoulders
    rounding, 38, 45
    upper body exercises for, 182–95
Shrimp
    Peruvian Seafood Stew, 84–85
    Rice Bowls with Shrimp and Bok Choy,
        86
    Special Shrimp Salad, 86
Side-lying clam, 262, **262**
Side-lying windmill, 157, **157**
Side pillar jack, 316, **316**
Side plank, 287, **287**
Side plank and rotate, 287, **287**
Side plank test, **123**, 123–24
Side plank with row, 294, **294**
Side-to-side pushup, 143, **143**
Single-arm dumbbell chest press, 149, **149**
Single-arm dumbbell front squat, 236, **236**
Single-arm dumbbell push press, 206, **206**
Single-arm dumbbell squat, 236, **236**
Single-leg barbell Romanian deadlift,
        254, **254**
Single-leg hip raise, 257, **257**
Single-leg pushup, 137, **137**
Single-leg pushup with shoulder touch,
        139, **139**
Single-leg squat, 267, **267**
Sitting posture, 50–51
Situp, 29
Skater jump, 233, **233**
Sleep, 11–12, 79
Slide out, 322, **322**
Smith, Jim, 29, 340, 342
Smoothies
    Chocolate-Peanut Butter Smoothie, 91
    High-Protein Blueberry Yogurt Shake,
        90
    Mint Chocolate Chip Smoothie, 91

    Mixed Fruit Breakfast Smoothie, 90
    Strawberry-Banana Protein Smoothie,
        91
Snacks
    calories in, 12–13
    eating plan, 59, 60–63
    overeating, 64
    role in diet plan, 74, 76, 78
Snatch grip deadlift, 251, **251**
Soda, 26, 54, 57
Spices, 59
Spiderman lunge, 268, **268**
Spiderman pushup, 153, **153**
Spinach
    Berry Goat Cheese Salad, 85
    Chicken with Walnuts and Spinach, 88
    Spinach and Feta Frittata, 83
    Tangy Turkey Ciabatta, 85
Spine
    bracing, 39
    normal alignment, **34**
    stress on, 38
Split jump, 243, **243**
Split squat, form for, 40, **40**
Split squat and overhead press, 221, **221**
Split stance cable chop, 312, **312**
Split stance single-arm cable row, 165, **165**
Sports hernia, 27
Sprints, 361
Squat, 27, 31
    barbell, 230, **230**
    barbell front squat, 232, **232**
    barbell hack squat, 271, **271**
    bodyweight, 231, **231**
    Bulgarian split squat, 250, **250**
    dumbbell Bulgarian split squat, 275,
        275
    dumbbell curl to squat to press, 200,
        200
    dumbbell front squat, 231, **231**
    dumbbell split squat, 235, **235**
    dumbbell squat jump, 240, **240**
    dumbbell squat thrust, 204, **204**
    form, 36, **36**
    goblet, 237, **237**
    goblet squat to press, 203, **203**
    kettlebell, 274, **274**

one-arm dumbbell sumo front squat, 240, **240**

overhead split squat, 242, **242**

single-arm dumbbell front squat, 236, **236**

single-arm dumbbell squat, 236, **236**

single-leg, 267, **267**

split squat and overhead press, 221, **221**

Squat and cable row, 220, **220**

Squat jump, 234, **234**

Squat tests, 124

Squat to press, 199, **199**

Squat to stand, 202, **202**

Stability ball front plank with mini rollout, 47, **47**

Stability ball jackknife, 304, **304**

Stability ball plank with mini rollout, 302, **302**

Stability ball reaching crunch, 306, **306**

Stability ball reverse leg lift, 305, **305**

Stability ball side crunch, 307, **307**

Standing hips flexed Ts and Ws, 43, **43**, 194, **194**

Standing overhead dumbbell triceps press, 177, **177**

Standing posture, 50

Starches, 65

Static back extension test, 124

Stepup, 260, **260**

Stir-fry

Beef, Vegetable, and Almond Stir-Fry, 88

Strawberries

Berry Goat Cheese Salad, 85

Peanut Butter Strawberry Wrap, 84

Strawberry-Banana Protein Smoothie, 91

Strength training. *See* Weight training

Strength workouts

Cardio-Strength Workout, 354–55

Heavy Training, 108–9, **108–9**, 114–15, **114–15**

Legs/Hips/Abs Strength Workouts, 371

Perfect Posture Workout A, 364

Perfect Posture Workout B, 364

Push/Pull Strength Workouts, 371

Stress

effect on eating, 16

on spine, 38

tension as, 35

Stroke, 13

Stubborn Fat Loss Workout, 360–61

Sugar, 57

Suitcase carry, 30, 226, **226**

Sulaver, Rob, 357

Summer Abs Workout, 352–53

Sumo deadlift, 255, **255**

Supersets, in 4-Day Core Transformation Plan, 371

Supplements

fat loss, 25, 71

fish oil, 14, 97

lactase, 95

to vegetarian diet, 97

Sweeteners, artificial, 26

Swiss ball body saw, 327, **327**

Swiss ball hip raise and leg curl, 259, **259**

Swiss ball mountain climber, 303, **303**

Swiss ball pike, 320, **320**

Swiss ball stir the pot, 319, **319**

T

Tall kneeling kettlebell halo, 300, **300**

TEF, 73

Tension, in muscle, 35

Tests

breathing, 122–23

plank, 123, **123**

pushup, **124**, 124–25

side plank, **123**, 123–24

squat, 124

static back extension, 124

Thermic effect of food (TEF), 73

Three-point dumbbell row, 167, **167**

Three-way ankle mobilization, 264, **264**

3-way ankle mobilization, 41, **41**

Tight rotation, 314, **314**

Total body exercises, 196–227

Total Body Jump Start, 340–45, **343–45**

T raise, 186, **186**

Trans fats, 15, 24

Trap bar deadlift, 273, **273**

Treadmill

in Summer Abs Workout, 353

in Warrior's Workout, 348–51

Triceps rope extension, 174, **174**

Triglycerides, 75

Triple plank, 30

Tumminello, Nick, 371

Turkey

Tangy Turkey Ciabatta, 85

Two-Exercise Abs Builder workout, 366–67

U

Underhand barbell bent-over row, 163, **163**

Upper back, self-myofacial release for, 343, **343**

Upper body

exercises for

arms, 172–81

back, 158–71

chest, 131–57

shoulders, 182–95

horizontal pulling (movement pattern), 42–43, **42–43**

horizontal pushing (movement pattern), 46–47, **46–47**

vertical pulling (movement pattern), 44–45, **44–45**

vertical pushing (movement pattern), 48–49, **48–49**

Utensils, 59

V

Valslide body saw, 332, **332**

Valslide hip raise and hamstring curl, 277, **277**

Valslide mountain climber, 333, **333**

Valslide reverse lunge, 278, **278**

Valslide side lunge, 279, **279**

Valslide spiderman pushup, 154, **154**

Vegetables, 56–57

Beef, Vegetable, and Almond Stir-Fry, 88

benefits of, 70

Vegetables (*cont.*)
    eating early in meal, 72
    role in diet plan, 70, 72
    shopping list, 65
Vegetarian diet, 96–97
Vitamin D, 18

W

Wall slide, 45, **45**, 192, **192**
Wall snow angel, 49, **49**, 195, **195**
Walnuts
    Chicken with Walnuts and Spinach, 88
Warmup
    for Abs Workout, 108
    benefits of, 339
    Cardio Workout, 120
    Total Body Jump Start, 340–45, **343–45**
Warrior's Workout, 348–51
    Category 1 Workout, 349
    Category 2 Workout, 350
    Category 3 Workout, 351
Water, 13, 69–70
Weighted wide grip pullup, 169, **169**
Weight gain
    after dieting, 64
    with eating fast, 16
    with less sleep, 11–12, 79
    processed foods and, 58
Weight loss. *See also* Fat loss
    fat loss *versus*, 22
    sources of
        fat in diet, 75
        protein in diet, 57

vegetables in diet, 56, 72
water consumption, 69–70
weight training, 24, 26
    without exercise, 22
Weight training
    benefits of, 55
    cardio compared, 24, 54–55, 56
    form (*see* Exercise movement
        patterns)
    lifting heavier weights, 14, 54, 106
    machine use compared, 14
    metabolism boost from, 14, 22, 55
    movement correction (*see* Exercise
        movement patterns)
Whey protein, 17, 18, 95
Whitfield, Mike, 361
Workouts, 346–83
    ab-centric, 19
    Athlete's Core Workout, 358–59
    Better Sex Workout, 372–73
    Bodyweight Training, 112–13, **112–13**,
        118–19, **118–19**
    Burn Your Spare Tire, 378–81
    cardio workouts
        Cardio-Strength Workout, 354–55
        high-intensity interval training
            (HIIT), 120
        20-minute moderate-intensity,
            121
    Descending Pyramids, 110–11, **110–11**,
        116–17, **116–17**
    eating after, 29
    4-Day Core Transformation Plan,
        368–71

Legs/Hips/Abs Strength Workouts,
    371
Metabolic Circuit, 370
Push/Pull Strength Workouts, 371
frequency of, 14, 28, 55, 56
Heavy Training, 108–9, **108–9**, 114–15,
    114–15
high-rep, 29–30
Hollywood Abs Workout, 382–83
intensity, 28, 55
No-Crunch Abs Workout, 356–57
Perfect Posture Workout, 362–65
Rapid Fat Loss Workout, 376–77
rules for, 339
schedule, 109
Stubborn Fat Loss Workout, 360–61
Summer Abs Workout, 352–53
Total Body Jump Start, 340–45,
    343–45
Two-Exercise Abs Builder, 366–67
Warrior's Workout, 348–51
    Category 1 Workout, 349
    Category 2 Workout, 350
    Category 3 Workout, 351

Y

Yogurt
    fat loss with, 95
    High-Protein Blueberry Yogurt Shake,
        90
    Mint Chocolate Chip Smoothie, 91
    as probiotic, 95
Y raise, 187, **187**